ILLUSTRATED TEXTBOOK OF

Paediatrics

Reader in Paediatrics

United Medical and Dental Schools of Guy's
and St Thomas's Hospitals

London, UK

M Mosby

London Philadelphia St. Louis Sydney Tokyo

D1344542

Illustration Manager:	Lynda Payne
Illustrations:	Marion Tasker
Publisher:	Richard Furn
Development Editor:	Jennifer Prast
Editorial Manager:	Kirsten Lees
Editorial Assistant:	Leslie Sinoway
Project Manager:	Peter Harrison
Production:	Gudrun Hughes
Index:	Anita Reid
Design:	Lara Last
Layout:	Rob Curran
Cover Design:	Lara Last
Cover Illustration:	Jimmy King, aged 5 years

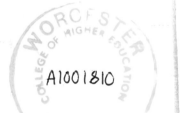

Copyright © 1997 Times Mirror International Publishers Limited

Published in 1997 by Mosby, an imprint of Times Mirror International Publishers Limited

Printed by Grafos, SA Arte sobre papel, Barcelona, Spain

Reprinted in 1997.

ISBN 0 7234 1657 5

For full details of all Times Mirror International Publishers Limited titles, please write to Times Mirror International Publishers Limited, Lynton House, 7–12 Tavistock Square, London WC1H 9LB, England.

A CIP catalogue record for this book is available from the British Library

Contents

Foreword

You are about to read a textbook unlike any you have ever read before. It is unique in its presentation, organization, graphics and design. I predict that the *Illustrated Textbook of Paediatrics* will become a standard by which all other medical textbooks will be judged. The plethora of information which every medical student is expected to absorb and integrate is unending. Therefore, it is incumbent on teachers and texts to be innovative and creatively selective in their presentation of information and wisdom. The editors, Tom Lissauer and Graham Clayden, have been successful in achieving this.

The information is presented in a clear, concise fashion and has been supplemented by original illustrations and colourful, easy-to-read charts and graphs.

Each section of the book deserves praise. The chapter on genetics is noteworthy because it does not present overwhelming details of biochemical/molecular biology, but presents a comprehensive compendium of the subject, the importance of which is undisputed in the 20th century. Perinatology and nutrition offer the student important information that has occasionally been slighted in older texts.

The reader will find both enjoyment and instruction in this new introduction to clinical paediatrics. The text is practical and the information is easily accessible.

In conclusion, I salute the authors and editors. I wish I had written this book.

Frank A. Oski, MD

Preface

This textbook has been written for undergraduates, but is also suitable for postgraduates approaching such examinations as the Diploma of Child Health (DCH) and Membership of the Royal College of Physicians (MRCP). We have focused on what we consider to be core knowledge. Basic physiology has not been included as it is amply covered in textbooks of physiology and adult medicine. The ever-increasing information about medical conditions has forced us to distil out what we believe is essential for doctors to know. Paediatrics includes many rare disorders. We have included only those which are important in the differential diagnosis of common clinical problems or are treatable.

In order to make learning from this book easier we have followed a lecture-note style using short sentences and lists of important features. Illustrations have been used to help the student recognise important signs or clinical features and to make the book more attractive and interesting to use. Key learning points have been identified for most topics. Case histories have been chosen to highlight points within their clinical context.

We have tried to ensure that this book focuses on the presentation and diagnosis of disorders rather than detailed specialised treatment. The introductory chapters therefore cover history and examination; child development; the care of the sick child and paediatric emergencies, and are followed by system-based chapters. Because community child health is rapidly changing and expanding, we have incorporated many of its principal aspects into the book. These include child surveillance, accidents and their prevention, child protection and the child with special needs. As we hope that this book will be used not only in the United Kingdom but also abroad, we have tried to keep to the principles of management and have avoided details about how services may be provided, as these vary widely between localities. For the same reason, we have kept discussion of the legal aspects of child health to a minimum.

The chapters in this book covering paediatric specialities have been written by specialists in those fields. We would therefore like to thank the many individuals involved both for their contributions and for their tolerance in permitting us to edit their texts.

We have removed the possessive 's' often placed after eponyms such as Down syndrome, as this conforms with current practice in the genetic literature. To be consistent, we have extended this to include all eponyms throughout the book.

The male gender for children has been used throughout the book for stylistic simplicity alone.

We would also like to thank Dr. Harvey Marcovitch for his constructive comments and for correcting our grammar. We are grateful to Mosby for helping us to achieve our aim to produce a textbook which is illustrated to the highest standards.

Drug dosages are included only for emergencies. The dosages used are correct at the date of publication, but it is imperative that they are checked beforehand.

We would welcome any comments about the book.

Tom Lissauer and Graham Clayden

Contributors

Dr. Lynne Ball
Formerly Consultant Paediatric Haematologist
Royal Liverpool Children's Hospital
Liverpool, UK
Ch. 19: Haematological Disorders

Prof. Ian Booth
Prof. of Paediatric Gastroenterology & Nutrition
Institute of Child Health
University of Birmingham
Birmingham, UK
Ch. 10: Nutrition and *Ch. 11: Gastroenterology*

Dr. Graham Clayden
Reader in Paediatrics
United Medical and Dental Schools of Guy's and
St. Thomas' Hospitals
London, UK
Ch. 1: History and Examination

Dr. Jon Couriel
Consultant in Paediatrics & Paediatric Respiratory Medicine
Booth Hall Children's Hospital
Manchester, UK
Ch. 13: Respiratory Disorders

Dr. Nigel Curtis
MRC Clinical Training Fellow in Paediatric Infectious Diseases
Imperial College School of Medicine at St Mary's
London, UK
Ch. 4: Paediatric Emergencies
Ch. 12: Infection and Immunity

Dr. Gill Du Mont
Consultant Paediatrician
St. Thomas' Hospital
London, UK
Ch. 21: Skin

Prof. Peter Hill
Foundation Professor
Department of Mental Health Sciences
St. George's Hospital Medical School
London, UK
Ch. 20: Emotions and Behaviour

Dr. Tony Hulse
Consultant Paediatrician
Maidstone Hospital
Kent, UK
Ch. 9: Growth and Puberty
Ch. 22: Endocrine and Metabolic Disorders

Dr. Deirdre A. Kelly
Consultant Paediatric Hepatologist
The Children's Hospital
Birmingham, UK
Ch. 17: Liver Disorders

Dr. Nigel Klein
Senior Lecturer in Paediatric Infectious Diseases and Immunology
Great Ormond Street Hospital for Children
London, UK
Ch. 4: Paediatric Emergencies
Ch. 12: Infection and Immunity

Dr. Tom Lissauer
Consultant Paediatrician
St. Mary's Hospital
London, UK
Ch. 1: History and Examination; Ch. 3: Care of the Sick Child;
Ch. 7: Perinatal Medicine and *Ch. 8: Neonatal Medicine*

Mr. Nicholas Madden
Consultant Paediatric Surgeon
Chelsea & Westminster Hospital and St Mary's Hospital
London, UK
Ch. 16: Genitalia

Dr. Richard Newton
Consultant Paediatric Neurologist
Royal Manchester Children's Hospital
Manchester, UK
Ch. 24: Neurological Disorders and *Ch. 25: The Child with Special Needs*

Dr. Angus Nicoll
Consultant Clinical Epidemiologist
Communicable Disease Surveillance Centre
London, UK
Ch. 2: Development, Language, Hearing and Vision

Dr. Andrew Redington
Consultant Paediatric Cardiologist
Royal Brompton & National Heart & Lung Hospital
London, UK
Ch. 14: Cardiac Disorders

Dr. Lesley Rees
Consultant Paediatric Nephrologist
Royal Free Hospital
London, UK
Ch. 15: Kidney and Urinary Tract

Prof. Jo Sibert
Professor of Community Child Health
University of Wales College of Medicine
Penarth, Wales, UK
Ch. 5: Environment

Dr. John Sills
Consultant Paediatrician
Royal Liverpool Children's Hospital
Liverpool, UK
Ch. 23: Bones and Joints

Dr. Karen Simmer
Staff Specialist in Neonatology
Flinders Medical Centre
Bedford Park, South Australia
Ch. 7: Perinatal Medicine and *Ch. 8: Neonatal Medicine*

Dr. Michael Stevens
Consultant Paediatric Oncologist
The Children's Hospital,
Birmingham, UK
Ch. 18: Malignant Disease

Dr. Elizabeth Thompson
Consultant Clinical Geneticist
South Australian Clinical Genetics Service
Women's and Children's Hospital
North Adelaide, Australia
Ch. 6: Genetics

CHAPTER 1

History and Examination

• *Taking a history* • *An approach to examining children* • *Examination* • *On completion of the history and examination*

The child's age is a key feature in the history and examination as it determines:
• the nature and presentation of illnesses, developmental or behaviour problems
• the way the history taking (Fig. 1.1) and examination is conducted
• the way in which any subsequent management is organised.

During the interview an assessment is also made of:
• the family (who is in it, its dynamics)
• the family's social circumstances
• the child's personality
• the family's community (culture, nursery/school).

Taking a history

Introduction
• When you welcome the child, parents and siblings, check that you know the child's first name and sex. Ask how the child prefers to be addressed.
• Introduce yourself.
• Avoid having desks or beds between you and the family.
• Eye contact with the parents and an older child is reassuring. Younger children need time to get to know you and it is best not to look at them directly until the history taking has been completed.

• Address questions to both the parents and child when appropriate.
• Have toys suitable for his and any siblings' ages. Observe how the child and any siblings play and their relationship with their parents.

Presenting symptoms
• Parents are astute observers of their children. Never ignore or dismiss what they say.
• Full details are required of the presenting symptoms: onset, duration, previous episodes, what relieves/aggravates them and any associated symptoms. Have they affected the child's or family's lifestyle? What has the family done about it?

Make sure you know:
• what prompted referral to a doctor
• what the parents think or fear is the matter.

The scope and detail of further history-taking is determined by the nature and severity of the presenting complaint and the child's age. Whilst the comprehensive assessment listed here is sometimes required, usually a selective approach is more appropriate (Fig.1.2).

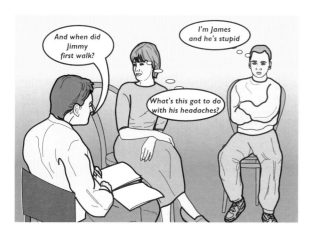

Fig 1.1 The history must be adapted to the child's age.

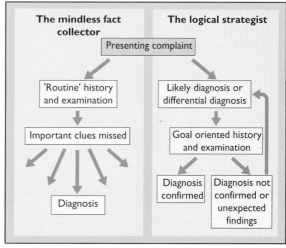

Fig 1.2 The history and examination should be goal-oriented, based on the presenting complaint. Comprehensive history taking is best reserved for training or for complex, multi-system disorders. (Adapted from Hutson JM, Beasley SW. The Surgical Examination of Children. Heinemann Medical Books 1988.)

Systemic enquiry

Check:
- general health: how active and lively?
- feeding/appetite
- breathing problems
- vomiting
- bowels
- any recent change in behaviour or personality.

Past medical history

Check:
- past illnesses
- maternal obstetric problems
- birth weight and gestation
- if admitted to special care baby unit
- immunisations (ideally from the personal child health record).

Medication

Check:
- past and present medications
- known allergies.

Family history

- Ask parents for the relevant information and draw family tree.
- Is there consanguinity?
- Have any members of the family or relatives had similar problems or any serious disorder?

Development

Check:
- child's temperament
- sleeping problems
- dry by day and night
- bowel control
- concerns and progress at nursery/school?
- key developmental milestones (Fig. 1.3)
- parental worries about vision, hearing and development
- previous child-health surveillance developmental checks

Look through the personal child health record.

Social history

Check:
- behaviour problems
- home relationships with siblings
- relationships at nursery/school
- relevant information about the family and its community: parental occupation, housing, family stresses.

An approach to examining children

Adequacy of the examination

- Whilst it may be difficult to examine young children fully, it is usually possible with resourcefulness and imagination on the doctor's part.

Obtaining cooperation

- Make friends with the child.
- Be confident but gentle.
- Avoid towering over the child.
- Short mock examinations, e.g. auscultating a teddy or the mother's hand may allay a young child's fears.
- When touching a young child, do so first on an area he feels is non-threatening, such as a hand or knee.
- A smiling, talking doctor appears less threatening, but this should not be overdone as it can interfere with

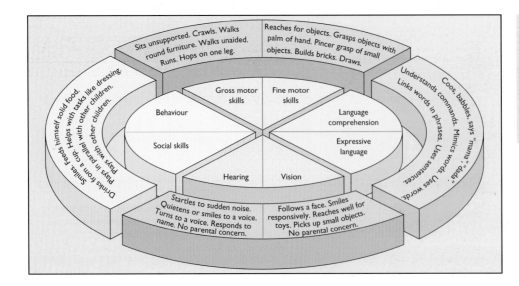

Fig 1.3 Some key developmental milestones in young children. These are considered in detail in Chapter 2.

one's relationship with the parents.
* Leave unpleasant procedures until last.

Developmental skills
A good overview of developmental skills can be obtained by watching the child play. A few simple toys, such as some bricks, a car, doll, ball, pencil and paper are all that are required, as they can be adapted for any age. If developmental assessment is the focus of the examination, it is advisable to play with the child before the physical examination, as cooperation may then be lost.

Explanation
Explain to the child what you are about to do and what you want him to do, in language he can understand. As the examination is essential, not optional, it is best not to ask his permission, as it may well be refused!

Adapting to the child's age
Adapt the examination to suit the child's age.
* Babies in the first few months are best examined on an examination couch with a parent next to them.
* A toddler is best initially examined on his mother's lap. Parents are generally reassuring for the child and helpful in facilitating the examination if guided as to what to do (Fig. 1.4).
* Pre-school children may initially be examined whilst they are playing.
* Older children and teenagers are often concerned about privacy. Teenage girls should normally be examined in the presence of their mothers or a nurse, if the examining doctor is male. Be aware of cultural sensitivities in families which differ from your own.

Undressing children
The area to be examined must be inspected fully. It is usually best to do this in stages and redress the child when each stage has been completed. It is easiest and kindest to ask the parent or child to do the undressing.

Warm, clean hands
Hands must be washed before examining a child. Warm hands and a warm stethoscope also help!

Examination

INITIAL OBSERVATIONS
Careful observation is usually the key to success in examining children. Look before touching the child. His general appearance and behaviour during the interview is instructive. It will provide information on:
* severity of illness
* growth and nutrition
* behaviour, social responsiveness and response to parental control
* level of hygiene and care.

Severity of illness
Make an initial assessment of the severity of the child's illness. Is there:
* pallor or cyanosis?
* dehydration or shock?
* altered level of consciousness?
The care of the critically ill child is described in Chapter 4.

GENERAL APPEARANCE
The face, head and neck and hands are examined. The general morphological appearance may suggest a chromosomal or dysmorphic syndrome. In infants palpate the fontanelle and sutures.

Measurements
As abnormal growth may be the first manifestation of illness in children, always measure and plot growth on centile charts for:
* weight, including previous measurements from personal child health record
* head circumference in infants
* length (in infancy) or height.

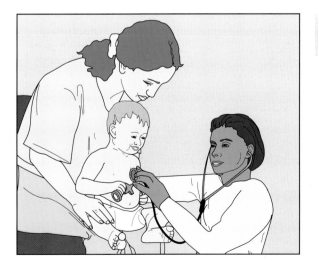

Fig 1.4 Distracting a toddler with a toy allows auscultation of the heart.

RESPIRATORY SYSTEM

Cyanosis
Central cyanosis is best observed on the tongue.

Clubbing of the fingers and/or toes
Clubbing (Fig. 1.5a) is usually secondary to chronic suppurative lung disease or cyanotic congenital heart disease. Occasionally it is associated with inflammatory bowel disease or chronic liver disease.

Tachypnoea (Fig. 1.5b)

Quality of breathing
Increased work of breathing is judged from:
- nasal flaring
- grunting on expiration – a sign of raised positive end-expiratory pressure
- use of accessory muscles, especially sternomastoids
- retraction of the chest wall, from use of suprasternal, intercostal and subcostal muscles
- difficulty feeding/speaking.

Chest shape
- Hyper-expansion or barrel-shape (Fig. 1.5c).
- Pectus excavatum (hollow chest) or pectus carinatum (pigeon chest).
- Harrison sulci (from diaphragmatic tug).
- Asymmetry of chest movements.

Palpation
- Chest expansion is 3–5 cm in school-aged children.
- Trachea: checking that the trachea is central is best left until last as it upsets children. It is seldom helpful. The position of the apex beat is helpful to establish the position of the mediastinum.

Percussion
Needs to be done gently. Seldom informative in infants.

Auscultation
Harsh breath sounds from the upper airways are readily transmitted to the upper chest in infants.
Hoarse voice–abnormality of the vocal cords.
Stridor–harsh, low pitched inspiratory sound from upper airways obstruction.
Wheeze–high pitched, expiratory sound from distal airway obstruction caused by mucosal oedema, mucus and bronchospasm (Fig. 1.5d).
Crackles–from the opening of bronchioles (Fig. 1.5d).

Respiratory system

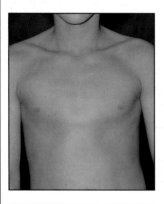

Fig 1.5a Clubbing of the fingers associated with cystic fibrosis.

Fig 1.5b Respiratory rate in children		
Age	**Normal respiratory rate (breaths/min)**	**Tachypnoea (breaths/min)**
Neonate	30–50	>60
Infants	20–40	>50
Young children	20–30	>40
Older children	15–20	>30

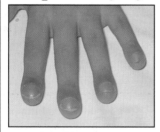

Fig 1.5d Chest signs of some common chest disorders of children			
	Chest movement	**Percussion**	**Auscultation**
Bronchiolitis	Laboured breathing Hyperinflated chest Subcostal recession	Hyper-resonant	Fine crackles in all zones Wheezes may/may not be present
Pneumonia	Reduced on affected side Rapid, shallow breaths	Dull	Bronchial breathing Crackles
Asthma	Reduced but hyperinflated Use of accessory muscles Chest retraction	Hyper-resonant	Wheeze

Fig 1.5c Hyper-expanded chest from chronic obstructive airways disease. This boy had severe asthma.

 Infants with pneumonia may have no abnormal signs on auscultation.

 Sputum is rarely produced by children as they swallow it. The main exception is suppurative lung disease from cystic fibrosis.

CARDIOVASCULAR SYSTEM

Clubbing of fingers or toes
Check if present.

Pulse
Check:
- rate (Fig. 1.6a), which is increased with fear, exercise, stress or arrhythmia
- rhythm
- volume: small volume in circulatory insufficiency or aortic stenosis; collapsing in patent ductus arteriosus.

Inspection
Look for:
- praecordial bulge
- ventricular impulse: visible if thin, hyperdynamic circulation or left ventricular hypertrophy.

Palpation
Thrill = palpable murmur.
Right ventricular tap = right ventricular hypertrophy or normal thin child.
Apex (4th intercostal space, mid-clavicular line):
- heave from left ventricular hypertrophy
- not palpable in some normal infants, plump children or dextrocardia.

Percussion
Cardiac border percussion is rarely helpful in children.

Auscultation
Heart sounds:
- splitting of second sound usually easily heard (Fig. 1.6b)
- fixed splitting in atrial septal defects
- third sound in mitral area is normal in young children.

Murmurs:
- timing–ejection systolic/ pansystolic/ continuous/ diastolic
- character
- loudness–systolic murmurs graded:
  1 (barely audible) to
  3 (easily audible, no thrill) to
  6 (extremely loud with thrill)
- site–mitral/pulmonary/aortic/tricuspid areas
- radiation:
  to neck in aortic stenosis
  to back in coarctation of the aorta or pulmonary stenosis.

Hepatomegaly
Important sign of heart failure in infants. An infant's liver is normally palpable 1–2 cm below the costal margin.

Femoral pulses
In coarctation of the aorta:
- decreased volume or absent in infants
- brachio-femoral delay in older children.

 Heart disease is more common in children with other congenital abnormalities or syndromes e.g. Down and Turner syndromes.

Cardiovascular system

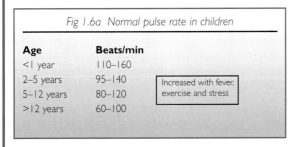

Fig 1.6a Normal pulse rate in children		
Age	**Beats/min**	
<1 year	110–160	
2–5 years	95–140	Increased with fever, exercise and stress
5–12 years	80–120	
>12 years	60–100	

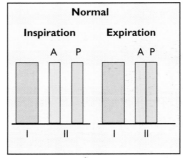

Fig 1.6b The splitting of the second heart sound is easily heard in children.

 Features suggesting a murmur is significant:
- *conducted all over praecordium*
- *loud*
- *thrill (equals grade 4–6 murmur)*
- *pansystolic*
- *any diastolic murmur*
- *accompanied by other abnormal cardiac signs.*

 Features of heart failure:
- *poor feeding/failure to thrive*
- *sweating*
- *tachypnoea*
- *tachycardia*
- *gallop rhythm*
- *cardiomegaly*
- *hepatomegaly*

ABDOMEN

The abdomen is often protuberant in young children. Abdominal wall muscles must be relaxed for palpation.

Associated signs

Examine the eyes for signs of:
- jaundice
- anaemia.

Examine the fingers for clubbing.

Inspection

Generalised abdominal distension (the 5 'F's):
- Fat
- Fluid (ascites, usually from nephrotic syndrome)
- Faeces (constipation/Hirschsprung disease)
- Flatus (intestinal obstruction)
- Fetus (not to be forgotten after puberty).

Localised abdominal distension:
- upper: pyloric stenosis, hepato/splenomegaly
- lower: obstructed bladder.

Peristalsis–pyloric stenosis, intestinal obstruction.

Inguinal region–inguinal hernia, lymphadenopathy

Genitalia–undescended testis (distinguish from retractile testes); hydrocele; phimosis. Genital area is examined routinely in young children but in older children only if relevant, e.g. suspected sexual abuse.

Anus–fissure, ectopic.

Palpation

Ask about tenderness. Watch the child's face for grimacing as you palpate. A young child may become more cooperative if you palpate first with his hand or putting your hand on top of his.

Tenderness

Location–localised in appendicitis, hepatitis, pyelonephritis; generalised in mesenteric adenitis, peritonitis. Guarding–often unimpressive on direct palpation in children. Pain on coughing is helpful. Pain on moving about/walking/bumps during car journey suggests peritoneal irritation. Back bent on walking may be from psoas inflammation in appendicitis.

Enlarged viscera

Hepatomegaly (Fig. 1.7a):
- palpate from left iliac fossa
- edge may be soft or firm
- cannot get above it
- moves with respiration
- measure size below costal margin .

Splenomegaly (Fig. 1.7c):
- palpate from right iliac fossa
- edge usually soft
- cannot get above it
- notch may be palpable
- moves on respiration
- measure size below costal margin (Fig. 1.7b).

Kidney (not usually palpable beyond neonatal period):
- palpate by balloting bimanually
- moves on respiration
- can get above it.

Abnormal masses

Wilms tumour: renal mass does not cross mid-line.
Neuroblastoma: irregular mass, may cross mid-line; the

Abdomen

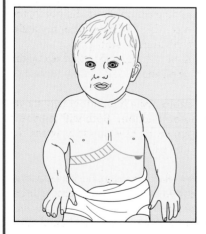

Fig 1.7b The liver edge is 1–2 cm below the costal margin in infants and young children. The spleen may be below the costal margin in infants.

Fig 1.7a Causes of hepatomegaly	
Infection	Congenital, hepatitis A, B or C, infectious mononucleosis, septicaemia, malaria
Malignancy	Leukaemia, lymphoma, hepatoblastoma
Liver disease	Neonatal liver disease, chronic liver disease, autosomal dominant polycystic liver/kidney disease
Metabolic	Carbohydrate–glycogen storage disorders, galactosaemia
	Protein–tyrosinaemia, α_1-antitrypsin deficiency
	Lipid–storage disorders e.g. Gaucher, mucopolysaccharidoses
Haematological	Sickle-cell anaemia, thalassaemia
Cardiovascular	Heart failure, tricuspid regurgitation (pulsatile)
Apparent	Chest hyperexpansion from bronchiolitis or asthma

Fig 1.7c Causes of splenomegaly	
Infection	Bacterial: septicaemia, infective endocarditis, typhoid
	Viral: infectious mononucleosis, CMV, etc.
	Protozoal: malaria, toxoplasmosis, leishmaniasis
Haematological	Haemolytic anaemia
Malignancy	Leukaemia, lymphoma
Other	Portal hypertension, Still disease (juvenile chronic arthritis)

child is usually very unwell.
Intussusception: most often palpable in right iliac fossa.
Faecal loading.

Percussion

Hepato/splenomegaly: dullness used to confirm size.
Kidney: not dull to percussion.
Ascites: shifting dullness.

Auscultation

Bowel sounds: increased in intestinal obstruction and
acute diarrhoea; absent in peritonitis, paralytic ileus or
severe sepsis in infancy.

Rectal examination

Rarely indicated in children unless obese as tenderness/
faeces can be detected on palpating the abdomen. Some
surgeons advocate it to identify a retrocaecal appendix, but
interpretation is problematic as most children will complain
of pain and dislike the procedure intensely. If intussusception is suspected, the mass may be palpable and stools
looking like redcurrant jam revealed on rectal examination.

 *A hyper-expanded chest in bronchiolitis or asthma
may displace the liver and spleen downward,
suggesting hepato/splenomegaly.*

NEUROLOGY/NEURODEVELOPMENT

Brief neurological screen

A quick neurological and developmental overview
should be performed in all children.

Higher mental function, hearing and language, vision
Is assessed by parents' description and observing the
child, noting language skills and speech, social interaction, copying, drawing and writing if old enough.
Does vision and hearing appear to be normal?

Motor function
Assess primarily by observation:

- in infants, observe posture and movements of the
limbs. When picking up the infant, note tone. The
limbs and body may feel normal, floppy or stiff. Head
control may be poor with abnormal head lag on
pulling the infant to sitting.
- beyond infancy, observe manipulative skills in play
and gait on walking.

More detailed neurological assessment is performed
only if indicated. Specific problems in development or
behaviour require detailed assessment.

More detailed neurological examination

Patterns of movement
Observe walking, running and tip-toe gait. A heel
coming off the ground on walking suggests a tight
tendo-achilles as in pyramidal tract dysfunction (particularly hemiplegia and diplegia), or a muscle disorder
such as Duchenne muscular dystrophy, but can be seen
intermittently in some normal children. A broad-based
gait may be due to an immature gait or secondary to a
cerebellar disorder.

Observe standing from lying down supine. Children up
to three years of age will turn prone in order to stand
because of poor pelvic muscle fixation. Beyond this age
children with neuromuscular weakness (e.g. Duchenne
muscular dystrophy) will push themselves off the
ground with straightened arms, and then climb up their
legs (Gower sign).

Coordination
Assess this by:

- asking the child to build one brick upon another or
using a peg-board
- asking the child to hold his arms out straight, close
his eyes, and observe for drift or tremor
- finger-nose testing (use teddy's nose to reach out
and touch if necessary)
- rapid alternating movements of hands and fingers
- touching tip of each finger in turn with thumb
- asking the child to walk heel–toe, jump and hop.

Inspection of limbs
Muscle bulk: wasting may be secondary to meningomyelocele, cerebral palsy or a muscle disorder or from
previous poliomyelitis; polio; increased bulk of calf muscles may indicate Duchenne muscular dystrophy.

Muscle tone
Tone in limbs– best assessed by taking the weight of the
whole limb and then bending and extending it around
a single joint. Testing is easiest at the knee and ankle
joints. Assess for the range of movement as well as the
feel of it. Increased tone in adductors and internal rota-
tors of the hips is usually the result of pyramidal dysfunction as are increased pronation of the forearms at
rest and clonus at the ankles. The posture of the limbs
may give a clue as to the underlying tone, e.g. scissoring
of the legs, pronated forearms.

Truncal tone–in pyramidal tract disorders the trunk and
head tend to arch backwards (extensor posturing). In
muscle disease and some central brain disorders, the
trunk may be hypotonic. The child feels floppy to handle
and cannot support the trunk in sitting.

Head lag–is best tested by pulling the child up by the
arms from the supine position.

Power
Difficult to test in babies. Watch for antigravity movements and note motor function. Both will tell you a
lot about power. From six months onwards, watch the
pattern of mobility and gait.

Reflexes
Test with the child in a relaxed position. Brisk reflexes may
reflect anxiety in the child or a pyramidal disorder. Absent
reflexes may reflect inexpert or anxious examiner, a neuromuscular problem or a lesion within the spinal cord.
Children will reinforce reflexes if asked.

Plantar responses
An overrated activity, unpopular with children, and in
any case unreliable under one year of age. When done,
the responses are often equivocal, but may provide

additional evidence of pyramidal dysfunction.

Sensation
Testing the ability to withdraw to tickle is usually adequate as a screening test. If loss of sensation is likely e.g. meningomyelocele, more extensive sensory testing is performed.

Cranial nerves
These can usually be tested formally from four years of age. Before then ingenuity is required.

I	Need not be tested in routine practice. Can be done by recognising the smell of a hidden mint sweet
II	Visual acuity–determined according to age. Direct and consensual pupillary response tested to light and accommodation
III, IV, VI	Full eye movement through horizontal and vertical planes. Is there a squint? Nystagmus: avoid extreme lateral gaze, as it can induce nystagmus in normal children
V	Clench teeth and waggle jaw from side to side against resistance
VII	Close eyes tight, smile and show teeth
VIII	Hearing. Ask parents, though unilateral deafness could be missed this way
IX	Laevator palatae - saying 'aagh'
X	Recurrent laryngeal nerve - listen for hoarseness or stridor
XI	Trapezius and sternomastoid power - shrug shoulders and turn head against resistance
XII	Put out tongue and waggle it from side to side.

BONES AND JOINTS
- Inspect for–restriction/pain on moving; swelling from synovial thickening or joint effusion; muscle wasting.
- Palpate for–warmth, tenderness.
- Movements–active first, then passive, taking care to avoid pain.
- Scoliosis–inspect the back. Ask older child/adolescent to touch his toes.

LYMPH NODES
- Small, multiple nodes in the neck, inguinal area and axillae: common in normal children.
- Small, multiple nodes in the neck: common after upper respiratory tract infections (viral/bacterial).
- Single, large, tender node, may be fluctuant: infected/abscess.
- Variable size and shape:
  –infections: viral e.g. infectious mononucleosis, or TB
  –rare causes: malignant disease, Kawasaki disease, cat-scratch.

BLOOD PRESSURE
Indications– must be closely monitored (Fig. 1.8) if critically ill; renal or cardiac disease or diabetes mellitus; receiving drug therapy which may cause hypertension e.g.

corticosteroids. Not measured often enough in children.
Technique–when measured with a sphygmomanometer:
- show the child that there is a balloon in the cuff and demonstrate how it is blown up
- use largest cuff which fits comfortably, covering at least two-thirds of the upper arm
- the child must be relaxed and not crying
- systolic pressure is the easiest to determine in young children and clinically most useful
- diastolic pressure is when the sounds become muffled. Cannot always be discerned in young children.

Measurement–must be interpreted according to a centile chart (see Appendix). Blood pressure is increased by tall stature and obesity. Charts relating blood pressure to height are available; for convenience, charts of blood pressure according to age are often used. An abnormally high reading must be repeated with the child relaxed on at least three separate occasions.

EYES
Examination–the eyes, pupils, iris, sclerae are examined. Are eye movements full and symmetrical? Is there a squint? Is nystagmus detectable? If so, may have ocular or cerebellar cause, or testing may be too lateral to the child.
Ophthalmoscopy:
- in infants, the red reflex is seen from a distance of about 20 cm. It is not observed if there is a cataract, corneal clouding or retinoblastoma. Fundoscopy is difficult. Mydriatics are required for a proper examination of the fundi, e.g. for retinopathy of prematurity, retinopathy in congenital infections, choroido-retinal degeneration or haemorrhages in suspected child abuse.
- in older children, e.g. with headaches, the fundi can be examined without mydriatics.

EARS AND THROAT
Examination–usually left until last as their examination is unpleasant. Parental help in holding the young child is required for success and to avoid possible injury (Figs 1.9 and 1.10).

Fig 1.8 Measuring blood pressure in children
Sphygmomanometer
Stethoscope in older children
Doppler ultrasound in infants
Oscillometric (e.g. Dynamapp)
Helpful in infants and young children
Invasive
Direct measurement from an arterial catheter is mandatory if critically ill

On completion of the history and examination

At the end of the history and examination:
- summarise the key problems (in physical, emotional, social and family terms if relevant)
- list the diagnoses or differential diagnosis
- draw up a management plan to address the problems
- provide explanations to both the parents and to the child, if old enough, and written information if available.
- consider if other professionals should be informed.

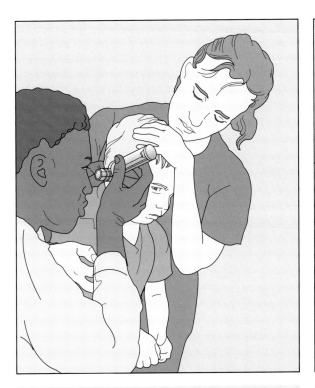

Fig 1.9 Holding a young child correctly is essential for successful examination of the ear with an auroscope. The mother has one hand on the head and the other holding the upper arm.

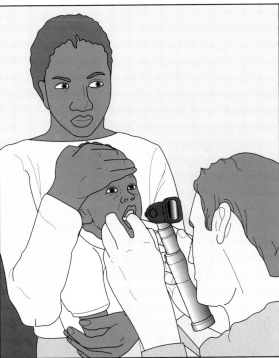

Fig 1.10 Holding a young child to examine the throat. The mother has one hand on the head and the other across the child's arms.

FURTHER READING

Gill D, O'Brien N. *Paediatric Clinical Examination*, Churchill Livingstone, Edinburgh 1993.

CHAPTER 2

Development, Language, Hearing & Vision

• The process of child development • Key developmental milestones • Surveillance reviews • Language and speech • Hearing • Vision

The main objectives of developmental paediatrics are:
- to help all children achieve their maximum developmental potential
- the early detection of delayed development including specific sensory impairments of hearing and vision; investigation of their cause and management including treatment of the condition. Even where there is no specific treatment, the effects of the condition can often be modified.
- to be the entry point for the care and management of the child with special needs.

The process of child development

A child's development represents the interaction of heredity and the environment. Heredity determines the potential of the child while the environment influences the extent to which he or she achieves that potential. For optimal development the environment has to meet the child's physical and psychological needs (Fig. 2.1). These vary with age and stage of development:
- an infant is physically totally dependent on parents and requires a limited number of carers to meet his psychological needs
- a primary school-age child can usually meet some of his physical needs and cope with many social relationships
- teenagers are able to meet most of their physical needs while experiencing increasingly complex emotional needs.

Any child whose development is delayed or sub-optimal needs assessment to determine the cause and how best to help (Fig. 2.2). Development may be disrupted by a neurological disorder in the child which affects development directly (e.g. cerebral palsy or visual impairment) or indirectly through ill-health (e.g. cystic fibrosis) or adverse environmental factors.

FIVE PERIODS OF DEVELOPMENT IN YOUNG CHILDREN

Development is most rapid in the first four years of life, which can be conveniently split into five periods:
- the newborn baby
- the supine infant (6–8 weeks old)
- the sitting infant (6–9 months old)
- the mobile toddler (18–24 months old)
- the communicating child (3–4 years old).

These periods correspond with child health promotion and surveillance reviews. There is considerable individual variation in the age at which a child passes through one developmental period to another.

EIGHT AREAS OF DEVELOPMENT

It is useful to subdivide development into eight functional skills (Fig. 2.3). These provide a framework for more detailed assessment. A child can have a deficiency in one skill area, although this can impact on other areas, e.g. a hearing impairment may result in poor language development and social skills.

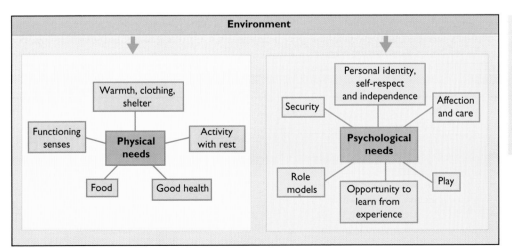

Fig. 2.1 Development can be impaired if the environment is lacking in physical or psychological needs.

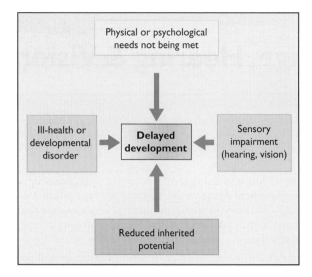

Fig. 2.2 If development is delayed, the cause should be determined.

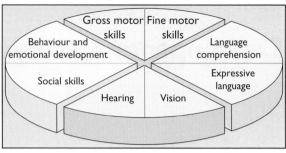

Fig. 2.3 The eight areas of child development.

3. Eventual level of attainment

This depends on heredity and environment.

Key developmental milestones

Parents naturally enquire if their child is progressing well. As part of child health surveillance, professionals need to decide whether every individual child under their care is within the range of normality for his age and stage of development. There is no simple answer to this question. Median ages, when half of a standard population of children have achieved a skill, are often quoted; for example, 50% of children are walking by their first birthday. Undoubtedly this information is useful and further median ages will be quoted below (data from the Denver Developmental Screening Test, a frequently used standard in developmental paediatrics). However, these figures can also be misleading if they are applied too rigidly, since by definition 50% of parents could feel their child is slow in development and it would be impractical to investigate every child who was doing less well than these median standards.

A child may achieve one skill at the expected age and yet need help with developmental progress in other areas. In addition, the quality of a child's development is also important. An older child may attain a developmental milestone in language, such as putting words and sentences together,

As the child grows, additional skills become increasingly important, for example attention and concentration and how well an individual child's skills are integrated.

THE RANGE OF NORMALITY AND INDIVIDUAL VARIATION

There is a remarkable consistency in the pattern of children's developmental progress. However, children vary greatly in:

1. Rate of development

Different children attain milestones at different ages and yet all may come within normal. For example, the percentage of children who are walking unsupported is:

- 25% by 11 months
- 50% by 12 months
- 75% by 13 months
- 90% by 14–15 months. At 14 months the majority of children not yet walking unsupported will be normal. At 18 months (two standard deviations from the mean) many will be normal late walkers but there will be a small percentage who will have an underlying medical problem such as Duchenne muscular dystrophy or mild cerebral palsy. Hence any child who is not walking by 18 months should be carefully examined. Thus 18 months is a 'limit age' for children not walking. Some other 'limit ages' are shown in Figure 2.4.

2. Pattern of development

Development is not always straightforward. All normal babies progress from immobility to walking but not all do so in the same way (Fig. 2.5). There is even more variation in the area of social skills and behaviour, e.g. from the age of six months most babies develop a fear of strangers, but a few never show this.

Fig. 2.4 Some developmental 'limit ages'	
Further assessment is indicated if these skills have not been acquired by this age	
Age	**Developmental sign**
8/52	Responsive smiling
3/12	Good eye contact
5/12	Reaches for objects
10/12	Sits unsupported
18/12	Walks unsupported
18/12	Says single words with meaning
30/12	Speaks in phrases

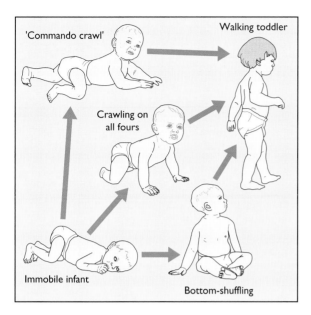

'Commando crawl'

Walking toddler

Crawling on all fours

Immobile infant

Bottom-shuffling

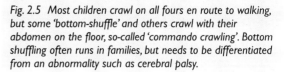

Fig. 2.5 Most children crawl on all fours en route to walking, but some 'bottom-shuffle' and others crawl with their abdomen on the floor, so-called 'commando crawling'. Bottom shuffling often runs in families, but needs to be differentiated from an abnormality such as cerebral palsy.

programme for young children with recommended ages is shown in Figure 2.6. There is a physical assessment at birth followed by a review in each key period of development (Figs 2.7–2.12). The ages at which these reviews are undertaken are not fixed, but are within age-bands, e.g. for the sitting child the review should be in the age-band six to nine months.

At each review, the individual areas of developmental skills are considered. Equally important is the child's overall development–how well are individual skills integrated and what is the quality of development? The emphasis on parental opinion of vision and hearing at every age is deliberate, as parents are usually excellent detectors of special sense problems. At these reviews the child's health and growth are also checked. Other aspects of health that need monitoring during the first five years of life as part of health promotion include immunisation and accident prevention. The timing of the immunisations is also shown as they can sometimes be given at the end of the review.

but be unskilled and clumsy in trying to converse with other children and adults.

 Developmental milestones–both attainment and quality are important

Surveillance reviews

A standard child health surveillance and immunisation

 Health surveillance and promotion should be provided for every child.

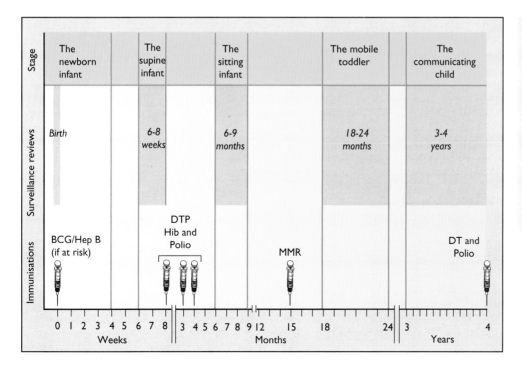

Stage	The newborn infant	The supine infant	The sitting infant		The mobile toddler	The communicating child
Surveillance reviews	Birth	6-8 weeks	6-9 months		18-24 months	3-4 years
Immunisations	BCG/Hep B (if at risk)	DTP Hib and Polio		MMR		DT and Polio

0 1 2 3 4 5 6 7 8 — Weeks
3 4 5 6 7 8 9 12 15 18 24 — Months
3 4 — Years

Fig. 2.6 A standard child health surveillance and immunisation programme in young children as performed in England and Wales. There is also a surveillance review at age 5½–6½ years (school entrance).

The newborn infant: surveillance at birth

Fig. 2.7a The newborn baby: surveillance at birth	
	Expected findings include:
Gross motor skills	Symmetrical and anti-gravity movements of all four limbs (Figs 2.7 b and c)
	Muscle tone normal
Language	Cries
Social skills	Responsive to being picked up
Hearing	Stills to voice; startles to loud noises
Vision	Looks at faces; responds to light
(This examination is described in more detail on page 80 in Chap. 7)	

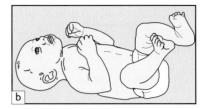

Fig. 2.7b
Supine — symmetrical posture, limbs flexed.

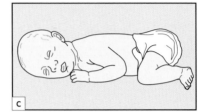

Fig. 2.7c
Prone — flexed posture with knees tucked under the abdomen.

The supine infant (6–8 weeks): surveillance review

Fig. 2.8a The supine infant age 6–8 weeks: surveillance review (Median ages are given in brackets)	
	Expected findings include:
Gross motor skills	Symmetrical movements of all four limbs
	Muscle tone normal (Fig. 2.8b)
Fine motor skills/vision	Eyes follow an object (six weeks) (Fig. 2.8c); show conjugate movement, no squint or nystagmus
Language/hearing	Normal cry; parents have observed response to sounds
Social skills	Smiles responsively (six weeks) (Fig. 2.8d)
Other components of review usually carried out by a doctor:	
Parents	Are there any concerns?
Growth	Measure weight and head circumference; chart centiles and review progress
Physical examination	Check for congenital dislocation of the hip (CDH)
	Inspect eyes including red reflex with ophthalmoscope to exclude congenital cataract and gross retinal lesion (retinoblastoma)
Special senses	Discuss with parents the checklist in the child's personal child health record (PCHR) on how to detect hearing loss
Health promotion	Discuss or commence immunisation, recognition of illness, sleeping position, nutrition, accident prevention
	Is BCG indicated (according to local and national guidelines), and if so has it been given?

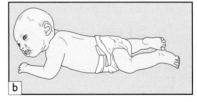

Fig. 2.8b
Prone — raises head to 45°.

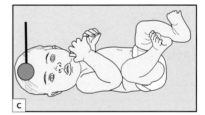

Fig. 2.8c
Follows a moving object or face, with turning of the head.

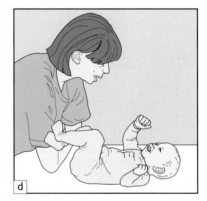

Fig. 2.8d
Smiles responsively.

If a baby has been born preterm (<37 weeks) this should be allowed for in assessing developmental progress. Developmental age is calculated from the expected date of delivery.

If this review takes place at eight weeks, the first immunisation (DPT, polio and Hib) can be given. In preterm infants, immunisations are given according to chronological age, i.e. not corrected for prematurity.

The sitting child (6–9 months): surveillance review

Fig. 2.9a The sitting child age 6–9 months: surveillance review (Median ages are given in brackets)

	Expected findings include:
Gross motor skills	Sits without support (six months) (Fig. 2.9b)
	Stands holding on (seven months)
	Pulls to standing (nine months)
Fine motor skills/vision	Reaches for small objects, holds them in a palmar grasp (Fig. 2.9c) and passes them from one hand to another (six months)
	Bangs together two toys held in either hand
	No squint
Language/hearing	Turns to a voice (seven months)
	Passes the distraction hearing test; babbles; says 'mama' or 'dada' non-specifically (10 months)
Social and self-help skills	Can put solid food in mouth (six months)

Surveillance review is usually undertaken by a health visitor and focuses on the following items:

Parents	Are there any concerns?
Growth	Measure weight; chart and review progress; measure head circumference and length if indicated
Physical examination	Check again for congenital dislocation of the hip (CDH) by inspecting for limited abduction or asymmetry of the hip
	Check for testicular descent in boys
Special senses	Review parental checklist on detection of hearing loss
	Perform distraction hearing test (requires two trained operators)
	Observe visual behaviour, look for and ask about squint
Health promotion	Check that primary immunisation is complete; discuss recognition of illness, nutrition, dental prophylaxis, developmental needs, sleeping position, safety in cars, passive smoking, accident prevention

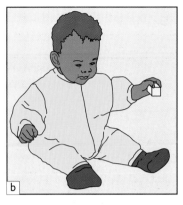

Fig. 2.9b Sits without support with a straight back and passes objects from one hand to another.

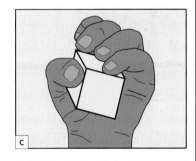

Fig. 2.9c Palmar grasp (six months).

The 1-year-old child

Fig. 2.10a The 1-year-old-child (this is not a standard surveillance review period, but is a time of rapid developmental progress). (Median ages are given in brackets)

	Expected findings include:
Gross motor skills	Walks holding on to furniture (nine months)
	Walking if led (Fig. 2.10b) and able to take a few steps unsupported (12 months)
Fine motor skills/vision	A good pincer (thumb and first or second finger) grip of a small object (10.5 months)
	No squint on observation and parental report
Language/hearing	Parents feel child can understand simple commands such as 'no','bring that here'; says 'mama' or 'dada' and one or two other words appropriately (13 months)
	Parents have no concern about hearing
Social and self-help skills/ behaviour	Drinks from a cup (12 months)
	Finger-feeds or uses a spoon
	Waves 'bye-bye' (8 months)
	Wary of strangers; socially responsive

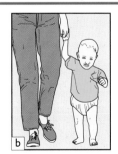

Fig. 2.10b Walks when led.

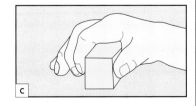

Fig. 2.10c Mature pincer grasp (10½ months).

The mobile toddler (18–24 months): surveillance review

Fig. 2.11a The mobile toddler age 18–24 months: surveillance review.
(Median ages are given in brackets)

	Expected findings include:
Gross motor skills	Walks well with normal gait (Fig 2.11b)
	Kicks a ball (20 months)
Fine motor skills/vision	Scribbles with a pencil (14 months)
	Builds a tower of six one-inch cubes (24 months)
Language/hearing	Combines two different words (20 months)
	Uses pivotal grammar, i.e. uses one word such as 'gimmee' and attaches others such as 'milk', 'toy', 'dat', etc (24 months)
Social and self-help skills/behaviour	Points to a named part of the body (Fig 2.11c)
	Shows symbolic play when playing with miniature toys such as a doll, brush, chair and spoon; plays as if they were life-size equivalents
	Can remove a garment (18 months)
	Feeds self with a spoon (Fig 2.11d)
	Asserts own wishes
Hearing	Parents satisfied with hearing
Vision	No squint; manipulates small objects well; parents satisfied with vision

Surveillance review is usually carried out by the health visitor, preferably at home where mother and child are more relaxed, and focuses on the following items:

Parents	Ask about any concerns, particularly regarding behaviour and special senses
Growth	Measure; chart and review progress
	Physical examination. Consider if the child is anaemic (highest prevalence at this age)
Special senses	Review checklist on detection of hearing loss with parents
	Observe visual behaviour; look for and ask about squint
Health promotion	Check that primary immunisation is complete, including MMR. Discuss nutrition and accident prevention and review safety of the home; discuss developmental needs, language and play, need to mix with other children, avoidance and management of behaviour problems

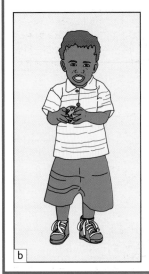
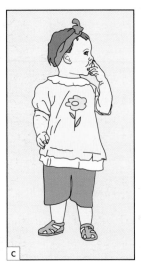
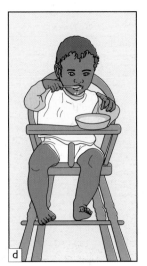

Fig. 2.11b Walks well carrying a toy.
Fig. 2.11c Points to a named part of the body.
Fig. 2.11d Holds a spoon and gets food safely to mouth.

The communicating child (3–4 years): surveillance review

Fig. 2.12a The communicating child age 3–4 years: surveillance review.
(Median ages are given in brackets)

	Expected findings include:
Gross motor skills	Hops on one foot (42 months)

Fine motor skills/vision	Manipulates small objects well
	Parents satisfied with vision; no squint
	Can draw a man of three parts
	  (four years)
	Can copy a circle (3 years)
	  or cross (4 years) (Fig. 2.12b)
	Builds a bridge or steps with one-inch
	  cubes when shown (Fig. 2.12c)

Language/hearing	Gives first and last name Recognises colours (three years) Speech fully comprehensible to strangers (48 months) Parents satisfied with hearing

Social and self-help skills/behaviour	Can name a friend
	Washes hands and brushes teeth
	  with help
	Eats with a knife and fork
	Vivid make-believe play
	Will play independently with other
	  children present
	Shows sympathy when appropriate,
	  e.g. with an injured child
	Likes hearing and telling stories (Fig. 2.12d)

Surveillance review is usually carried out by the health visitor and can be combined with pre-school immunisation. This review aims to ensure that the child is physically fit and that there are no medical, developmental or behavioural problems that will impede education.

Parents	Ask about parental concerns, particularly
	  regarding development, language,
	  behaviour and special senses

Growth	Measure and plot on centile chart

Physical examination	Check for testicular descent in boys
	Complete primary immunisation with
	  pre-school booster
	  (diphtheria/tetanus and polio) and
	  MMR if not previously given

Special senses	Arrange hearing test if concern about
	  hearing or language
	Arrange ophthalmological assessment if
	  concern about vision or squint

Health promotion	Discuss accident prevention, fires,
	  drowning and road safety
	Discuss developmental needs and
	  preparation for school;
	  review nutrition and dental care

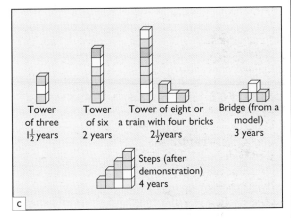

Circle
3 years

Cross
4 years

Square
4½ years

Triangle
5 years

Fig. 2.12b Hand skills. Ability to copy (draw without seeing how it is done). Children can usually imitate (draw after seeing it done) 6 months before they can copy

Tower of three 1½ years

Tower of six 2 years

Tower of eight or a train with four bricks 2½ years

Bridge (from a model) 3 years

Steps (after demonstration) 4 years

Fig. 2.12c Hand skills. Building with bricks showing the age of copying.

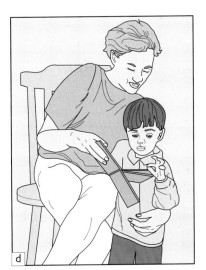

Fig. 2.12d Likes being read to and telling stories.

Language and speech

It is necessary to distinguish between:
- language – the underlying complex series of rules and codes governing communication and
- speech – the actual sounds that are made.

These are two separate entities. Children may have an isolated language disorder where they make speech sounds perfectly but are unable to communicate, or they can have a speech disorder, in which they can use the underlying rules for speech but are unable to communicate effectively because others cannot understand what they say.

Language is further divided into language comprehension and expressive language, and a child may have a deficit in either. As in other developmental areas, language comprehension and expressive language go through a developmental progression.

Many language problems are first suspected by parents or primary health professionals. However, diagnosis and treatment are specialist areas, the province of speech and language therapists and paediatricians with an interest in communication disorders. Therapy, though, may be performed by parents, teachers and others under the direction of therapists.

LANGUAGE TESTS AND ASSESSMENT

There is considerable overlap between language development and general intellectual development. 'Performance' or 'non-verbal' intelligence tests try to disregard the language component. However, the opposite is not the case and language tests, especially those for the younger child, assess general development levels as well as language.

Language tests are many and varied and usually applied by speech and language therapists. Some tests are:
- the symbolic toy test–assesses essential pre-language development. This test may be applied without specialist training
- the Reynell test–for the pre-school child. It has separate sections for comprehension and expression and is administered by specially trained professionals, usually speech and language therapists.

LANGUAGE AND SPEECH DELAY

Common causes include:
- hearing loss
- environmental deprivation
- general developmental delay.

There may be a family history of delay in language or speech which is transient. Once delay is identified and the child's hearing checked, a therapy programme may be initiated for the parents under the therapist's direction.

LANGUAGE AND SPEECH DISORDERS

These are more serious conditions and require specialist diagnosis and treatment. There may be a disorder of speech and speech sounds, such as stammering, incompre-

hensible speech or dysarthria. There may be receptive aphasia (inability to comprehend language) and expressive aphasia (inability to speak). Intensive therapy and even special schooling may be needed. Related but broader conditions are autism and also Asperger syndrome, where there is a specific communication and emotional disorder.

Hearing

At birth, a baby reacts to sound, but there is a marked preference for voices. The ability to locate and turn towards sounds comes later in the first year. The early detection of deafness is important (Figs 2.13 and 2.14). If left untreated, the child will have impaired speech, language and learning and behavioural problems stemming from difficulty in communication.

HEARING LOSS

The causes of hearing loss are listed in Figure 2.15. They can be divided into sensorineural and conductive.

Sensorineural hearing loss

This type of hearing loss is uncommon (1 in 1000 of all births, 1 in 100 in extremely low birthweight infants). It is usually present at birth or develops in the first few months of life. The loss of hearing is usually due to abnormalities of or damage to the cochlea and/or central neural

Fig. 2.13 Hearing checklist for parents.	
Shortly after birth	Startles and blinks at a sudden noise, e.g. slamming of door
By one month	Notices sudden prolonged sounds, e.g. a vacuum cleaner, and pauses and listens when they begin
By four months	Quietens or smiles to the sound of your voice even when he cannot see you. He may also turn his head or eyes towards you if you come up from behind and speak to him from the side
By seven months	Turns immediately to your voice across the room or to very quiet noises made on each side so long as he is not too occupied with other things
By nine months	Listens attentively to familiar everyday sounds and searches for very quiet sounds made out of sight. Should also show pleasure in babbling loudly and tunefully
By 12 months	Shows some response to his own name and to other familiar words. May respond when you say 'no' and 'bye-bye' even when he cannot see any accompanying gesture

If you suspect that your baby is not hearing normally, seek advice from your health visitor or doctor.
(Used by permission of Dr Barry McCormick, Children's Hearing Assessment Centre, Nottingham)

pathways. The hearing loss can be of any severity, including profound.

In newborn infants, hearing impairment can be identified using auditory evoked potentials, which detect brainstem responses to sounds, or the auditory response cradle, which relies on detecting a variety of behavioural responses to sound, such as turning of the head and changes in respiration. These tests require sophisticated equipment but can be applied if there are risk factors for hearing impairment, though routine screening is performed in some centres. More recently, otoacoustic emission testing has been introduced as a screening test and is relatively easy to perform. An earpiece is inserted into the ear canal and produces a sound which evokes an echo or emission from the ear if cochlear function is normal.

At seven to nine months of age, the distraction test is used for screening infant hearing in most parts of the UK (Fig. 2.16). This test relies on the baby locating and turning appropriately towards sounds. High- and low-frequency sounds are presented out of the infant's field of vision. Testing is unreliable if it is not carried out by properly trained staff since it can be difficult to identify hearing-impaired infants as they are particularly adept at using non-auditory cues.

Performance testing using high and low-frequency stimuli and speech discrimination testing using miniature toys can be used among children with suspected hearing loss at 15 months to four years of age (Fig. 2.17). Threshold

Fig. 2.14 Tests of hearing and auditory function.

Age	Test	Indication
Birth	Otoacoustic emission Brain stem evoked potential Auditory response cradle	Children at high risk, e.g. children of affected parents, preterm, received neonatal intensive care. Screening of all newborn infants in a few centres
6–9 months	Distraction test (using sounds)	Screening of all children except for a few areas
15 months –4 years	Threshold audiometry (>3 yrs) Speech discrimination test Impedance audiometry	Children with suspected hearing loss
4 years and upwards	Threshold audiometry	Screening of all children at school entry. Suspected hearing loss

Fig. 2.15 Causes and management of hearing loss.

	Sensorineural	Conductive
Causes	Genetic Perinatal congenital infection preterm, birth asphyxia hyperbilirubinaemia Postnatal meningitis/encephalitis head injury drugs, e.g. aminoglycosides	Wax (only rarely a cause of hearing loss) Secretory otitis media (glue ear)
Hearing loss	May be profound (20–120 dB hearing loss)	Maximum of 20-60 dB hearing loss
Natural history	Does not improve/ progresses	Intermittent/resolves
Management	Amplification/ cochlear implant	Conservative/ medical/surgery

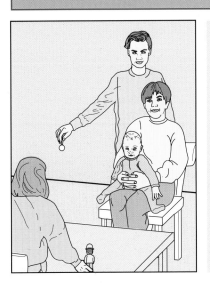

Fig. 2.16 Distraction hearing test. The test is hard to perform reliably as babies with hearing disability learn to compensate by using shadows, smells and guess-work to locate the presenter. The test must be done by well-trained professionals.

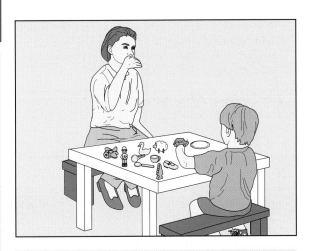

Fig. 2.17 Speech discrimination testing using miniature toys to detect hearing loss in children between 15 months and four years of age.

audiometry can be used to detect and assess the severity of hearing loss in children from four years old (Fig. 2.18a–d).

Sensorineural hearing loss is irreversible. The child with severe bilateral hearing impairment will need early amplification with hearing aids for optimal speech and language development. Hearing aid use requires careful supervision, beginning in the home together with the parents and continuing into school. Children often resist wearing hearing aids because background noise can be amplified unpleasantly. Cochlear implants may be required where hearing aids give insufficient amplification. Intensive specialist teaching and support is provided by peripatetic teachers for children with hearing impairment.

Children with hearing impairment should be placed in the classroom so that they can readily see the teacher. Gesture, visual context and lip movement will also allow children to develop language concepts. Many children with moderate hearing impairment can be educated within the mainstream school system or in partially hearing units attached to mainstream schools. Speech may be delayed, but with appropriate therapy can be of good quality. Schools for children with severe hearing impairment still perform a vital role when a child's needs cannot be met through mainstream education. Modified and simplified signing such as Makaton can be helpful for children who are both hearing impaired and learning disabled.

Conductive hearing loss

Conductive hearing loss from middle ear disease can be up to 60 decibels, but is usually less. It is much more common than sensorineural hearing loss. In association with upper respiratory tract infections, many children have episodes of hearing loss which are usually self-limiting but can be prolonged. Conductive hearing loss is often acquired in the first few years of life and may be recurrent.

In most affected children there are no risk factors present, but children with Down syndrome and cleft palate and atopy are particularly prone to middle ear disease. Any

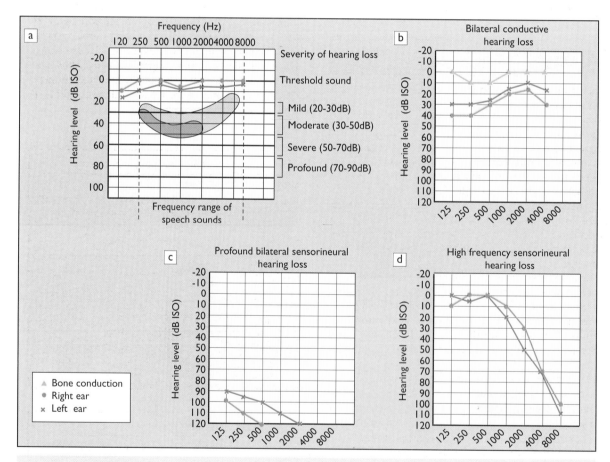

Fig. 2.18a Audiogram showing normal hearing and the loudness of normal speech. The light blue area represents the consonants (high frequency sounds); the green area the vowels (low frequency sounds)
Fig. 2.18b Audiogram showing bilateral conductive hearing loss. There is a 20–40 dB hearing loss in both the right and left ears.
Fig. 2.18c Audiogram showing bilateral profound sensorineural hearing loss.
Fig. 2.18d Audiogram showing bilateral high-frequency sensorineural hearing loss.

concern about hearing loss should be taken seriously. Any child with delayed language or speech, learning difficulties or behavioural problems should have his hearing tested, as a mild hearing loss can be the underlying cause without parents or other carers being aware.

Detection is by the same methods as for sensorineural loss, except electrical stimulation tests are not useful. Impedance audiometry tests whether the middle ear functions normally. If the condition does not improve spontaneously, medical treatment (decongestant or a long course of antibiotics) can be given. If that fails, then surgery is considered, with insertion of tympanostomy tubes (grommets) with or without the removal of adenoids. The role of surgery remains controversial.

In this condition two children may have the same degree of hearing loss and one manage well, the other poorly. The decision whether to intervene should be based on the degree of functional disability rather than on absolute hearing loss.

 Any child with poor or delayed speech or language must have his hearing checked.

Vision

A newborn infant's vision is limited: the visual acuity is only about 6/200. The retina is well developed but the fovea is immature. Well-focused images on the retina are required for the acquisition of visual acuity and any obstacle to this, e.g. from a cataract, will interfere with the normal development of the optic pathways and visual cortex unless corrected early in life.

Most newborn infants can fix and follow horizontally. There is a preference for looking at faces. Initially the eyes may move independently and the baby may appear to squint; this is particularly noticeable when the baby tries to look at near objects and the eyes overconverge.

By around six weeks of age both eyes should move together when following a light source and no squint should be present. Babies slowly develop the ability to focus at different distances and visual acuity improves from 6/60 at three months to adult levels at around three years. Testing for abnormalities has to allow for this.

Visual impairment may present in infancy with:
- lack of following and fixation
- random eye movements
- nystagmus
- not smiling responsively by six weeks post-term
- delayed development and visual inattention
- squint
- photophobia
- loss of red reflex from a cataract
- a white reflex in the pupil; may be due to retinoblastoma, cataract or retinopathy of prematurity.

The assessment of vision at different ages is shown in Figure 2.19.

ABNORMALITIES OF VISION
Severe visual impairment
This affects 1 in 3000 births but is important to detect early. A family history of severe visual impairment or extreme prematurity places the infant at an increased risk. In developed countries about 50% of severe visual impairment is genetic (Fig. 2.20). The eye examination may be normal when visual impairment is of cortical origin resulting from cerebral damage.

Although few causes of severe visual impairment can be treated, much can be done to help the child and his parents. Parents of a partially sighted or severely visually impaired child need appropriate advice on how to provide non-visual stimulation using speech and touch, on providing a safe home environment and how to build the child's confidence. In the UK this is usually provided by peripatetic teachers for the visually impaired. Partially sighted children may be able to attend a mainstream school but require special assistance with low vision aids which include filtered lenses, high-powered magnifiers and small telescopic devices and computers. Severely visually impaired children often need special schooling. They will usually need to be taught Braille to enable them to read. While many severely visually impaired children have a visual disability only, at least half have additional neurodevelopmental problems.

Age	Test
Birth	Face fixation and following demonstrated
	Preferential looking–preference for patterned objects to plain ones
Six weeks	Optokinetic nystagmus demonstrated on looking at a moving, striped target
Six months	Reaches well for toys
Two years	Can identify specific pictures of reducing size
Three years onwards	Letter matching using single letter charts, e.g. Sheridan Gardiner
Five years onwards	Can identify a line of letters on a Snellen chart by name or matching

Fig. 2.19 Testing vision at different ages.

Genetic	Antenatal and perinatal	Postnatal
Cataract	Congenital infection	Trauma
Albinism	Retinopathy of prematurity	Infection
Retinal dystrophy	Hypoxic-ischaemic encephalopathy	
Retinoblastoma	Cerebral abnormality/damage	

Fig. 2.20 Causes of visual impairment.

Squints (strabismus)

In this common condition there is misalignment of the visual axes. The history may be helpful as squints may be intermittent and parents are usually correct if they report deviation of the eyes. There may be a history of squint in the family.

Newborn babies often give the appearance of having a squint because of over-convergence. In older infants and young children marked epicanthic folds may cause confusion (pseudosquint). Any infant with a fixed squint or any squint persisting beyond two months of age should be referred for a specialist ophthalmological opinion. A squint is usually caused by failure to develop binocular vision due to refractive errors, but cataracts, retinoblastoma and other intraocular causes must be excluded.

Squints are commonly divided into:

- Concomitant (common) – usually due to a refractive error in one or both eyes which is often treated by correction with glasses but may require surgery. Squints are common in children with neurodevelopmental delay. The squinting eye most often turns inwards (convergent), but there can be outward (divergent) or rarely vertical deviation
- paralytic (rare) – due to paralysis of the motor nerves. When rapid in onset this can be sinister because of the possibility of a space-occupying lesion such as a brain tumour.

Corneal light reflection test

For the non-specialist, the light reflection test is used to detect squints (Fig. 2.21). It is easiest to use a pen torch held at a distance to produce reflections on both corneas simultaneously. The light reflection should appear in the same position in the two eyes. If it does not, a squint is present. However, a minor squint may be difficult to detect.

Cover test

When a squint is present and the fixing eye is covered, the squinting eye moves to take up fixation (Fig. 2.22).

The child's interest can be attracted with a toy or light. The test should be performed with the object near (33 cm) and distant (at least 6 metres) as certain squints are present only at one distance. Occlusion should be with a card or plastic occluder. To obtain reliable results, this test should be performed by an orthoptist or ophthalmologist.

Refractive errors

Hypermetropia

This is the most common refractive error in young children and should be corrected early to avoid irreversible damage to vision (amblyopia). This is more likely if accompanied by a squint but may occur without.

Myopia

Is uncommon in young children and is less likely to cause amblyopia unless it is severe or only one eye is affected. All children in the UK are screened for visual acuity and squint at school entry. In some parts of the UK pre-school children (at $3^{1}/_{2}$–4 years) are screened.

Amblyopia

This is a loss of visual acuity and the eye is often referred to as a 'lazy eye'. In most cases it affects one eye; rarely both are involved. Any obstacle to visual development may cause amblyopia, such as unilateral or bilateral refractive errors, squint or visual deprivation, e.g. ptosis or cataract. Treatment is with correction of any refractive error followed by patching of the 'good' eye for specific periods of the day until the vision no longer improves. Glasses are worn if required. The longer treatment is delayed, the less likely it is that normal vision will be obtained. Early treatment is essential as after seven years of age improvement is unlikely. Considerable encouragement and support are often needed, as young children usually dislike having their eye patched, particularly if vision in the unpatched eye is poor.

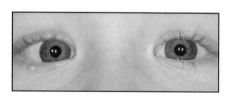

Fig. 2.21 Corneal light reflection test to detect a squint. The reflection is in a different position in the two eyes because of a small convergent squint of the right eye.

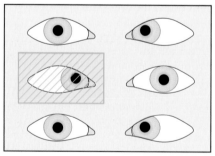

Fig. 2.22 The cover test is used to identify a squint. If the fixing eye is covered, the squinting eye moves to take up fixation. This diagram shows a left convergent squint.

FURTHER READING

Hall DMB (ed). *Health For All Children,* 3rd ed. Oxford University Press, Oxford, 1996. Describes child health promotion and surveillance, its potential and limitations.

Hall DMB, Hill P, Elliman D. *The Child Surveillance Handbook,* 2nd ed. Radcliffe Medical Press, Oxford, 1994. A practical guide to child development and surveillance.

Illingworth RS. *Basic Developmental Screening: 0–4,* Blackwell Scientific, Oxford, 1988. A short guide to child development.

McCormick B. *Hearing Screening 0–5 years,* 2nd ed. Croom Helm, London, 1994. A practical guide to hearing screening.

CHAPTER 3

Care of the Sick Child

• Primary care • Hospital care

Most sick children are cared for by their parents at home. Medical management is initially given by general practitioners or, in some countries, primary care paediatricians. Most hospital admissions are at secondary care level. A smaller number of children will require tertiary care in a specialist centre e.g. paediatric intensive care, cardiac or oncology unit. There are a few national centres for very rare and complex treatments, e.g. organ transplantation, craniofacial surgery (Fig. 3.1).

Primary care

GENERAL PRACTITIONER

The majority of acute illness in children is mild and transient or readily treatable. Although serious conditions are uncommon, they must be identified promptly. A sick baby's condition may deteriorate rapidly, and parents require rapid access for consultation from their general practitioner, who in turn requires ready access to secondary care, both inpatient and outpatient, in a wide range of services for children.

Hospital care

ACCIDENT AND EMERGENCY

Approximately 1 in 4 children attend an Accident and Emergency Department each year in England and Wales. The services which should be provided for children are shown in Figure 3.2. Unfortunately, many departments fail to meet these expectations.

HOSPITAL ADMISSION

In England and Wales, 1 in 11 children are admitted to hospital each year. This is 16% of all hospital admissions. About 42% of acute admissions are under the care of paediatricians, the remainder are surgical. Most paediatric admissions are of infants and young children and are emergencies, whereas surgical admissions peak at five years of age and one-third are elective (Fig. 3.3). The reasons for medical admissions are shown in Figure 3.4.

Although primary and community health services for children have improved markedly over the last decade, the hospital admission rate has continued to rise (Fig. 3.5). The reasons for this are unclear, but probably include:
- increased hospital admission rate for asthma, one of the commonest causes for inpatient treatment
- lower threshold for admission. In infants with respiratory disorders, this may be because of increased awareness of the risk of sudden infant death syndrome (SIDS). There also appears to be an increased expectation of hospital admission by parents and medical staff in case the child's clinical condition deteriorates as well as increased staff awareness of poor social circumstances
- repeated hospital admission of children with complex con-

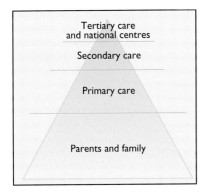

Fig. 3.1 Schematic representation of the provision of care for sick children. (Adapted from Audit Commission, Children First)

Fig. 3.2 Services which should be available for children attending an Accident and Emergency Department		
Environment	**Staff**	**Medical care**
Separate waiting area, play facilities, treatment and recovery areas	Medical and nursing staff trained and experienced in the care and treatment of children	Resuscitation and other equipment for children
Access for parents to examination, X-ray and anaesthetic rooms	Non-paediatric staff trained in communicating with children and families	Priority for prompt treatment
		Rapid transfer if inpatient admission is needed
		Child protection policies
	Effective communication with other health professionals	Procedures and counselling following the sudden death of a child

(Adapted from Welfare of Children in Hospital)

ditions who would have died in the past but are now surviving, e.g. very low birthweight infants from neonatal intensive care units, children with cancer or major organ failure.

Strenuous efforts are being made to reduce the rate and length of hospitalisation.

Day case surgery has been instituted for many operations which used to require overnight stay. Day units are used for complex procedures and investigations.

Home care teams aim to provide care in the child's home and thereby reduce the need to attend hospital and/or the length of stay in hospital. Most teams comprise community paediatric nurses, but some include doctors, and they either cover all aspects of paediatric care within a geographical area or are for a specific condition, e.g. cystic fibrosis or malignancy, usually centred round a tertiary referral centre. The problems managed at home by such teams include:

• changing postoperative wound dressings or managing burns
• day to day management and family support for chronic illnesses, e.g. diabetes, asthma and eczema

• specialist care, e.g. home oxygen therapy, intravenous infusions via a central venous catheter (e.g. antibiotics or chemotherapy), or peritoneal dialysis
• symptom and pain control and emotional support of terminally ill children (Fig. 3.6).

Some teams provide a 'hospital at home' service for children who are acutely ill to avoid hospitalisation.

CHILDREN IN HOSPITAL

Children should only be admitted to hospital if their care cannot be provided safely at home. Removing young children from their familiar environment to a strange ward is stressful and frightening for the child, parents and family. It also disrupts family routines, not only of the child on the ward, but also of siblings who may still need to be transported to and from school or nursery, fed and looked after.

Family-centred care

Care in hospital should be child- and family-centred. Parents and siblings should be involved in the child's care, which should be appropriate for the child's physical and emotion-

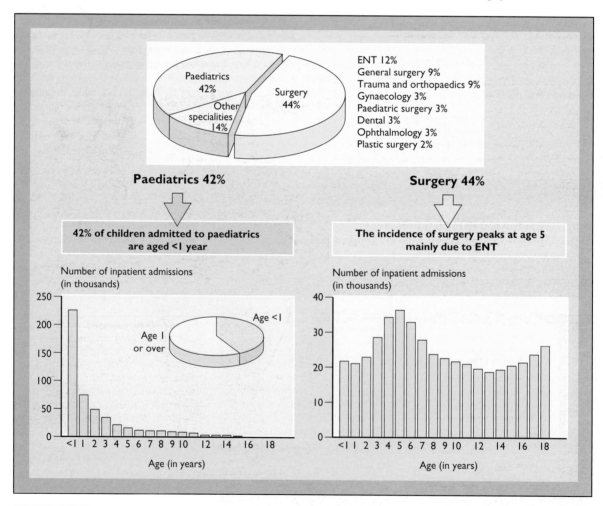

Fig. 3.3 *Hospital inpatients of children aged 0–18 years in England and Wales in 1990–91. (Adapted from Audit Commission,* Children First)

al maturity and needs. A holistic approach should be taken to the child and his family rather than simply focusing on the child's medical condition. Young children may interpret the pain experienced in hospital and separation from their home or parents as punishment. In general, the distress arising from separating children from their mothers is greatest in young children, and increases the longer the length of stay and the more often the child is admitted. Parents should be encouraged to continue to provide the care and support they would give at home. Parents know best about their child's usual behaviour and habits and due attention must be paid to their worries or comments. Many parents rapidly learn some of the nursing skills, e.g. tube feeding required by their child.

Good communication is needed between staff and parents to arrive at a mutually agreed plan of responsibilities for looking after the child. This will avoid parents either feeling pressurised to accept responsibilities they are not confident about or feeling brushed aside and underestimated by staff. Parents should be able to stay overnight with their child.

Child-orientated environment

Children should be cared for within a children's ward. Adolescents should be with others of their own age and not forced to accept ward arrangements designed for babies or adults. Education should be provided.

Information and psychosocial support

Detailed information should be provided, given personally and preferably written. This should be available in ethnic community languages. Staff should be sensitive to the family's individual needs according to their social, educational, ethnic and religious background. Play specialists should be part of the ward team because they can help children understand their illness and its treatment through play. Emotional and psychological support should be given to all. For elective admissions, children and their families should be offered an advance visit and have details of proposed treatment and management explained to them at a level appropriate to their understanding.

Fig. 3.4 Reasons for paediatric medical admissions to a district general hospital.	
Respiratory 31%	Asthma 11%
	URTI 6%
	Croup 4%
	Bronchiolitis 4%
	Pneumonia 3%
	Tonsillitis 2.5%
Environment 22%	Head injury 12%
	Poisoning 8%
	Child protection 1.5%
Gastroenterology 15%	Gastroenteritis 7%
	Constipation/soiling 2%
	Abdominal pain/vomiting 2%
	Failure to thrive 1%
Infection 10%	Viral infection 6%
	Septicaemia/meningitis 1.5%
Neurology 8%	Febrile convulsions 3%
	Epilepsy 3%
	Apnoea/cyanotic attacks 2%
Kidney and urinary tract 3%	Urinary tract infection 2.5%
Other 11%	

(Data based on 2160 consecutive admissions to Pinderfields Hospital, Wakefield. Courtesy of Dr Roddy MacFaul.)

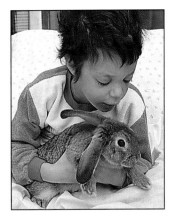

Fig. 3.6 Providing terminal care in a child's home. Although Georgina required a subcutaneous morphine infusion to control her pain from malignant disease, she was able to remain at home and enjoyed playing with her pet rabbit. (By kind permission of her parents and Dr Ann Goldman).

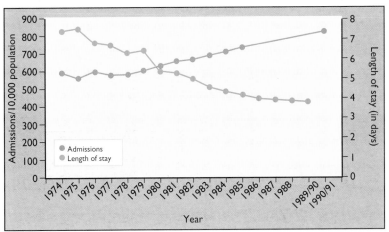

Fig. 3.5 Inpatient admission rates for children aged 0–14 years in England. There has been a marked increase in the paediatric admission rate, whereas the surgical admission rate has remained unchanged. In both, there has been a marked reduction in the average length of stay. (From Audit Commission, Children First)

Skilled staff

Children in hospital should be cared for by specially trained medical, nursing and support staff. Every child admitted to hospital should be supervised by a children's physician or surgeon. Children constitute only a relatively small proportion of the workload in acute surgical specialties, so surgeons and anaesthetists should treat a sufficient number of children to maintain their skills. There should be a 'named nurse' responsible for planning and coordinating care by other nurses, to ensure that families receive all the information they need and provide a link with staff involved in discharge planning and post-discharge arrangements.

Multidisciplinary care

Successful management of paediatric conditions often relies on a network of multidisciplinary care, with all the professionals working well together as a coordinated team. If this breaks down, particularly when dealing with complex issues such as child protection, the consequences may be disastrous for the child, family and professionals involved. Child psychiatrists, the community paediatric team and social services are important members of the team.

PAIN

It is easy to ignore or underestimate pain in children. Pain should ideally be anticipated and prevented.

Acute pain

May be caused by:
- tissue damage, e.g. burns/trauma
- disease, e.g. sickle cell crisis
- medical intervention – investigations/procedures
- surgical intervention.

Chronic pain

In children, chronic pain sometimes occurs as a result of disease, such as juvenile chronic arthritis or progressive malignancy. Chronic persistent pain, such as backache is uncommon, in contrast to the recurrent episodic pain of headaches, abdomen or limbs in otherwise healthy children.

Older children can describe the nature and severity of the pain they are experiencing. In younger children, assessing pain is more difficult. Observation and parental impression are commonly used and a number of self-assessment tools have been designed for children over three years old (Fig. 3.7).

Management

The approaches to pain management are listed in Figure 3.8. For severe pain, there was reluctance in the past to use morphine in children for fear of depressing breathing. This should not occur when morphine is given in appropriate dosage under nursing supervision to children with a normal respiratory drive. Intravenous morphine can be given using a patient-controlled delivery system in older children or a nurse-controlled system in young children.

PRESCRIBING DRUGS

There are marked differences in the absorption, distribution and elimination of drugs between children and adults.

Absorption

In the neonate and infant, oral formulations of drugs can be given as liquids. However, their intake cannot be guaranteed and absorption is unpredictable as it is affected by gastric emptying and acidity, gut motility and the effects of milk in the stomach. Rectal administration can be used for some drugs; absorption is more reliable but the route is not popular in the UK. In acutely ill neonates and infants drugs are given intravenously to ensure reliable and adequate blood and tissue concentrations. Intramuscular injections should be avoided if possible as there is little muscle bulk available for injection, absorption is variable and they are painful. Significant systemic absorption can occur across the skin, particularly in preterm infants. Occasionally this can be used therapeutically, but is also a potential cause of toxicity, e.g. alcohol and iodine absorption of cleansing solutions applied to the skin for procedures.

Young children find it difficult to take tablets and a liquid formulation is required. Most are glucose-free. Persuading children to take medicines is often a problem. Compliance is improved when medicines are only required once or twice a day.

Distribution

Water comprises a larger percentage of the body in the neonate (80%) than older children and adults (55%). Drugs which distribute within the extracellular fluid will require a larger dose relative to body weight in infants than adults. As extracellular fluid correlates with body surface area, this is used when accurate drug dosage is required,

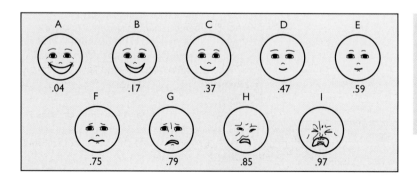

Fig. 3.7 An example of a scoring system for pain assessment in children. (From Mc Grath PA, DeVeber LL, Hearn MT. Multidimensional pain assessment in children. In: Fields H, Dubner R, Cervero F (eds). Advances In Pain Research and Therapy. *Raven Press, New York, 1985; 387–393*)

Fig. 3.8 Approaches to pain management

Explanation and information

Psychological, by the parent, doctor or nurse
- behavioural
- distraction
- hypnosis

Medical
- local: anaesthetic cream, local infiltration, nerve blocks, warmth or cold, physiotherapy, transcutaneous electrical nerve stimulation (TENS)
- general analgesics:
    mild – paracetamol, NSAID
    moderate – codeine, NSAID
    strong – morphine

Consider the route for analgesics – oral if possible, otherwise intravenous, subcutaneous or rectal.

---

e.g. cytotoxic agents. Body weight is used for drugs with high therapeutic indices as it is easier to measure. Alternatively, dosage may be based on age using an average-sized child. Weight dosages should not be extrapolated to older children as the dosage will be excessively large.

In the first few months of life the plasma protein is low. More of the drug may be unbound and pharmacologically active. In jaundiced infants, bilirubin may compete with some drugs e.g. sulphonamides for albumin binding sites.

Elimination

In neonates, drug biotransformation is reduced as the microsomal enzymes in the liver are immature. This leads to a prolonged half-life of drugs metabolised in the liver e.g. theophylline. Renal excretion is reduced by the low glomerular filtration rate which increases the half-life of some drugs, e.g. gentamicin. Measuring the plasma drug concentration is necessary under these circumstances.

Dosage of intravenous drugs:
Easy to miscalculate in children as it varies widely with size and drugs are often diluted. All dosages and dilutions of drugs that have potentially serious side-effects must be checked independently by two trained members of staff.

CONSENT

Informed consent of both child and parent should be obtained, except in an emergency. In the UK, the age of consent is 16 years. In principle, if a child below 16 years has sufficient understanding, the child may consent or refuse to consent to be examined or treated. In practice, problems occur only when the child and parents have strongly opposing views. This is rare and legal advice may then be needed. Younger children should be provided with as much information as possible in language they can understand, and their wishes determined and taken into account. Consent must always be obtained for children to

take part in medical research. Guidance is available on the ethics of research involving children.

BREAKING BAD NEWS

Doctors often face the difficult task of imparting bad news to parents and children. In paediatrics it is often because there is:
- a serious congenital abnormality at birth, e.g. spina bifida, chromosomal disorder
- the diagnosis of a disabling condition, e.g. cerebral palsy, neurodegenerative disorder, gross intracranial abnormality seen at ultrasound in preterm infants
- a serious illness, e.g. meningitis or malignant disease, or an accident, e.g. head injury
- the sudden death of a child, e.g. sudden infant death syndrome (SIDS).

Initial interview

The manner in which the initial interview is conducted is very important. It may have a profound influence on the parents' ability to cope with the problem and their subsequent relationship with health professionals. Parents often continue to recall and recount for many years details of the initial interview when they were informed that their child had a serious problem. Parents of children with life-threatening illnesses have said that what they valued most was open, sympathetic, direct and uninterrupted discussion in private that allowed sufficient time for doctors to repeat and clarify information (Fig. 3.9).

DISCHARGE FROM HOSPITAL

Children should be discharged from hospital as soon as clinically and socially appropriate. Although there is increasing pressure to reduce the length of hospital stay to a minimum, this must not allow discharge planning to be neglected. Before discharge from hospital, parents and children should be informed of:
- the reason for admission and its implications for the future
- details of medication and other treatment
- any clinical features which should prompt them to seek medical advice, and how this should be obtained
- the existence of any voluntary self-help groups if appropriate
- problems or questions likely to be asked by other family members or in the community. These should be anticipated by the doctor and discussed. What does the nursery/school, baby sitters or friends need to know? What about sports etc?

In addition:
- suitability of home circumstances needs to be assessed, particularly when the home requires adaptation for special needs
- social support may need to be arranged, especially in relation to child protection
- medical information should be added to the personal child health record

Fig. 3.9 *How parents wish to be told the diagnosis of a life-threatening illness. This may take several interviews.*

Setting	In private
	Uninterrupted
	Unhurried
	Both parents (or friend/relative) present
	   if possible
	Senior doctor
	Nurse or social worker present
		Address feelings	Be prepared to tolerate reactions of shock,
			   especially anger or weeping
			Acknowledge uncertainty
			How is it likely to affect the family?
			What and how to tell other children, relatives
			   and friends?

Establish contact	Find out what the family knows or suspects
	Respect family's vulnerability
	Use the child's name
	Do not avoid looking at them
	Be direct, open, sympathetic
		*Concluding the
		interview*
			Elicit what parents have understood
			Clarify and repeat
			Acknowledge that it may be difficult for parents
			   to absorb all the information
			Mention sources of support
			If available, give parents contact telephone
			   number
			Give address of self-help group

Provide information	Flexibility is essential
	Pace rather than protect from bad news
	Name the illness
	Describe symptoms relevant to child's
	   condition
	Discuss aetiology – parents will usually want
	   to know
	Anticipate and answer questions. Don't avoid
	   difficult issues because parents have not
	   thought to ask
	Explain long-term prognosis
	If child is likely to die, listen to concerns about
	   time, place and nature of death
	Outline the support/treatment available
		Follow-up	Offer early follow-up
			Suggest to families that they write down
			   questions in preparation for next appointment
			Ensure adequate communication of content of
			   interview to :
			   • other members of staff
			   • general practitioner and health visitor
			   • other professionals, e.g. a referring
			     paediatrician

(Adapted from Woolley H, Stein A, Forrest GC, Baum JD. Imparting the diagnosis of life-threatening illness in children, Br Med J, *1989;* **298***: 1623–1626)*

- consider who else should be informed about the admission and what information is relevant for them. This must be done before or at the time of discharge. The aim is to provide a seamless service of care, treatment and support, with the family and all the professionals fully informed (Fig. 3.10). This can be facilitated for children with a chronic illness or disability and their family by having a key worker to coordinate their care.

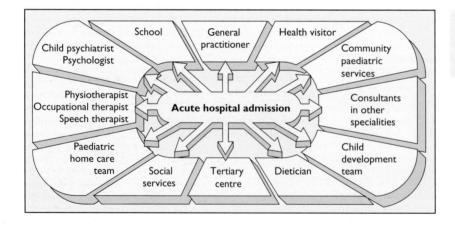

Fig. 3.10 *Some of the professionals who may need information about an acute hospital admission.*

FURTHER READING

Audit Commission. *Children First. A study of hospital services.* HMSO, London, 1993.

Schechter NL, Berde CB, Yaster M. *Pain in Infants, Children and Adolescents.* Williams and Wilkins, Baltimore, 1993. Comprehensive book.

Welfare of Children and Young People in Hospital. HMSO, London, 1991. Details of hospital services for children.

CHAPTER 4

Paediatric Emergencies

• The critically ill child • Shock • Diabetic ketoacidosis • Status epilepticus • The febrile child • Septicaemia • Bacterial meningitis • Viral encephalitis • The death of a child

There are few situations that provoke greater anxiety in doctors than being called to see a child who is critically ill. This chapter outlines a basic approach to the emergency management of critically ill children. A number of important anatomical and physiological differences influence emergency management (Fig. 4.1).

The critically ill child

The approach to the critically ill child must address the dual needs of treating the immediate medical problems and discovering the underlying cause. In practical terms

this means obtaining a history from the parents or those accompanying the child, at the same time as assessing and treating the child (Figs 4.2–4.4).

CARDIOPULMONARY RESUSCITATION (CPR)

Whatever the underlying cause of the child's condition, if a child's airway, breathing or circulation are inadequate a number of basic measures need to be taken.

Airway and breathing

Airway obstruction may be due to excessive secretions or an inhaled foreign body which should be removed. An appropriate-sized oral airway should be inserted. Correct

	Fig. 4.1 Important anatomical and physiological differences in young children	
	Features in young children	**Consequence**
Anatomical	Large head, short neck	
	Small face and mandible	Influence size and shape of the airway.
	Large tongue	Where the airway is narrow, obstruction is more likely
	Narrow nasal passages	
	Adenotonsillar hypertrophy	
	Trachea short and soft	Trachea is easily compressed if the neck is over-extended.
		This is important in maintaining airway patency during resuscitation and at tracheal intubation.
	Larger surface area to weight ratio relative to adults	Greater fluid and heat loss needs to be allowed for when calculating fluid replacement, e.g. after burns.
		Influences drug dosage.
		Hypothermia occurs more readily.
Physiological	Different baseline physiological parameters	Normal ranges vary with age (see Fig. 4.2).
	Lungs have a relatively small alveolar surface area	Less respiratory reserve than adults
	Compliant chest wall	Sternal recession and use of accessory muscles of respiration are early signs of increased respiratory effort
	Greater metabolic rate and oxygen consumption	Faster respiratory rate in children
	Small stroke volume	Higher heart rates (Cardiac Output = Stroke Volume × Heart Rate)
	Cannot rely on specific response to commands to assess level of consciousness	Modified Glasgow Coma Scale for children (see Fig. 4.3)

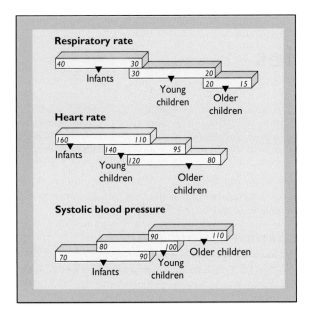

Fig. 4.3 Glasgow Coma Scale		
Glasgow Coma Scale (4-15 years)		
	Response	**Score**
Eyes	Open spontaneously	4
	Verbal command	3
	Pain	2
	No response	1
Best motor response	Spontaneous or obeys verbal command	6
	Painful stimulus:	
	Localises pain	5
	Flexion with pain	4
	Flexion abnormal	3
	Extension	2
	No response	1
Best verbal response	Orientated and converses	5
	Disorientated and converses	4
	Inappropriate words	3
	Incomprehensible sounds	2
	No response	1
Children's Coma Scale (<4 years)		
	Response	**Score**
Eyes	Open spontaneously	4
	Reacts to speech	3
	Reacts to pain	2
	No response	1
Best motor response	Spontaneous or obeys verbal command	6
	Painful stimulus:	
	Localises pain	5
	Withdraws in response to pain	4
	Abnormal flexion to pain (decorticate posture)	3
	Abnormal extension to pain (decerebrate posture)	2
	No response	1
Best verbal response	Smiles, orientated to sounds, follows objects, interacts	5

	Crying	Interacts	
	Consolable	Inappropriate	4
	Inconsistently consolable	Moaning	3
	Inconsolable	Irritable	2
	No response	No response	1

A score of < 8 out of 15 means that mechanical ventilation is required.

positioning of the head in relation to the neck is essential for optimal ventilation. Over-extension of the neck may worsen rather than relieve the obstruction (Fig 4.5 a, b). If ventilation remains inadequate, a correctly sized face mask and rebreathing bag should be used to assist with breathing. If this fails tracheal intubation and artificial ventilation will be necessary (Fig. 4.6).

Circulation

Cardiopulmonary resuscitation is performed at a ratio of five compressions to one breath aiming for 20 cycles per minute (i.e. 100 compressions and 20 breaths per minute). The optimal position for chest compression in children of different sizes is shown in Figure 4.7a–c.

Circulatory support with intravenous fluids
Many critically ill children are hypovolaemic. Intravenous access should be established at the earliest possible opportunity. If there is delay in establishing intravenous access, an intraosseous infusion can be established with a needle inserted directly into the tibia. Very large volumes of fluid may be needed.

Drugs
Management of asystole or ventricular fibrillation is instituted if the circulation has not been restored despite adequate cardiopulmonary resuscitation (Figs 4.8 and 4.9). Drug treatment and defibrillation have a lesser role in the resuscitation of children as myocardial ischaemia is much less common than in adults.

CLINICAL PRESENTATION AND CAUSES OF CRITICAL ILLNESS
There are four main modes of clinical presentation of critical illness in children (Fig. 4.10):
- shock
- respiratory distress
- the drowsy/unconscious child
- surgical emergencies.

The initial management of some specific emergencies is described in this chapter. Appropriate early management will improve their outcome. The other disorders listed in Fig. 4.10 are described in the relevant chapters.

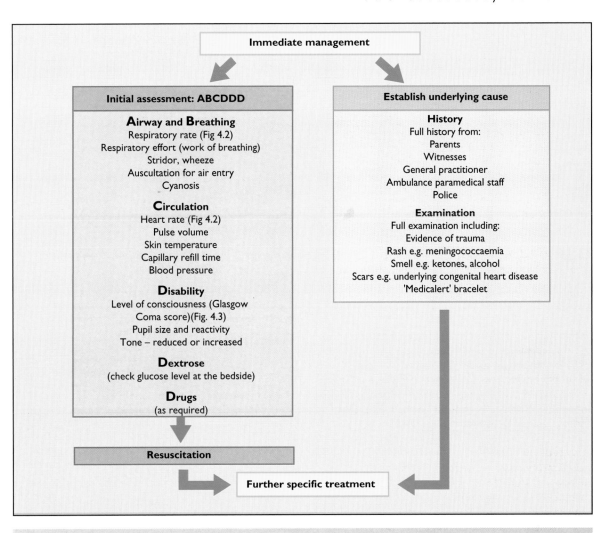

Fig. 4.4 The dual approach to the critically ill child.

Airway and Breathing

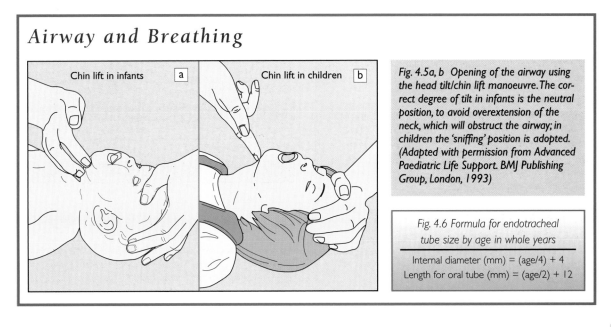

Chin lift in infants [a]

Chin lift in children [b]

Fig. 4.5a, b Opening of the airway using the head tilt/chin lift manoeuvre. The correct degree of tilt in infants is the neutral position, to avoid overextension of the neck, which will obstruct the airway; in children the 'sniffing' position is adopted. (Adapted with permission from Advanced Paediatric Life Support. BMJ Publishing Group, London, 1993)

Fig. 4.6 Formula for endotracheal tube size by age in whole years

Internal diameter (mm) = (age/4) + 4
Length for oral tube (mm) = (age/2) + 12

Circulation

Chest compression in children of different ages. (Published with permission from Advanced Paediatric Life Support. *BMJ Publishing Group, London, 1993*)

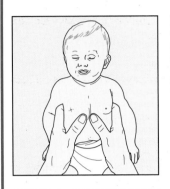

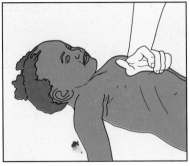

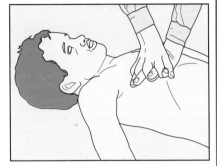

Fig. 4.7a Infant: one finger's breadth below nipple line.

Fig. 4.7b Small child: one finger's breadth above xiphisternum.

Fig. 4.7c Large child: two finger's breadth above xiphisternum.

Drugs

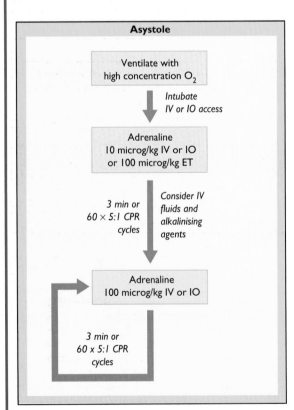

Fig. 4.8 Management of asystole. IO = intraosseous, IV = intravenous, ET = endotracheal tube. (Published with permission from Advanced Paediatric Life Support. *BMJ Publishing Group, London, 1993.*)

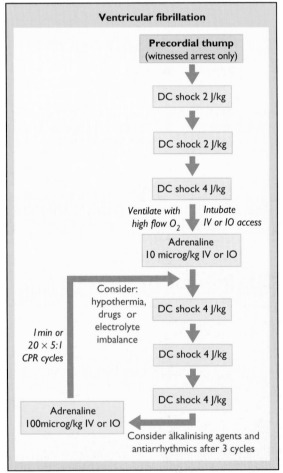

Fig. 4.9 Management of ventricular fibrillation. (Published with permission from Advanced Paediatric Life Support. *BMJ Publishing Group, London, 1993.*)

Shock

Critically ill children are often in shock.

Why children are so susceptible to fluid loss

Children have a much higher fluid requirement per kg body weight than adults (Fig. 4.11).

They will therefore rapidly become dehydrated if:
- they are unable to take fluids
- there are additional fluid losses from vomiting, diarrhoea, capillary leak as in septicaemia, through the skin, e.g. fever, sweating burns.

Clinical signs (Fig. 4.12)

In shock, dehydration is marked, with >10% loss of body weight (see Chapter 11).

MANAGEMENT PRIORITIES

Fluid resuscitation (Fig. 4.13)

The type of fluid is less critical than rapid restoration of the intravascular circulating volume. When there is evidence of capillary leak it is preferable to use colloids.

Fig. 4.10 The principal causes of the four main modes of clinical presentation of critically ill children.

1. Shock

Hypovolaemia	Dehydration – gastroenteritis, diabetic ketoacidosis
	Blood loss – trauma
	Plasma loss – burns, nephrotic syndrome
Maldistribution of fluid	Septicaemia
	Anaphylaxis
	Bowel obstruction
Cardiogenic	Arrhythmias
	Heart failure

2. Respiratory distress

Upper airway obstruction (stridor)	Foreign body
	Croup (laryngotracheobronchitis)/ epiglottitis
	Congenital malformations
	Trauma
Lower airway disorders	Asthma
	Bronchiolitis
	Pneumonia
	Pneumothorax

3. The drowsy/unconscious or fitting child

Post ictal/status epilepticus	
Infection	Meningitis/encephalitis
Metabolic	Diabetic ketoacidosis,
	Hypoglycaemia,
	Electrolyte disturbances (calcium, magnesium, sodium),
	Reye syndrome,
	Inborn errors of metabolism
Head injury	Trauma/non-accidental injury
Drug/poison ingestion	
Intracerebral haemorrhage	

4. Surgical emergencies

Acute abdomen	Appendicitis, perforation
Intestinal obstruction	
Trauma	

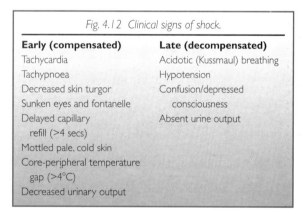

Fig. 4.11 Fluid intake at different ages	
Infants	100–120 ml/kg/24h
Young children (>1 yr)	90–120 ml/kg/24h
Older children (2–15 yr)	50–90 ml/kg/24h
Adult (> 15 yr)	20–35 ml/kg/24h

Fig. 4.12 Clinical signs of shock.	
Early (compensated)	**Late (decompensated)**
Tachycardia	Acidotic (Kussmaul) breathing
Tachypnoea	Hypotension
Decreased skin turgor	Confusion/depressed
Sunken eyes and fontanelle	consciousness
Delayed capillary refill (>4 secs)	Absent urine output
Mottled pale, cold skin	
Core-peripheral temperature gap (>4°C)	
Decreased urinary output	

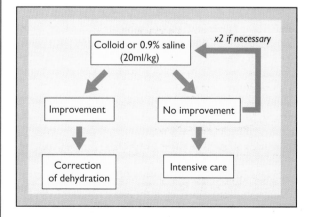

Fig. 4.13 Initial fluid resuscitation.

SUBSEQUENT MANAGEMENT

If there is no improvement or there is evidence of multi-organ failure, the child should be transferred to a paediatric intensive care unit for:

- mechanical ventilation
- intensive monitoring, including central venous pressure (CVP) and arterial pressure
- inotropic support
- correction of haematological and biochemical derangements.

 Fluid therapy is the key element to the successful treatment of shock.

Diabetic ketoacidosis

INITIAL ASSESSMENT AND INVESTIGATIONS (See Figs 4.14 and 4.15).

MANAGEMENT PRIORITIES

This regimen is initiated if there is vomiting, dehydration or reduced level of consciousness. Otherwise, even if newly presenting with diabetes, subcutaneous insulin alone can be given.

1. Fluids

Initial resuscitation of shock with colloid or normal saline, followed by correction of dehydration over 48 h (*see* Fig. 4.13). Avoid over-rapid rehydration as it may lead to cerebral oedema. Monitor neurological state with Glasgow Coma Scale (*see* Fig. 4.3). Monitor fluid balance:

- fluid input and output
- regular check of electrolytes, creatinine and acid-base status
- CVP and urinary catheterisation if required.

A nasogastric tube is passed for acute gastric dilation if there is vomiting or depressed consciousness.

2. Insulin

Insulin infusion (0.05–0.1 unit/kg/h), titrating the dose according to the blood glucose. Do not give a bolus. Monitor the blood glucose regularly. Aim for a gradual reduction of blood glucose of about 2 mmol/h as rapid reduction is dangerous. Change to 4% dextrose/0.18% saline when the blood glucose has fallen to 10 mmol/l to avoid hypoglycaemia.

3. Potassium

Although the initial plasma potassium concentration is usually high, plasma potassium will drop following treatment with insulin. Potassium replacement must be instituted as soon as urine is passed.

4. Acidosis

Although a degree of acidosis is inevitable, bicarbonate should be avoided unless the pH <is 7.0 or is not improving. The acidosis will self-correct with fluid and insulin therapy.

5. Identification and treatment of an underlying cause

Infection may need antibiotics.

6. Re-establish oral fluids, subcutaneous insulin and diet

Do not stop the intravenous insulin infusion until after the subcutaneous insulin has been given. If the child was known to have diabetes, consider the reason for developing ketoacidosis.

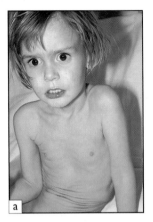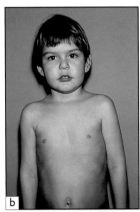

Fig. 4.14a Severe dehydration and weight loss from diabetic ketoacidosis. Fig. 4.14b Four months later. (Courtesy of Dr Jill Challener)

Fig. 4.15 Initial assessment and investigation of diabetic ketoacidosis	
History	Polyuria
	Polydipsia
	Weight loss
	Vomiting
	Abdominal pain
	Lethargy
Examination	Dehydration (>10%)
	Smell of ketones on the breath
	Deep sighing (Kussmaul) breathing
	Confusion
	Coma
Essential initial investigations	Blood glucose (>15 mmol/l)
	Urea and electrolytes, creatinine (dehydration)
	Blood gas analysis (severe metabolic acidosis)
	Urinary glucose and ketones (both are present)
	Evidence of a precipitating cause; e.g. infection(blood and urine cultures performed)
	Cardiac monitor for T-wave changes of hypokalaemia
	Consider salicylate level (similar presentation)
	Weight

Status epilepticus

This is a seizure lasting more than 30 minutes. See Fig. 4.16 for assessment and Fig. 4.17 for management.

Fig. 4.16 Initial assessment and investigation of status epilepticus.

History
Previous seizures
Past medical history:
   birth/neonatal problems
   meningitis/encephalitis
   neurological disorders
     e.g. neurocutaneous syndrome
     or neurodegenerative disorder
   developmental delay
   trauma
Recent head injury
Ingestion of drugs

Examination
Nature of convulsion – generalised
   or focal
Fever
Evidence of trauma:
   accidental/non-accidental
Level of consciousness

Investigations
Blood glucose
Electrolytes:
   sodium, potassium, calcium,
   magnesium
Drug levels if on anticonvulsants
   or ingestion suspected
Further investigations as indicated:
   septic screen, liver function tests,
   coagulation screen, acid–base status,
   blood ammonia, toxicology screen,
   skull X-ray, cranial ultrasound,
   CT scan
More complex investigations
   may be required e.g. EEG.

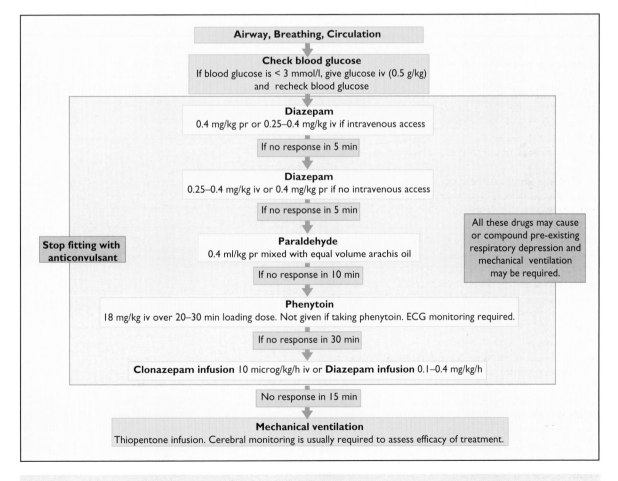

Fig. 4.17 Management protocol for status epilepticus.

The febrile child

Most febrile children have a brief, self-limiting viral infection, either of the respiratory tract or one of the common infectious diseases, e.g. human herpes virus 6 (HHV6). Mild localised bacterial infections, e.g. otitis media or tonsillitis, may be diagnosed clinically and treated with oral antibiotic therapy. The problem lies in identifying the relatively few children with a serious illness which needs prompt treatment.

Factors which need to be considered are:
- past medical history
- illness of other family members
- if a specific illness is prevalent in the community
- immunisation status
- recent travel abroad, e.g. malaria, typhoid
- contact with animals, e.g. brucellosis
- predisposition to infection e.g. nephrotic syndrome, sickle cell disease, HIV infection, chemotherapy for malignant disease or, rarely, a primary immunodeficiency.

INITIAL ASSESSMENT, INVESTIGATIONS AND MANAGEMENT

Infants and toddlers often present with non-specific signs. Some diagnostic clues to evaluating the febrile child are shown in Figure 4.18. If a severe bacterial infection is suspected, urgent investigation, which is called a septic screen (Fig. 4.19) and immediate intravenous antibiotic therapy are required to avoid the illness becoming more severe and to prevent rapid spread to other sites of the body (Fig. 4.20). Treatment is re-evaluated according to the results of the investigations and the clinical course of the child's illness. Less severely ill children will require continuous review, either in hospital or at home by the parents, who need to be given absolutely clear instructions about any signs of improvement or deterioration. This is important because the child may not be particularly unwell if he has been seen early in the course of a serious illness. If the child has a mild illness, reassurance or specific treatment can be given.

Fig. 4.18 Some diagnostic clues to evaluating the febrile child

Upper respiratory tract infection

Very common, may be coincidental with another more serious illness

Otitis media

Always examine tympanic membranes in febrile children

Tonsillitis

Erythema or exudate on the tonsils

Stridor

Epiglottitis?

Viral croup?

Bacterial tracheitis?

Pneumonia

In infants, only raised respiratory rate and increased respiratory effort may be present, with no abnormality on auscultation – diagnosis will then require chest X-ray

Urinary tract infection

Urine sample needed for any seriouly ill young child or any febrile illness that does not settle

Septicaemia

Can be difficult to recognise before shock develops

Need to start antibiotics on clinical suspicion without waiting for culture results

Meningitis/encephalitis

Lethargy, loss of interest in surroundings, drowsiness/unconscious?

Neck stiffness, arching of the back, bulging fontanelle, positive Kernig sign (neck pain on leg straightening)?

Only non-specific symptoms and signs may be present in young children (<18 months)

Osteomyelitis or septic arthritis

Suspect if painful bone or joint or asymmetrical movement in young children

Periorbital cellulitis

May spread to orbit of the eye

Rash

Viral exanthem?

Purpura from meningococcal infection?

Abdominal pain

Appendicitis?

Pyelonephritis?

Hepatitis?

Diarrhoea

Gastroenteritis?

Fever with blood and mucus in the stool:

  Shigella?

  Salmonella?

  Campylobacter?

Seizure

Febrile convulsion?

Meningitis?

Encephalitis?

Prolonged fever

Bacterial infection e.g. UTI, bacterial endocarditis

Other infections – viral, fungal, protozoal

Kawasaki disease

Drug reaction

Malignant disease

Connective tissue disorder (e.g. Still disease)

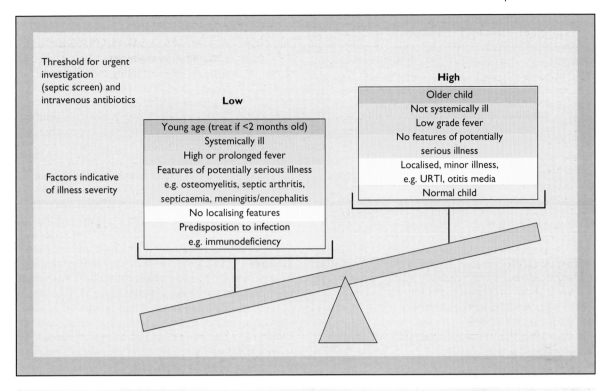

Fig. 4.20 Evaluation of the need for urgent investigation and treatment in the febrile child.

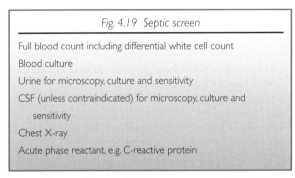

Fig. 4.19 Septic screen

Full blood count including differential white cell count

Blood culture

Urine for microscopy, culture and sensitivity

CSF (unless contraindicated) for microscopy, culture and
    sensitivity

Chest X-ray

Acute phase reactant, e.g. C-reactive protein

 *If severe bacterial infection is suspected in infants
and young children, a septic screen and intravenous antibiotic therapy is indicated*

Septicaemia

In bacterial infections, the organism may cause a focal
infection or it may spread systemically to cause septicaemia. In septicaemia the host response includes the
release of inflammatory mediators and activation of
inflammatory cells which lead to shock. The commonest causes of septicaemia in childhood are also the main
causes of meningitis, with meningococcal sepsis the most
severe. *Pneumococcus* is the commonest organism causing
bacteraemia, but it is unusual for it to cause severe sepsis.

INITIAL ASSESSMENT AND INVESTIGATIONS
See Figure 4.21.

MANAGEMENT PRIORITIES

1. Antibiotics
Choice depends on the child's age, any predisposition to
infection and the likely source of infection.

2. Fluids and capillary leak
Significant hypovolaemia is common and is made worse
by the loss of intravascular proteins and fluid which may
occur due to 'capillary leak'. CVP monitoring and urinary
catheterisation are often required to guide resuscitation,
which frequently requires a large volume of colloid. When
pulmonary oedema is present mechanical ventilation is
needed.

3. Circulatory support
Inotropic support may be required to maintain an adequate cardiac and urine output and tissue perfusion.

4. Correcting clotting derangement
Disseminated intravascular coagulation (DIC) should be
corrected with fresh frozen plasma and/or cryoprecipitate.
If there is active bleeding, platelet transfusions may be
needed; however, they rarely compensate for the underlying consumptive coagulopathy.

5. Steroids
There is no evidence that steroids are of benefit in gram-
negative shock. They may be beneficial in staphylococcal
or streptococcal toxic shock syndrome.

Fig. 4.21 Initial assessment and investigation of septicaemia

History	Examination	Essential investigations
Fever	Fever	Blood glucose
Poor feeding	Purpuric rash (meningococcal septicaemia)	Full blood count and differential white count
Miserable	Irritability	Screen for likely cause of infection -
Lethargy	Shock	culture of blood, urine, CSF, suspected
History of focal infection, e.g. meningitis, osteomyelitis, gastroenteritis, cellulitis	Multi-organ failure	infected sites
Predisposing conditions, e.g. sickle-cell disease, immunodeficiency		Rapid bacterial antigen detection tests
		Acute phase reactant e.g. C-reactive protein
		Blood gases
		Plasma creatinine and electroytes
		Coagulation screen

Bacterial meningitis

INITIAL ASSESSMENT AND INVESTIGATIONS

See Figure 4.22. For neonatal meningitis, *see* Chapter 8; for meningitis, *see* Chapter 24.

MANAGEMENT PRIORITIES

1. Antibiotics

Choice depends on age. An example of a drug regimen is:
- ≤ 3 months of age: ampicillin iv with either cefotaxime or ceftriaxone iv
- > 3 months of age: cefotaxime or ceftriaxone iv alone.

2. Steroids

In children over one month old, if *Haemophilus influenzae* meningitis is suspected, dexamethasone (0.6 mg/kg/day) should be given as soon as possible. The benefit of steroids in other forms of bacterial meningitis is unproven but steroids are widely used as they are are thought to reduce inflammatory complications, e.g. deafness.

3. Fluids

If shock is present, resuscitation with colloid is essential. Inotropes and vasodilators may be required, as guided by haemodynamic monitoring. Fluid restriction to about 70% maintenance may be beneficial to reduce cerebral oedema and counteract inappropriate antidiuretic hormone (ADH) secretion. However, this should not be at the expense of an adequate intravascular volume. Fluid balance must be monitored continuously.

4. Cerebral monitoring

Mechanical ventilation should be instituted if the child has evidence of respiratory impairment, intractable seizures or raised intracranial pressure. Seizures should be treated with anticonvulsants. Although intracranial pressure monitoring has been popular, current practice is to focus on maintaining metabolic, respiratory and haemodynamic parameters within the normal range. Mannitol, an osmotic diuretic, may be given. Hyperventilation is no longer recommended as it may further reduce cerebral blood flow.

5. Public health notification and antibiotic prophylaxis of contacts

---

Fig. 4.22 Initial assessment and investigation of bacterial meningitis

History	Examination	Essential investigations
Fever	Fever	Blood glucose
Headache	Purpuric rash (meningococcal septicaemia)	Blood gases
Photophobia	Photophobia	Full blood count and differential white count
Poor feeding/vomiting	Neck stiffness/Kernig sign positive	Blood culture
Irritability	Papilloedema (uncommon)	Acute phase reactant e.g. C-reactive protein
Hypotonia	Convulsions	Blood and urinary rapid bacterial antigen detection tests
Drowsiness		Coagulation screen
Coma		CSF (unless contraindicated) for microscopy, culture, glucose, protein and bacterial antigens
		Consider CT or MR scan, EEG, chest X-ray, Mantoux test

Viral encephalitis

The diagnosis of viral encephalitis needs to be considered in any drowsy/unconscious or fitting child and treatment given until this or an alternative diagnosis is reached. No virus can be identified in half the children diagnosed clinically as having viral encephalitis.

INITIAL ASSESSMENT AND INVESTIGATIONS
See Figure 4.23 and encephalitis/encephalopathy in Chapter 24.

MANAGEMENT PRIORITIES
1. Antiviral and antibiotic therapy
Acyclovir iv is given to treat herpes simplex encephalitis. Erythromycin iv is added if mycoplasma is suspected.

Antibiotics are given as for bacterial meningitis until a viral aetiology is confirmed.
2. Mechanical ventilation
If there is evidence of raised intracranial pressure, depressed consciousness or abnormal breathing.
3. Cerebral monitoring
EEG monitoring may be diagnostic and prognostic. Temporal lobe abnormalities are often seen on EEG and CT or MR scan in herpes simplex encephalitis. Intracranial pressure monitoring has been used when there is evidence of raised intracranial pressure, but it has not been shown to improve clinical outcome.

 Early treatment with acyclovir dramatically reduces the morbidity and mortality associated with herpes encephalitis

History	Examination	Essential investigations
Fever	Fever	Full blood count
Headache	Papilloedema (rare)	Blood, urine and stool culture
Focal neurological deficit	Focal neurological signs	Serology – viral and other causes including
Disturbed consciousness	Convulsions – often focal	Mycoplasma IgM,
	Coma	bacterial rapid antigen detection tests
		CSF (unless contraindicated) for microscopy,
		culture (bacterial and viral), viral PCR
		glucose, protein
		CT or MR scan, EEG, chest X-ray

Fig. 4.23 Initial assessment and investigation of viral encephalitis

The death of a child

The main causes of unexpected death in infants are sudden infant death syndrome (SIDS) and undiagnosed congenital abnormalities, such as congenital heart disease. In older children, road traffic or other accidents are the commonest cause.

Sudden Infant Death Syndrome (SIDS)
This is defined as the sudden and unexpected death of an infant or young child for which no adequate cause is found after a thorough post-mortem examination. Sudden unexpected death from inherited metabolic disorders, e.g. fatty acid oxidation defects (notably medium chain acyl CoA dehydrogenase deficiency), is rare. Although death by suffocation by parents has received considerable attention in the medical literature and media, it is uncommon.

There is marked variation in the incidence of SIDS in different countries, suggesting that environmental factors are important (Fig. 4.24). SIDS occurs most commonly at 2–4 months (Fig. 4.25). The risk for subsequent children is slightly increased.

In the UK, the incidence of SIDS has fallen dramatically during the last few years (Fig. 4.26), coinciding with a national campaign advocating that infants should sleep on their back or side, to avoid overheating and not to smoke near infants.

Following the sudden death of a child
The sudden death of a child is one of the most distressing events that can happen to a family. If close family members are absent, arrangements should be made for them to come, if this is possible. The family should be told sympathetically and in private (*see* Fig 3.9 in Chapter 3).

Most families will wish to see and hold their dead child, and the opportunity to do this should be offered to them. This should be encouraged as it helps them accept the reality of their child's death. Even if the child has visible injuries, parents should be supported in seeing their child, as their fantasies in the future are usually worse than the reality. They may wish to see the child again within the next few days. The family may wish a minister of religion to be called.

In the UK, the coroner has to be notified of all unexpected deaths and will arrange for a postmortem to be performed. The parents should be informed of this, and that details will automatically be passed on to the police, who will conduct their own inquiry. This will include interviewing the parents and whoever was looking after the child at the time of death. The parents need to know that this does not imply that they are being blamed or are responsible for their child's death. The general practitioner, health visitor and other relevant health professionals should be informed, and any appointments for the health clinic or hospital cancelled.

Parents should be given written information about the condition and given advice about talking about what has happened to siblings and other family members.

Follow-up needs to be arranged, to provide the family with an opportunity to discuss the results of the postmortem and consider its implications for future pregnancies. Genetic counselling may be indicated.

The grief following the sudden death of a child will profoundly affect all the members of the family. Bereavement counselling is increasingly available from health professionals in the hospital or community. Parents should be given information about bereavement support from other agencies e.g. the Foundation for the Study of Infant Deaths, Child Death Helpline and CRUSE.

 Sudden infant death syndrome (SIDS) is the commonest cause of death in children aged 1 month to 1 year

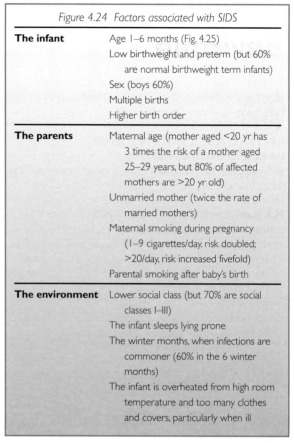

Figure 4.24 Factors associated with SIDS	
The infant	Age 1–6 months (Fig. 4.25) Low birthweight and preterm (but 60% are normal birthweight term infants) Sex (boys 60%) Multiple births Higher birth order
The parents	Maternal age (mother aged <20 yr has 3 times the risk of a mother aged 25–29 years, but 80% of affected mothers are >20 yr old) Unmarried mother (twice the rate of married mothers) Maternal smoking during pregnancy (1–9 cigarettes/day, risk doubled; >20/day, risk increased fivefold) Parental smoking after baby's birth
The environment	Lower social class (but 70% are social classes I–III) The infant sleeps lying prone The winter months, when infections are commoner (60% in the 6 winter months) The infant is overheated from high room temperature and too many clothes and covers, particularly when ill

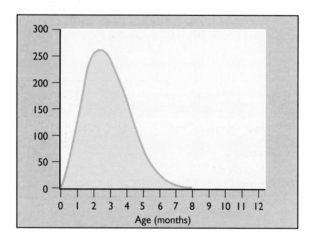

Fig. 4.25 Age distribution of SIDS. (From data for England and Wales, 1988–92)

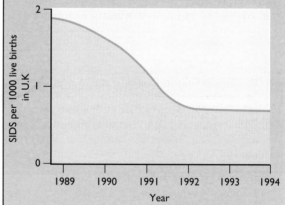

Fig. 4.26 Decline in the number of deaths from SIDS in the UK from 1.9/1000 live births in 1989 to 0.7 in 1993. The incidence remained at 0.7/1000 live births in 1994.

FURTHER READING

Advanced Paediatric Life Support. The practical approach. BMJ Publishing Group, London, 1993. The core text for the Advanced Paediatric Life Support (UK) course.

Goldman A. *Care of the Dying Child.* Oxford Medical Publications, Oxford, 1994. Medical, psychological and practical issues of caring for terminally ill children and their families.

CHAPTER 5

Environment

• *Accidents* • *Poisoning* • *Child abuse*

Children need a safe, healthy and loving environment to achieve their full potential. Hazards in their environment include accidents, poisons and abuse. As far as possible, children should be protected from harm. This involves not only parents and families but also doctors and many other professionals and institutions in our society. The risk of environmental hazards is increased by:
- poverty
- poor quality, overcrowded homes
- poor parenting skills, which may be due to parental psychiatric illness, violent temperament, poor education or lack of social support.

Accidents

Accidents are extremely common. In the UK, 1 in 5 children attend an Accident and Emergency Department each year following an accident. Most accidents, especially after falls, cause only minor injury, but some are fatal. Accidents are by far the most common cause of death in children over one year old (Figs 5.1 and 5.2). Accidents also cause significant

disability and suffering to children, and may result in post-traumatic stress disorders. Head injuries are the major cause of disability from accidents. Children may also suffer brain damage following near drowning or suffocation. Cosmetic damage following burns, scalds and other accidents may cause the child profound psychological harm.

 Accidents are the commonest cause of death in children over one year old.

TYPES OF ACCIDENTS AFFECTING CHILDREN

Childhood accidents depend on the child's age and stage of development. Toddlers constantly explore their immediate environment, usually the home, and are unaware of the consequences of their actions. They are prone to falls, scalds, ingest potentially harmful substances and drown in the bath, ponds or pools. Babies and toddlers need to be constantly supervised by adults. Most serious accidents in young children can be anticipated by an observant adult and prevented. Older children experience a different range of accidents, mainly as pedestrians or cyclists, while playing sport or from falls while climbing.

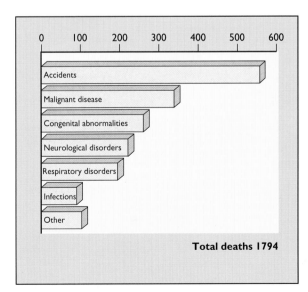

Fig. 5.1 Causes of death in children 1–14 years in England and Wales (1992).

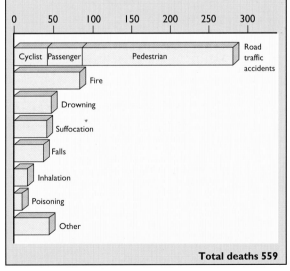

Fig. 5.2 Causes of fatal accidents in children in England and Wales (1992). The most common cause is road traffic accidents.

ACCIDENT PREVENTION

The prevention of childhood accidents is clearly important. Doctors who treat children and see the effects of accidents are particularly well placed to provide the community with advice on appropriate preventive measures (Fig. 5.3).

In order to prevent accidents:

* the relationship between an individual type of accident and the child's developmental level must be considered
* specific solutions based on detailed epidemiology, e.g. child-resistant containers for medicines, are more successful than health education.

Changes backed by legislation are the most successful.

 The number of children killed in accidents has declined markedly.

ROAD TRAFFIC ACCIDENTS

Road traffic accidents (RTAs) are the most common cause of accidental death in childhood and can be divided into several types.

Pedestrian road traffic accidents

Children's involvement in road traffic accidents is mostly as pedestrians. Boys between the ages of five and nine years are at maximum risk, particularly after school. They are unable to estimate the speed or dangers of traffic and to foresee dangerous situations. Although it is important to make children aware of the dangers, education about road safety has proved of little value in reducing the number of accidents. Primary prevention needs to be done by modifying the environment.

Child passengers in cars

Unrestrained children become missiles inside cars during crashes, even at low speeds. There is good evidence that child restraint systems prevent injury and death.

Bicycle accidents

Bicycle accidents are common. A boy has a 1 in 80 chance of having a cycling-related head injury severe enough to warrant admission to hospital during childhood.

HEAD INJURIES

Minor head injuries in childhood are common, and the vast majority of children recover without suffering any ill effect. However, about 1 in 800 of these children develop serious problems. The aim of the management

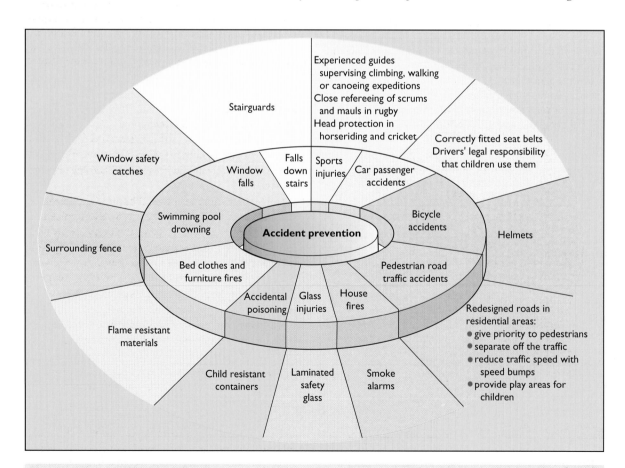

Fig. 5.3 Examples of accident prevention.

of head injuries is to identify those children requiring treatment and to avoid secondary damage to the brain from hypotension, hypoxia, infection and raised intracranial pressure (Fig. 5.4a, b). In infants, as their skull sutures have not fused, their cranial volume may increase from an extradural or subdural bleed before neurological signs or symptoms develop. Their haemoglobin concentration may fall and they may become shocked. In young children, unexplained head injuries may result from child abuse. The presence of retinal haemorrhages is highly suggestive of a shaking injury.

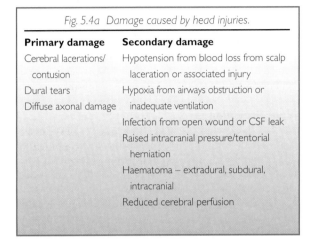

Fig. 5.4a Damage caused by head injuries.

Primary damage	Secondary damage
Cerebral lacerations/ contusion	Hypotension from blood loss from scalp laceration or associated injury
Dural tears	Hypoxia from airways obstruction or inadequate ventilation
Diffuse axonal damage	Infection from open wound or CSF leak
	Raised intracranial pressure/tentorial herniation
	Haematoma – extradural, subdural, intracranial
	Reduced cerebral perfusion

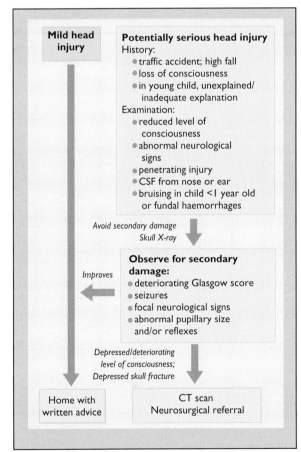

Fig. 5.4b Outline of the initial management of head injuries. The aim is to prevent secondary damage.

INTERNAL INJURIES

Children may suffer internal injuries associated with severe trauma. These include:

- abdominal injuries including a ruptured spleen, ruptured liver, kidney and bowel. A high index of suspicion should be kept for these injuries if there has been blunt abdominal trauma. The child needs close observation. Abdominal ultrasound and X-rays may be helpful. If there is any doubt a laparotomy is undertaken.
- chest injuries, including pneumothorax and haemopericardium, which may require emergency treatment.

These children should be managed in a paediatric intensive care unit.

BURNS AND SCALDS

Burns and scalds are the second most common cause of death from accidents. Most deaths occur in house fires, from gas and smoke inhalation rather than by thermal injury. Scalds in toddlers are common, from knocking over cups of hot liquid or grabbing the handle of a saucepan of boiling water on a cooker, or from bath water which is too hot.

Management

Initial assessment is for severity:

- any smoke inhalation. If this has occurred, there is a danger of subsequent respiratory complications. All affected children should be observed and managed in hospital
- depth of the burn. In superficial burns, the skin will be epithelialised from surviving cells. In partial thickness burns there is some damage to the dermis with blistering, and the skin is pink or mottled. In deep (full thickness) burns, the skin is destroyed down to and including the dermis and healing is from the margins. The skin is white or charred and is painless. Deep burns need assessment and treatment in hospital
- surface area of the burn. This should be calculated from a surface area chart (Fig. 5.5). The palm and adducted fingers cover about 1% of the body surface. Burns covering more than 10% need assessment and treatment in hospital, while children with burns involving more than 50% have a limited chance of survival
- involvement of special sites. Burns to the face may be disfiguring, to the mouth may compromise the airway from oedema, to the hand may cause functional loss from scarring and to the perineum are prone to infection.

Treatment

Should be directed at:

- relieving pain with the use of strong analgesics such as intravenous morphine
- treating shock with intravenous fluids, preferably plasma expanders, and close monitoring of haematocrit and urinary output. Children with more than 10% burns will require intravenous fluids
- providing wound care. Burns should be covered with sterile towels, which reduces pain from contact with cold air and reduces the risk of infection. Blisters should be left alone. Irrigation with cold water should only be used briefly to superficial or partial thickness burns covering less than 10% of the body as it may rapidly cause excessive cooling.

Severe burns or significant burns to special sites are best dealt with in specialist units. Plastic surgeons will often

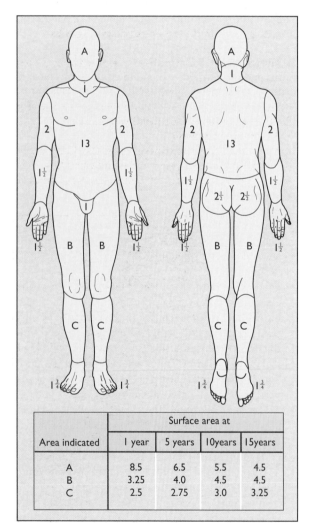

Area indicated	Surface area at			
	1 year	5 years	10 years	15 years
A	8.5	6.5	5.5	4.5
B	3.25	4.0	4.5	4.5
C	2.5	2.75	3.0	3.25

Fig. 5.5 Method of calculating the surface area of a burn (Lund and Browder chart).

need to embark on a programme of skin grafts and treatment of contractures. The psychological sequelae of severe burns are often marked and long lasting and appropriate psychological support is required.

DROWNING AND NEAR DROWNING

Drowning is the third most common cause of accidental death in children in the UK. Most victims are young children. Three times as many boys drown as girls. Warmer countries have a higher incidence of drowning than the UK. Children may drown as babies in the bath, as toddlers by wandering into domestic ponds or swimming pools or as older children in public swimming pools, rivers, canals, lakes and in the sea.

Near drowning

Up to 30% of fatalities can be prevented by skilled on-site resuscitation. Even children who are unconscious with fixed dilated pupils can survive near drowning episodes, particularly if they are very cold. This is because of the protective effect of hypothermia. Children who are unconscious with fixed dilated pupils should therefore be fully resuscitated until their temperature is nearly normal. Immediate management at the waterside is with mouth to mouth resuscitation. Heat loss should be prevented by covering and warming. Children who may have inhaled water should be admitted to hospital to observe for signs of secondary drowning and cardiac arrhythmias. Severely ill children require artificial ventilation in a paediatric intensive care unit. It was thought that there was a difference in outlook for fresh and salt water drowning but in practice this does not appear to be the case. Some children who nearly drown aspirate water and develop a pneumonia with secondary infection. Respiratory deterioration can also occur, with apparent pulmonary oedema, between 1 and 72 hours after the original incident. This is due to surfactant deficiency.

CHOKING, SUFFOCATION AND STRANGULATION

Children may choke on vomit, toys or food. Some children may strangle themselves accidentally on curtain cords, bedding and necklaces. Most are accidents but some are inflicted deliberately as a form of child abuse. Some older boys deliberately hang themselves whilst emotionally disturbed.

In airway obstruction from an aspirated foreign body, the Heimlich manoeuvre can be used in older children to expel the foreign body by suddenly raising intra-abdominal pressure (Fig. 5.6). Back blows and chest thrusts are recommended in infants and young children as abdominal thrusts may cause intra-abdominal injury (Fig. 5.7).

DOG BITES

One in a 100 children present to the Accident and Emergency Department with dog bites. Most dog bites are minor but severe lacerations, particularly to the face, do occur particularly in the toddler age group. Dog bites usually need only simple wound toilet. However, more serious injuries, particularly on the face, need careful debridement and skilled suturing to avoid unsightly scars. Antibiotics are not usually necessary. Although there has been much publicity about fierce dog breeds such as Rottweilers attacking children in parks or public places, most attacks are by dogs known to the child.

Poisoning

Most poisoning in children is accidental. Poisoning in children may be:
- accidental – the vast majority
- deliberate self-poisoning in older children
- non-accidental as a form of child abuse
- iatrogenic.

ACCIDENTAL POISONING

Although many thousands of young children are rushed to doctors' surgeries or hospital for urgent medical attention following accidental ingestion, most children do not develop serious symptoms as they ingest only a small quantity of poison. However, a small percentage of children become seriously ill and a very few children die from poisoning each year.

Most accidental poisoning is in young children, with a peak age of 30 months. Inquisitive toddlers are unaware of the potential danger of taking medicines, household products and eating plants. Most ingestions occur in the child's own home, while the child is not adequately supervised. Supervision entails not only reacting to a dangerous situation but prevention through anticipation.

The aim of management should be to prevent unnecessary admissions to hospital while maintaining safety. There has been a marked reduction in the hospital admission rate for poisoning. Reasons for this include:
- the introduction of child-resistant containers. In the UK they must be used for paracetamol and salicylate preparations and certain household products such as white spirit. An alternative container for tablets is opaque blister packs.
- a reduction in prescribing potentially harmful medicines, e.g. aspirin and iron.

Education campaigns have not proved to be successful in preventing accidental child poisoning.

Management
This comprises:
1. Identification of the agent
Parents usually know the identity or provide containers or tablets.
2. Assessment of the agent's toxicity (Fig. 5.8)
- low – allow home
- intermediate – observe for 6 hours, then home unless symptoms develop
- high – admit to hospital

Contact the Regional Poisons Information Centre if in doubt about a substance's identity or toxicity.
3. Removal of a poison
Ipecac is given to induce emesis unless the drug ingested is of low toxicity or its use is contraindicated (Fig. 5.9). More recently, doubt has been cast on the use of ipecac as

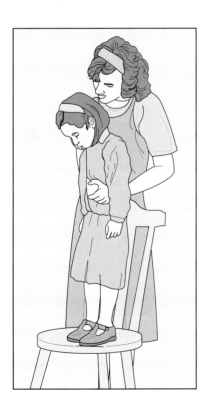

Fig. 5.6 Heimlich manoeuvre in older children to expel an inhaled foreign body. One hand is formed into a fist and placed against the child's abdomen above the umbilicus and below the xiphisternum. The other hand is placed over the fist. Both hands are thrust into the abdomen. This is repeated up to ten times. The child can be standing, or kneeling, sitting or supine.

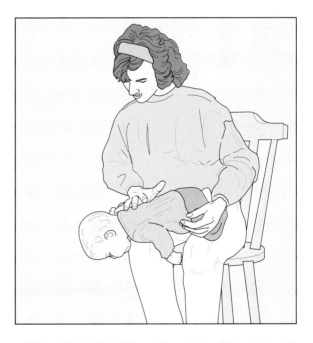

Fig. 5.7 In young children, back blows and chest thrusts are recommended to expel an inhaled foreign body.

Fig. 5.8 Potential toxicity in accidental poisoning in children.

Toxicity	Medicines	Household products	Plants
Low	Oral contraceptives, most antibiotics	Chalk and crayons, washing powder	Cyclamen, sweet pea
Intermediate	Paracetamol elixir, salbutamol	Bleach, disinfectants, window cleaners	Fuchsia, holly
High	Alcoholic drinks, digoxin, iron, salicylate, tricyclic antidepressants	Acids, alkalis, petroleum distillates, organophosphorus insecticides	Deadly nightshade, laburnum, yew

it is unpleasant, there is relatively little evidence that it significantly reduces drug absorption, few children develop toxic symptoms and it may cause persistent vomiting, diarrhoea, lethargy and drowsiness. Its use is likely to be reserved for large ingestions of drugs of high toxicity.

4. Activated charcoal
This is used to absorb a wide range of toxic drugs by offering alternative binding sites. It is an alternative to ipecac or used after vomiting has been induced. Children often find it difficult to take. It can be instilled by nasogastric tube.

5. Antidotes or specific therapy
These are available for only a limited number of poisons (Fig. 5.10). Observation and supportive care is required.

6. Social assessment
This is required in order to prevent further poisoning or accidents. The general practitioner and other health professionals should be contacted.

DELIBERATE POISONING IN OLDER CHILDREN
These children form one end of the age spectrum of overdose in adults and are more likely to take significant amounts of poison than younger children. Substances that can be regarded as having intermediate toxicity when taken accidentally should be regarded as potentially toxic when taken deliberately. Poisoning in older children should be recognised as a serious symptom and an indication of child and family dis-

turbance. Many of the children are depressed. All children who take poisons deliberately should be admitted to hospital and should be assessed by a child or adolescent psychiatrist. Many will also need education or social work assessment.

CHRONIC POISONING
Children can be poisoned by chronic exposure to chemicals and pollutants. An example from the past is mercury poisoning from teething powders, which used to cause 'pink disease', so called because it resulted in red painful extremities. It also caused anorexia, weight loss and hypotonia. Now the commonest chronic poisoning is from lead ingestion and from smoking.

Lead poisoning
In the past, certain paints contained lead. Children are liable to be poisoned from chewing paintwork or from inhalation when the paint is removed. This is still a problem in parts of the US. Lead fumes from burning batteries, lead shot for fishing and lead from old water pipes are other potential sources. Children from the Indian subcontinent may be poisoned by surma, the lead-containing eye make-up sometimes used even on young babies. Lead from vehicle exhaust fumes results in higher blood levels in children living in urban than rural areas. The change to unleaded petrol has been in response to concern about its potential as an environmental hazard.

Fig. 5.9 Removal of a poison.

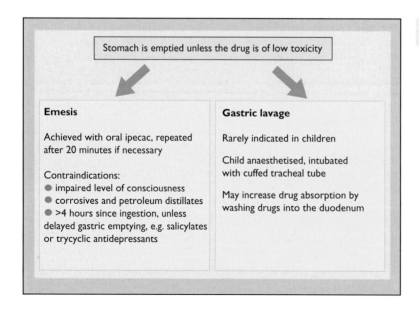

Stomach is emptied unless the drug is of low toxicity

Emesis

Achieved with oral ipecac, repeated after 20 minutes if necessary

Contraindications:
- impaired level of consciousness
- corrosives and petroleum distillates
- >4 hours since ingestion, unless delayed gastric emptying, e.g. salicylates or trycyclic antidepressants

Gastric lavage

Rarely indicated in children

Child anaesthetised, intubated with cuffed tracheal tube

May increase drug absorption by washing drugs into the duodenum

Children who are poisoned by lead acutely from ingestion or inhalation are likely to present with pica (compulsive eating of substances other than food), anorexia, colicky abdominal pain, irritability and failure to thrive and pallor from anaemia. Severe lead poisoning may present with neurological symptoms including drowsiness, convulsions and coma from lead encephalopathy. Raised intracranial pressure with papilloedema may be present. There is increasing evidence that chronic exposure to relatively low lead levels may be harmful to mental development.

Fig. 5.10 Potentially harmful poisons		
Poison	**Adverse effects**	**Management**
Alcohol (accidental in toddlers, experimenting by older children)	Hypoglycaemia	Monitor blood glucose. Intravenous glucose if necessary. Blood alcohol levels for severity
Acids and alkalis	Inflammation and ulceration of upper gastrointestinal tract leading to stenosis (pylorus – acids; oesophagus – alkalis)	No emesis/gastric lavage. No chemical antidotes as they produce heat. Early endoscopy. Steroids to suppress inflammation
Bleach (problems seldom arise in children)	Local lesions	No emesis. Milk/antacids orally. Endoscopy to identify oesophageal inflammation if indicated. Ventilatory support if required
Digoxin	Arrhythmias. Hyperkalaemia	ECG monitoring. Serum digoxin concentration is a guide to toxicity. Purified specific Fab antibody–binding fragments are available for life-threatening toxicity
Diphenoxylate (Lomotil)	Depressed respiration – opioid-like action. Also atropine-like effects	Naloxone. Observe for at least 36 h
Disc or button batteries	Mild gastrointestinal symptoms. Oesophageal stricture with large batteries (>20 mm). Corrosion of gut wall and perforation. Breaking open with release of mercury – rare	Monitor progress with chest and abdominal X-rays–almost all are passed within 2 days and do not cause symptoms. Remove if signs of disintegration. Some authorities recommend removal if not passed within 48 h to avoid danger of disintegration
Iron	Initial: vomiting, diarrhoea, hae-matemesis, melaena, acute gastric ulcerations. Latent period of improvement. Some hours later: drowsiness, coma, shock, liver failure with hypoglycaemia, convulsions. Long-term complications: gastric strictures. Serious toxicity if >60 mg/kg elemental iron ingested	Abdominal X-ray to count the number of tablets. Serum iron levels. Ipecac (gastric lavage considered in severe cases if <1 hr after ingestion). Intravenous desferrioxamine
Paracetamol – serious ingestion is uncommon as tablets difficult to swallow and elixir too sweet	Gastric irritation. Liver failure after 3–5 days	Check plasma concentration after 4 h after ingestion. If >150 mg/kg paracetamol is thought to have been taken, or the plasma concentration is high, start iv acetylcysteine. Monitor prothrombin time, liver function tests and plasma creatinine
Petroleum distillates (paraffin/kerosene, white spirit)	Aspiration causing pneumonitis	Emesis contraindicated. Usually no treatment required. Prophylactic antibiotics and steroids to reduce inflammation – no clear evidence of benefit. Additional inspired oxygen and intensive care for aspiration
Salicylates	Tinnitus, deafness. Nausea, vomiting. Dehydration. Hyperventilation, respiratory alkalosis. Metabolic acidosis. Hypoglycaemia. Disorientation	Measure plasma salicylate concentration. Empty stomach even if delay of up to 12 h and give activated charcoal. Monitor fluid and electrolyte balance. Correct dehydration, electrolyte imbalance and acidosis. Give vitamin K. Forced alkaline diuresis (difficult to achieve without fluid overload). Dialysis.
Tricyclic antidepressants	Sinus tachycardia. Conduction disorders. Dry mouth. Blurred vision. Agitation, confusion. Convulsions, drowsiness. Coma, respiratory depression. Hypotension	Emesis even if presentation delayed. Activated charcoal. Cardiac monitoring. Treat arrhythmias conservatively with sodium bicarbonate. Correct metabolic acidosis. Sedate/treat convulsions with diazepam

The diagnosis is confirmed by elevated blood lead levels. There may be a hypochromic anaemia and basophil stippling of neutrophils. Radiographs of the knee or wrist may show 'lead lines', dense metaphyseal bands. The source of lead should be identified and removed. Chelating agents are used to form non-toxic lead compounds. In mild cases D-penicillamine is given orally, and in severe cases sodium calciumedetate (EDTA) is indicated.

Smoking

The harmful effects of smoking are well documented. For the smoker the risk of developing chronic bronchitis, lung cancer and cardiovascular disease is greatly increased. Unfortunately, many children become regular smokers while still at school. Children should be given appropriate health education, but its effectiveness is limited by the poor example set by the widespread smoking of adults.

When parents or carers smoke, children have been shown to have a higher incidence of bronchitis, asthma, pneumonia and serous otitis media (glue ear). This particularly applies to babies and young children. Maternal smoking places the infant at increased risk of sudden infant death syndrome (SIDS).

 Parents' smoking adversely affects their children's health.

Child abuse

Children require protection and care. The concept that parents or carers might abuse their children was first recognised as a medical problem only in the 1950s. Although this caused great concern at the time, child abuse is not a new phenomenon. Children have been physically harmed, neglected and subjected to sexual abuse throughout history. What has changed is that society is no longer prepared to accept that parents or care-givers can do whatever they please to their children. Children are now afforded the right to receive recognised and accepted patterns of child care and rearing. Professionals, whether doctors, health visitors, social workers, teachers or others involved in the care of children now have duties to ensure this. Recognising potential child abuse has to be weighed against the damage of falsely accusing parents of abusing their children. This requires fine judgment and courage.

Types of child abuse

Initially, attention was focused on the 'battered baby', where severe physical injury was inflicted on babies. We now appreciate that in addition to inflicting physical injuries, adults may harm children in a number of different ways. These can be divided into:

- physical abuse (non-accidental injury, NAI) - bruises, burns, lacerations, fractures and internal injuries
- neglect

- emotional abuse
- sexual abuse, including the use of children for pornography
- non-accidental poisoning – where children are deliberately poisoned
- Munchausen syndrome by proxy – where symptoms or signs of illness are fabricated by the carer.

Although children may present with a single type of abuse, it is more common for children to suffer from a combination of several forms, e.g. physically abused children are often neglected and emotionally abused. Abuse of all types is very damaging to the emotional development of the child. Sexual abuse may also damage the future sexual responses of a girl or boy. Intervention should aim not only to prevent further injuries but to also provide therapy for any emotional damage inflicted.

Diagnosis

The diagnosis of child abuse is based on assessing the probability that individual injuries or harm have occurred non-accidentally. Serious injuries to children are rarely the initial presentation – they are almost always preceded by minor injuries. It is also known that if a particular child in the household has been subjected to abuse, further episodes are more likely to be directed towards the same child.

Adults who abuse children do not usually suffer from mental illness although alcohol, drugs and post-natal depression sometimes contribute. More often, the abuser has a personality disorder, may have experienced poor parenting and abuse as a child and is often immature. Factors in the child which may predispose to abuse include disability, low birthweight, the child's age and a demanding personality.

PHYSICAL ABUSE

Most injuries follow genuine accidents and must be differentiated from those which are inflicted deliberately. They can usually be differentiated by taking a full history and examining the whole child. It is vital to try to understand exactly how an accident happened and the circumstances surrounding the event. In child abuse there may be:

- a history which is not consistent with the injury
- delay in reporting the injury
- inconsistent histories from care givers
- inappropriate reaction of parents or care givers who are vague, elusive, unconcerned or excessively distressed or aggressive
- recurrent injuries
- injuries inconsistent with the child's stage of development.

Presentation of physical abuse
Bruises

These are the commonest mode of presentation (Fig. 5.11a–d). Whereas bruises on the forehead and shins are common in toddlers learning to walk they are exceptional

Fig. 5.11a–d Some clinical features of physical abuse.

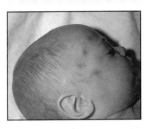

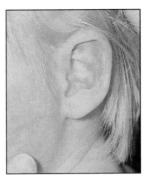

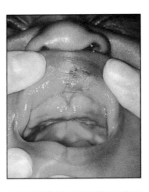

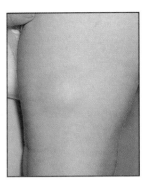

5.11a Bruising from finger-tips on a baby's head.

5.11b Bruising within the pinna is uncommon in accidental injury. Bruising behind the ear may be from blows to the ear.

5.11c A torn frenulum. This may be from forcing a bottle into the mouth or from a blow to the mouth.

5.11d A bite mark on an infant's leg. Adult bite marks may be seen in abuse, but bites from other children are not uncommon.

in non-mobile babies. Bruises on the face, back and buttock are uncommon in accidental injury.

Some patterns of bruising are suggestive of particular injuries. Bruises from finger tips gripping with excessive force are mostly on the trunk, often on either side of the spine, but may also be seen around the mouth to try and stop a baby's crying, or on the arms from shaking. Slap marks resembling hand prints may be seen on the face or buttocks. Bruises may outline a particular object, e.g. a hand, belt or flex used in beating.

Head and abdominal injuries

Head injuries follow whiplash injuries or, less often, from direct blows to the head. Vigorous shaking of babies may rupture the small vessels crossing the subdural space causing a subdural haemorrhage. There may be a similar injury if the child's head is hit against a soft object such as a bed. There may be no signs of bruising on the surface of the skull. Retinal haemorrhages are often present and are an important sign of non-accidental injury. Clinical features include irritability, poor feeding, increasing head circumference, convulsions, reduced level of consciousness and a full fontanelle.

Direct blows to the head are usually less of a diagnostic problem as there is bruising and there may be an underlying skull fracture. Visceral injuries, particularly to the spleen and liver, may follow blows to the abdomen. They are uncommon and often difficult to diagnose.

Burns or scalds

It is difficult to distinguish burns and scalds inflicted deliberately from those that are accidents. Accidental hot water burns tend to be asymmetrical and spare the flexures. Scalds on the back are uncommon in accidents. The shape of the scald may be suggestive of an iron or radiator or of a cigarette burn. Burns on the buttocks are unusual but may result from punishment during potty training.

Fractures

Fractures can be categorised according to their likelihood

of being caused by non-accidental injury. The most specific are fractures in infants which require violent handling or shaking (Fig. 5.12). When assessing fractures it is the child's age, mobility and development and the history which are the crucial features in distinguishing accidental from non-accidental injuries. In infants, relatively little force is required to produce a linear skull fracture, but accidental fractures of the long bones are uncommon. In mobile children, most long-bone fractures are accidental.

Investigation

Fractures in young children may not be detectable clinically. A radiographic skeletal survey should be performed in all infants with suspected physical abuse. Some lesions may be inconspicuous initially but can be identified on a radionuclide bone scan or can become evident on a repeat X-ray 1–2 weeks later (Fig. 5.13a,b). In children over one year old, a radionuclide bone scan can be substituted for the skeletal survey. In children over five years old skeletal surveys are of limited value.

Fig. 5.12 Likelihood of a fracture being due to non-accidental injury.	
High	Metaphyseal fractures
	Posterior rib fractures
Moderate	Multiple fractures
	Fractures of different ages
	Complex skull fracture
Low	Clavicular fractures
	Long bone shaft fractures
	Linear skull fractures

Adapted from Kleinman PK. Current Concepts: a categorical course in paediatric radiology. SPR, 1994.

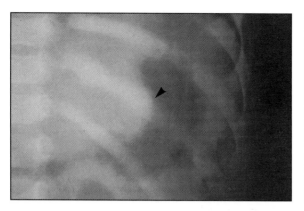

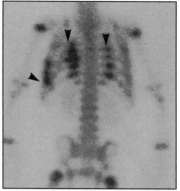

Fig. 5.13b A radionuclide bone scan is more sensitive in detecting fractures in the early stages. This scan shows the multiple rib fractures. (Courtesy of Dr Cathy Owens)

Fig. 5.13a Posterior rib fractures are usually from squeezing rather than direct trauma. They can be seen here in the healing phase with callus formation. Rib fractures are often difficult to identify on an x-ray.

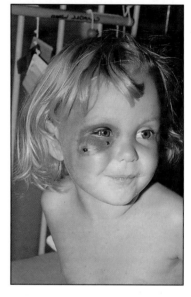

Fig. 5.14 A thorough medical assessment is required in all children when non-accidental injury is suspected. This girl's large bruise followed what was said to be a minor bump. Non-accidental injury was suspected, but examination showed multiple bruises and petechiae. She had idiopathic thrombocytopenic purpura (ITP).

Other medical conditions which need to be considered and excluded in suspected child abuse are:
- coagulation disorders – may result in bruising (Fig. 5.14). Occasionally abuse and a coagulation disorder may coexist
- osteogenesis imperfecta – predisposes to fractures. Features that characterise this uncommon condition are generalised osteoporosis, ligamentous laxity, skin fragility, blue sclerae and defective dentition. There may be a family history. Expert assessment of the X-rays is required. Fractures usually affect the shaft of the long bones
- copper deficiency – predisposes to fractures. It is rare, but can occur in a preterm or malnourished children
- bullous impetigo and scalded skin syndrome – caused by staphylococcal or streptococcal infection; may be mistaken for scalds or cigarette burns.

NEGLECT
Gross neglect of a child's developmental needs may present clinically as:
- failure to thrive
- inadequate hygiene including severe nappy rash or infestation
- poor development of emotional attachment to the child's care giver
- development and speech delay
- poor attendance for immunisations and school.
This will improve if the child's environment is changed to provide adequate food, shelter, affection and stimulation.

EMOTIONAL ABUSE
Emotional abuse includes:
- the withdrawal of love by rejecting the child
- malicious criticism, threats and ridicule
- scapegoating.

Children who have been repeatedly emotionally abused usually present with emotional or behavioural disturbances. There may be excessive compliance or aggressive defiance, poor self-esteem, poor ability to enjoy things or sustain self-occupation or they may exhibit pseudomature behaviour. Emotional abuse is often associated with physical or sexual abuse.

NON-ACCIDENTAL POISONING
These children are deliberately poisoned by their parents. They present with bizarre symptoms such as:
- hyperventilation after aspirin
- unexplained drowsiness after hypnotics, tranquillisers or alcohol.
The diagnosis is often difficult but can frequently be made by identifying the drug in the blood or urine.

MUNCHAUSEN SYNDROME BY PROXY
In this uncommon variant of physical abuse, illness in the child is fabricated by a parent, usually the mother. Many of the mothers have connections with health care services. The abuse appears to be a way in which these disturbed

parents obtain satisfaction from close association with hospital care. Examples include:
- putting blood in vomit, stool and urine
- placing sugar in the urine so that a diagnosis of diabetes is made
- contaminating microbiological specimens.

A clue may be that the condition only occurs when the parent is present or following a visit. The condition can be extremely difficult to diagnose, but may be suspected if the child has frequent unexplained illnesses and multiple hospital admissions with symptoms that only occur in the mother's presence and are not substantiated by clinical findings. This disorder can be very damaging to the child, as unnecessary investigations and potentially harmful treatment are likely to be given. The child also learns to live with a pattern of illness rather than health.

MANAGEMENT OF SUSPECTED CHILD ABUSE

Abused children may present to doctors in the hospital or to medical or nursing staff in the community. They may also be brought for a medical opinion by social services or the police. In all cases the procedures of the local area child protection committee should be followed. The medical consultation should be the same as for any medical condition, with a full history and total body examination. It is usually most productive when this is conducted in a sensitive and concerned way without being accusatory or condemning. Any injuries or medical findings should be carefully noted, measured, recorded and drawn on a topographical chart. They may need to be photographed with parental consent. The height, weight and head circumference should be recorded and plotted on a centile chart. The interaction between the child and parents should be noted. All notes should be dated, timed and signed. Treatment of specific injuries should be instigated and blood tests and X-rays undertaken.

If abuse is suspected or confirmed, a decision needs to be made whether immediate treatment is required and if the child needs immediate protection from further harm. If this is the case, this may be achieved by admission to hospital, which also allows investigations and multidisciplinary assessment. If sympathetically handled, most parents are willing to accept medical advice for hospital admission for observation and investigation. Occasionally this is not possible and legal enforcement is required. If medical treatment is not necessary and it is felt that it is unsafe for the child to return home, placement may be in a foster home or children's home.

In addition to a detailed medical assessment, evaluation by social workers and other health professionals will be required. A child protection conference under the child protection procedure of the area child protection committee will be convened. A conference will be chaired by a senior member of the Social Services Department or of the National Society for the Prevention of Cruelty to Children

(NSPCC). Members of the conference may include social workers, health visitor, police, general practitioner, paediatricians and nurses, teachers and lawyers. Increasingly, parents attend all or part of the case conference. Details of the incident leading to the conference and the family background will be discussed. Good communication and a trusting working relationship between the professionals are vital as it can be extremely difficult to evaluate the likelihood that injuries were inflicted deliberately and the possible outcome of legal proceedings. The conference will decide:
- whether to place the child's name on the Child Protection Register
- whether there should be an application to the court to protect the child
- what follow-up is needed.

If the child is placed on the Child Protection Register, the Social Services Department will produce a child protection care plan which will include medical follow-up in many instances.

Case history

CHILD ABUSE

A seven-month-old boy was noted by a relative to have a large, unexplained bruise over the side of the head. His mother took him to the nearest A&E department where a skeletal survey showed a normal skull x-ray but this metaphyseal fracture (Fig. 5.15). His mother thought that this must have occurred when he had fallen off his parents' bed the previous day. His mother was training to be a nursery school teacher. Her partner had recently been discharged from prison for burglary. Both parents were interviewed by social services and the police. A child protection conference was held, which the mother attended. The findings were suggestive of non-accidental injury, but definite evidence was lacking. The case conference considered the child to be at risk of significant harm and placed him on the Child Protection Register, with close supervision by the health visitor and social services.

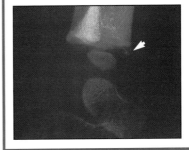

Fig. 5.15 A metaphyseal fracture, usually caused by wrenching, is highly suggestive of non-accidental injury.

SEXUAL ABUSE

A common definition of child sexual abuse is 'involvement of dependent, developmentally immature children and adolescents in sexual activities that they do not fully comprehend, are unable to give informed consent to and that violate social taboos of family roles'. It includes a variety of acts:

- genital exposure
- fondling
- genital, anal or oral sexual activity or intercourse, including rape
- involvement in pornography.

Victims can be of any age and of either sex, but girls outnumber boys. Risk factors in the family are listed in Figure 5.16. Children may be abused by:

- someone in the family
- a trusted adult, such as a baby-sitter
- someone outside the family, but this is much less common.

Male abusers are more common, but female abusers are being recognised with increasing frequency.

Sexual abuse usually presents as an incidental disclosure by a child, either spontaneously to a trusted adult or as the result of a crisis, such as running away or taking an overdose. It may also present with:

- genital trauma or infection
- sexually transmitted disease
- highly sexualised behaviour towards adults or children
- unexplained pregnancy
- inexplicable change in behaviour or school work.

When child sexual abuse is suspected, the need for and urgency of a medical examination should be assessed. The examination should be conducted by a senior doctor skilled in paediatric examination for child sexual abuse. Assessment of growth, behaviour and development should be made. Examination of the genitalia, which is usually only a detailed inspection and not an internal examination, is done as part of the general clinical examination. Clinical features include:

- bruising around the thighs, genitalia, anus, perineum and buttocks and lower abdomen
- tears and abrasions to the male genitalia
- tears and abrasions to the female genitalia. In particular, the hymen may be torn. However, vulval soreness is common in young girls and is rarely due to abuse
- anal fissures (may be associated with constipation)

Fig. 5.16 Family risk factors for child sexual abuse.

Poor parental sexual relationship
Maternal depression or physical illness
Mother sexually abused in childhood
Father/abuser either inadequate or aggressive
Family chaotic, disorganised or socially isolated
Parentified daughter who has taken over mother's role

- reflex anal dilation, where the buttocks are parted for 30–45 seconds. In a positive test the anus opens and the rectum can be seen because of incompetence of the internal sphincter. Reflex anal dilation and anal fissures in isolation are not reliable signs of child sexual abuse as they may have other causes, e.g. constipation.

If appropriate, a forensic physician should also be present to avoid having to repeat the examination. This allows agreement to be reached about the significance of any minor abnormalities, and forensic swabs and samples to be taken. Ideally this should be done within 72 hours of the incident.

The examination should be with the knowledge and agreement of the parent, though it may occasionally be performed at the request of the court. Adolescent girls must give their consent and all children should be accompanied by a trusted adult. In the case of young children this is usually a parent. It should be performed in privacy, calmly and in a non-threatening environment. The medical examination is rarely diagnostic and significant physical findings are present in less than 30% of abused children. Physical signs must be interpreted in conjunction with the history. There is considerable variation in the normal appearance of the female genitalia. This is partly age-dependent. A normal examination does not exclude abuse.

If sexual abuse is suspected, the procedures of the local area protection committee should be followed. Further information may be obtained from the child during an interview held jointly by a social worker and police officer experienced in child sexual abuse work. Psychological damage secondary to sexual abuse frequently occurs and may need specialist treatment. Post-traumatic stress disorder is a recognised sequel and can persist into adult life.

 At presentation, significant clinical abnormalities are present in less than 30% of sexually abused children.

FURTHER READING

Hobbs C, Hanks H, Wynne J. *Child Abuse and Neglect: A Clinician's Handbook.* Churchill Livingstone, London, 1993.
Meadow R (ed). *ABC of Child Abuse. (*2nd edn.) BMJ, London, 1993. Collection of review articles.
Sibert J (ed). *Accidents and Emergencies in Childhood.* Royal College of Physicians, London, 1992. Short review.

CHAPTER 6

Genetics

• *Chromosomal abnormalities* • *Mendelian inheritance* • *Polygenic or multifactorial inheritance* • *DNA analysis* • *Presymptomatic testing* • *Gene therapy* • *Genetic counselling* • *Syndrome diagnosis*

New techniques in molecular biology and cytogenetics have resulted in an explosion of knowledge about the genetic basis of diseases (Fig. 6.1). Clinical application of these advances is now available to parents through specialist genetic counselling and by antenatal diagnosis of an ever widening range of disorders. Gene therapy trials are underway, bringing hope of improved treatment in the future.

Genetic disorders are:
• common, with 2% of liveborn babies having a significant congenital malformation and about 5% a genetic disorder
• burdensome to the affected individual, family and society, as many are associated with severe and permanent disability.

Genetically determined diseases include those resulting from:
• chromosomal abnormalities
• the action of a single gene (Mendelian disorders)
• interaction of genetic and environmental factors (multifactorial or polygenic disorders).

Chromosomal abnormalities

Genes are composed of DNA which is wound around a core of histone proteins and packaged into a succession of supercoils to form the chromosomes. The human chromosome complement was confirmed as recently as 1956. Following the recognition in 1959 of the chromosome abnormalities in Down, Klinefelter and Turner syndromes, many hundreds of chromosome defects have now been documented. Chromosomal abnormalities are either numerical or structural (Fig. 6.2). They usually, but not always, cause multiple congenital anomalies and learning difficulties.

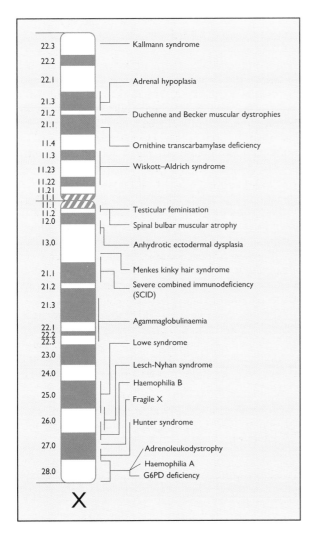

Fig. 6.1 Idiogram of the X chromosome, showing the position of some of the many genes for disorders located on it.

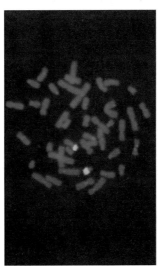

Fig. 6.2 Fluorescent in situ hybridisation (FISH), in which labelled DNA probes can be detected under fluorescent light. It is increasingly used to recognise chromosomal rearrangements, deletions and amplifications not visible using standard cytogenetic methods. Here a Y-specific probe shows additional material on the short arm of a chromosome 15 (the larger one). (Courtesy of MT Rebello, St Mary's Hospital Medical School, London.)

DOWN SYNDROME (TRISOMY 21)

This is the most common autosomal trisomy and the most common genetic cause of severe learning difficulties. The incidence in liveborn infants is about 1 in 650.

Clinical features

Down syndrome is usually suspected at birth because of the baby's facial appearance, but it can be difficult to be certain when relying on clinical characteristics alone.

Fig. 6.3 Characteristic clinical manifestations of Down syndrome.

Typical facial appearance:
  Round face
  Epicanthic folds
  Brushfield spots in iris
  Protruding tongue
  Small ears

Other anomalies:
  Flat occiput
  Abnormal creases on palms and soles (dermatoglyphics)
  Hypotonia
  Congenital heart defects (40%)
  Duodenal atresia

Later medical problems include:
  Severe learning difficulties
  Small stature
  Recurrent respiratory infections
  Hearing impairment from secretory otitis media
  Visual impairment from cataracts, squints
  Increased risk of leukaemia
  Risk of atlantoaxial instability (rare)
  Hypothyroidism
  Alzheimer disease

Chromosome analysis takes several days and sufficient certainty about the diagnosis is needed even to take blood for karyotyping. An incorrect suggestion that their baby may have Down syndrome is potentially damaging for parents, and therefore clinical suspicion should be confirmed by a senior paediatrician. In addition to the facial appearance, the flat occiput, abnormal dermatoglyphics and hypotonia are helpful diagnostic features (Figs 6.3 and 6.4a-c).

Parents need information about the short- and long-term implications of the diagnosis and of the assistance that is available from both professionals and self-help groups. Parents often find a written explanation of the condition a valuable adjunct to the discussion. They will have a chance to read it with their families and use it as a cue for asking more questions in subsequent discussions. Counselling may also be required to help the family deal with feelings of disappointment, anger or guilt. They will want to understand how and why the condition has arisen, the risk of recurrence and about antenatal diagnosis for future pregnancies.

It is important to note that parents appreciate reference to their baby not as a diagnostic category ('a Down's baby') but as an individual ('a baby with Down syndrome').

Cytogenetics

The extra chromosome 21 may result from non-disjunction, translocation or mosaicism:

1. Non-disjunction – 94%

- most cases result from an error at meiosis
- the pair of chromosomes 21 fails to separate, so that one gamete has two chromosomes 21 and one has none (Fig. 6.5).
- fertilisation of the gamete with two chromosomes 21 gives rise to a zygote with trisomy 21
- the incidence of trisomy 21 due to non-disjunction rises with increasing maternal age (Fig. 6.6), but is independent of paternal age, despite the fact that 10% of non-disjunctions are paternally derived.

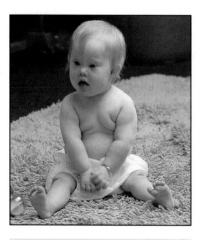

Fig. 6.4a Characteristic facies seen in Down syndrome. Her posture is due to hypotonia.

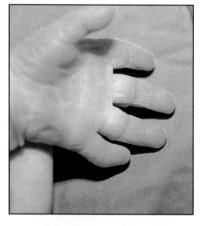

Fig. 6.4b Single transverse palmar crease.

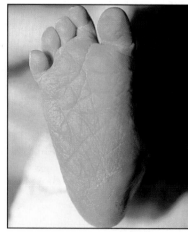

Fig. 6.4c Pronounced 'sandal gap' between the big and first toe.

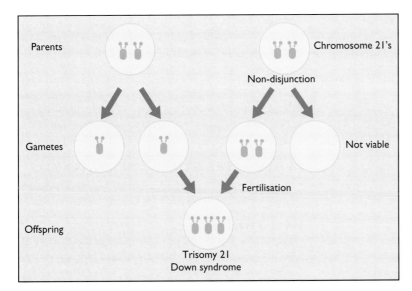

Fig. 6.5 Non-disjunction in Down syndrome.

Fig. 6.6 Risk of Down syndrome (live births) with maternal age at delivery.

Maternal age (years)	Risk of Down syndrome
All ages	1 in 650
30	1 in 900
35	1 in 380
37	1 in 240
40	1 in 110
44	1 in 37

Although the incidence of Down syndrome rises in babies of women over the age of 35 years, a smaller proportion of pregnancies occurs in women over this age and so most affected babies are born to younger mothers.

After having one child with trisomy 21 due to non-disjunction, the risk of recurrence of Down syndrome is 1 in 200 under 35 years and twice the age-specific risk at and above 35 years.

2. Translocation – 5%
A chromosome 21 is translocated onto a chromosome 14, or more rarely on to a chromosome 15, 22 or 21, and is known as a Robertsonian translocation. In about one-quarter of these, one parent has a balanced translocation, appearing to have only 45 chromosomes, but one chromosome 21 is attached to another chromosome. The affected child has three copies of chromosome 21 (Fig. 6.7).

In translocation Down syndrome:
- the risk of recurrence is 10–15% if the mother is the translocation carrier and about 2.5% if the father is the carrier
- if a parent carries the rare 21:21 translocation, all the offspring will have Down syndrome
- if neither parent carries a translocation, the risk of recurrence is <1%.

3. Mosaicism – 1%
In mosaicism some of the cells are normal and some have trisomy 21. This usually arises after the formation of the zygote, by non-disjunction at mitosis. The phenotype may be milder in mosaicism.

The chromosomes of a baby with Down syndrome must always be examined. If there is free trisomy 21, parental chromosomes need not be examined. If the baby has a

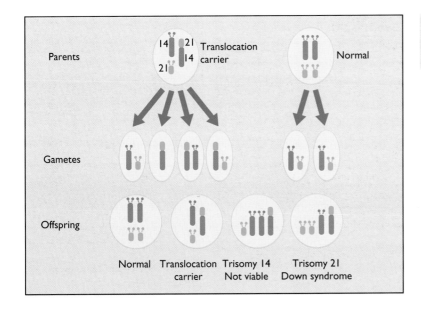

Fig. 6.7 Down syndrome with a translocation between chromosomes 21 and 14 inherited from a parent.

translation, then the parents' chromosomes should be studied, and if one carries a balanced translocation other relatives should also be offered genetic counselling.

> *Non-disjunction is the commonest cause of Down syndrome.*

EDWARDS SYNDROME (TRISOMY 18) AND PATAU SYNDROME (TRISOMY 13)

Although rarer than Down syndrome (1 in 8000 and 1 in 14000 livebirths respectively), the constellation of severe multiple abnormalities suggests the diagnosis at birth and most die in infancy (Figs 6.8–6.10).

TURNER SYNDROME (45, X)

Most (> 95%) result in early miscarriage. Occasional cases may be detected by ultrasound antenatally when a cystic hygroma and other evidence of fetal oedema may be present. In liveborn females, the incidence is about 1 in 2500.
Clinical features are listed in Figure 6.11.
Treatment is with:

- growth hormone therapy
- oestrogen replacement for development of secondary sexual characteristics at the time of puberty (but infertility persists).

Fig. 6.8 Clinical features of Edwards syndrome.
Small chin
Low-set ears
Overlapping of fingers (thumb across palm, overlapping middle and ring fingers)
Rocker bottom feet
Cardiac and renal malformations

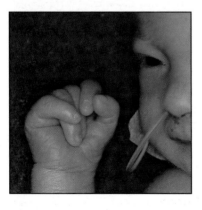

Fig. 6.9 Overlapping of the fingers in Edwards syndrome.

Fig. 6.10 Clinical features of Patau syndrome.
Structural defect of brain
Scalp lesions
Small eyes (microphthalmia) and other eye defects
Polydactyly
Cardiac and renal malformations

Cytogenetics

In about 50% of girls with Turner syndrome, there are only 45 chromosomes, with only one sex chromosome, the X. The others have either a deletion of the short arm of one X chromosome or an isochromosome which has two long arms but no short arm, or a variety of other structural defects of one of the X chromosomes. The incidence does not increase with maternal age and risks of recurrence are very low.

KLINEFELTER SYNDROME (47, XXY)

This occurs in about 1–2 per 1000 liveborn males. For clinical features see Figure 6.12.

DELETIONS

Deletions are one type of structural abnormality. Loss of a part of a chromosome usually results in physical abnormalities and learning difficulties. The deletion may involve loss of the terminal or, less commonly, the interstitial part of the chromosome.

An example of a deletion syndrome in man involves loss of the tip of the short arm of chromosome 5, hence the name 5p- or monosomy 5p. Because affected babies have a high-pitched mewing cry in early infancy, it is also known as *cri du chat* syndrome. Parental chromosomes should be checked to see if one parent carries a balanced chromosomal rearrangement.

FRAGILE X SYNDROME

This is an important syndrome since it is the second most common genetic cause of severe learning difficulties after Down syndrome. Prevalence estimates range from 1 in 1000 to 1 in 2250 males.

Fig. 6.11 Clinical features of Turner syndrome.
Lymphoedema of hands and feet in neonate
Short stature
Neck webbing
Wide carrying angle (cubitus valgus)
Widely spaced nipples
Congenital heart defects (particularly coarctation of the aorta)
Ovarian dysgenesis resulting in infertility
Normal intellectual development

Fig. 6.12 Clinical features of Klinefelter syndrome.
Infertility – most common presentation
Hypogonadism with small testes
Pubertal development apparently normally but some may benefit from testosterone therapy
Gynaecomastia in adolescence
Tall stature
Intelligence – usually in the normal range, but may have educational and psychological problems.

The diagnosis is made on the basis of the appearance of a gap in the distal part of the long arm of the X chromosome (at Xq27.3) in a proportion of lymphocytes. Special conditions are required for culturing cells, and so the cytogenetic laboratory must be aware that the diagnosis is suspected.

Although it is inherited as an X-linked disorder, affecting males primarily (Figs 6.13 and 6.14), there are some unusual features:

- one-third of obligate female carriers have learning difficulties, usually mild
- one-fifth of males who have inherited the mutation are phenotypically normal with normal chromosomes, and are referred to as 'normal transmitting males'. They may pass the disorder on to their grandsons through their daughters.

Unlike other X-linked disorders in which some are fresh mutations whose mothers are not carriers, all mothers of fragile-X males are carriers, but only about half of obligate female carriers express the fragile site cytogenetically. This, together with the other unusual features of the inheritance of this syndrome already mentioned, have made genetic counselling difficult for relatives of affected boys.

Recently the fragile X gene and its mutation were identified. The mutation involves amplification of a small segment of DNA in the gene. The expansion may become greater during transmission through females. This finding has improved the accuracy of carrier detection and antenatal diagnosis. Specialist genetic counselling and investigation using DNA analysis should be offered to affected families.

Fragile X syndrome is the second most common genetic cause of severe learning difficulties.

Mendelian inheritance

These patterns of inheritance, described by Mendel in 1865, are rare individually, but are collectively numerous, with several thousand single gene traits described.

For many disorders, the Mendelian pattern of inheritance is known. If the diagnosis of a condition is uncertain, its pattern of inheritance may be evident on drawing a family tree (pedigree), an essential part of clinical genetics (Fig. 6.15). It is important to ask specifically about abortions, stillbirths, infant deaths, multiple marriages and consanguinity.

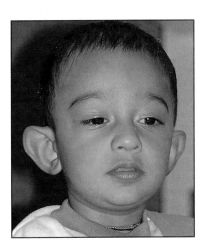

Fig. 6.13
A child with fragile X syndrome. At this age, the main feature is often the prominent ears.

Fig. 6.14 Clinical findings in males with fragile X syndrome.

Moderate learning difficulty (IQ 20–80, mean 50)

Macrocephaly

Macro-orchidism – more common post-pubertal than pre-pubertal

Characteristic appearance – long face, large everted ears, prominent mandible and large forehead, most evident in affected adults. Affected children may not appear to be dysmorphic facially.

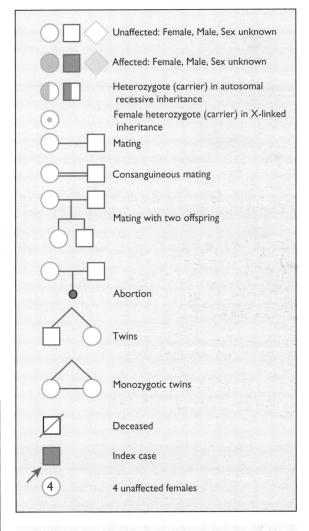

Fig. 6.15 Pedigree symbols.

AUTOSOMAL DOMINANT INHERITANCE

This is the most common mode of Mendelian inheritance (Fig. 6.16). An affected individual carries the abnormal gene on one of a pair of autosomes (chromosomes 1–22). In autosomal dominant disorders the heterozygote, carrying one copy of the abnormal gene, manifests the condition. The affected person passes to each offspring either the abnormal or the normal allele (form of the gene). Each offspring has a 1 in 2 (50%) chance of inheriting the abnormal gene (Fig. 6.17). Affected offspring are equally likely to be male or female (Fig. 6.18). The risk remains the same for each of any successive pregnancies. This is straightforward! However complicating factors include:

1. Variation in expression

Even in one family, some affected individuals may manifest the disorder mildly and others more severely. For example, a parent with tuberous sclerosis may have mild skin abnormalities only, but his affected child may have, in addition, epilepsy and learning difficulties.

2. Non-penetrance

Refers to the lack of clinical signs and symptoms in an individual who must have inherited the abnormal gene. An example of this is otosclerosis, in which about 40% of gene carriers develop deafness (Fig. 6.19).

3. No family history of the disorder

May be due to:

- a new mutation in one of the gametes which led to the conception of the affected person. This is the most common reason for absence of dominant disorders in a family history, e.g. >80% of individuals with achondroplasia have normal parents. New dominant mutations are more likely in children of older fathers. The risk of recurrence in siblings is likely to be low, provided that the parents have been examined carefully to exclude a mild form of the disorder. The risk to the offspring of the affected individual is still 1 in 2
- gonadal mosaicism – very occasionally a healthy parent carries in the gonad a number of gametes harbouring the mutation (gonadal mosaicism). This can account for recurrences of autosomal dominant disorders in siblings born to apparently normal parents. It has been described in congenital lethal osteogenesis imperfecta
- non-paternity – if the apparent father is not the biological father.

AUTOSOMAL RECESSIVE INHERITANCE

Several hundred disorders resulting from this type of inheritance are known (Fig. 6.20). An affected individual has inherited an abnormal allele from each parent, both of whom are heterozygous carriers for the same abnormal gene. Unlike in autosomal dominant inheritance, the heterozygote is healthy, because the abnormal allele is recessive in its effect to the normal allele. The affected

---

Fig. 6.16 Examples of autosomal dominant disorders.

Achondroplasia

Ehlers-Danlos syndrome

Familial hypercholesterolaemia

Huntington disease

Marfan syndrome

Myotonic dystrophy

Neurofibromatosis

Noonan syndrome

Osteogenesis imperfecta

Otosclerosis

Polyposis coli

Tuberous sclerosis

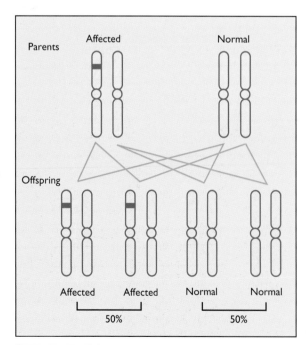

Fig. 6.17 Autosomal dominant disorder.

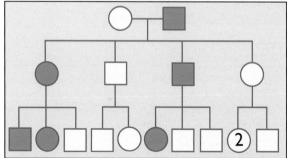

Fig. 6.18 Typical pedigree of an autosomal dominant disorder.

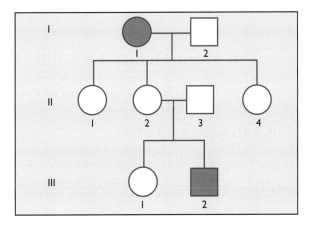

Fig. 6.19 Example of non-penetrance. I1 and III2 have otosclerosis. II2 has normal hearing but must have the gene. The gene is non-penetrant in II2.

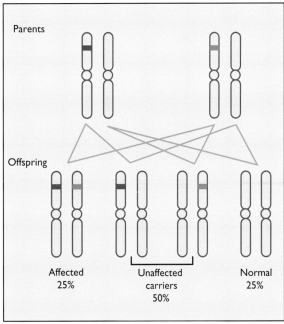

Fig. 6.21 Autosomal recessive inheritance.

person is homozygous for the abnormal allele and so has no 'working copy' of the normal gene.

The risk of each child of two carrier parents being affected is 1 in 4 (25%) (Fig. 6.21). Males and females are equally likely to be affected since the abnormal gene is on an autosome. Although the abnormal gene may be transmitted from one generation to the next there is usually no positive family history outside the sibship. This is because other carriers in the family usually will not have carrier partners (Fig. 6.22). All offspring of affected individuals will be carriers.

Consanguinity

It is thought that we all carry at least one abnormal recessive gene; fortunately, our spouse usually carries a different one. Marrying a cousin or other relative increases the chance of a couple carrying the same abnormal autosomal recessive gene, since they could inherit it from a common ancestor. A couple who are cousins therefore have a small increased risk of having a child with a recessive disorder.

Whereas autosomal dominantly inherited conditions often involve structural defects, autosomal recessive disorders are often metabolic disorders resulting from enzyme deficiences and are more often life-threatening.

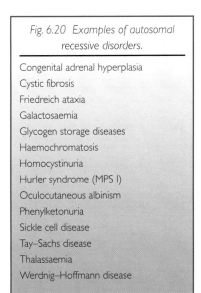

Fig. 6.20 Examples of autosomal recessive disorders.

Congenital adrenal hyperplasia

Cystic fibrosis

Friedreich ataxia

Galactosaemia

Glycogen storage diseases

Haemochromatosis

Homocystinuria

Hurler syndrome (MPS I)

Oculocutaneous albinism

Phenylketonuria

Sickle cell disease

Tay–Sachs disease

Thalassaemia

Werdnig–Hoffmann disease

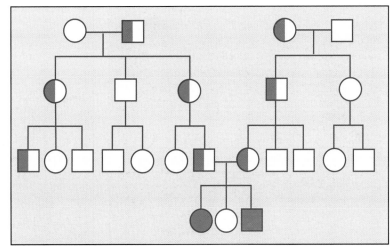

Fig. 6.22 Typical pedigree of an autosomal recessive disorder.

Recessive gene frequencies may vary between racial groups (Fig. 6.23). When the gene occurs sufficiently frequently and the gene or its effect can be detected, carrier detection and antenatal diagnosis can be performed.

 Autosomal recessive disorders are often metabolic, autosomal dominant are usually structural.

X-LINKED RECESSIVE INHERITANCE

At least 250 of these disorders have been described (Fig. 6.24). The abnormal gene is carried on the X chromosome. In the carrier female, the normal allele on her other X chromosome 'protects' her from the disease. In the male however, the abnormal allele on his X chromosome is not balanced by a normal allele and he manifests the disease. In X-linked recessive inheritance:

- males are affected
- females can be carriers but are usually healthy
- occasionally a female carrier shows mild signs of the disease
- each son of a female carrier has a 1 in 2 (50%) risk of being affected (Fig. 6.25)
- each daughter of a female carrier has a 1 in 2 (50%) risk of being a carrier
- daughters of affected males will all be carriers. Sons of affected males will not be affected, since a man passes a Y chromosome to his son (Fig. 6.26).

The family history may be negative however, since new mutations are fairly common. Identification of carrier females in the family requires interpretation of the pedigree, looking for mild clinical manifestations and specific tests such as biochemical markers, e.g. creatine kinase levels and DNA analysis in Duchenne muscular dystrophy.

X-LINKED DOMINANT INHERITANCE

Although dominantly inherited X-linked disorders occur, e.g. a variant of vitamin D-resistant rickets, they are rare. Males and females can be affected.

Y-LINKED INHERITANCE

No serious genetic defects, apart from some rare forms of intersex and a gene for azoospermia have been located to the human Y chromosome, which seems reasonable given that half the population live happily without a Y chromosome!

MITOCHONDRIAL OR CYTOPLASMIC INHERITANCE

Although rare and not strictly Mendelian, these disorders deserve mention. Unlike sperm, the egg contains cytoplasm in which are found mitochondria with their own chromosomes. These are maternally derived. In Leber hereditary optic neuropathy and some mitochrondrial myopathies, mutations in mitochondrial DNA have been reported, and these disorders show maternal transmission only.

IMPRINTING AND UNIPARENTAL DISOMY

In the past, it was accepted that the activity of a gene is the same regardless of whether it is inherited from the mother or father. Recently, however, there is evidence that some genes only express the copy derived from a parent of a given sex. This is called 'imprinting'. An example involves

Fig. 6.23 Examples of carrier frequencies in various ethnic groups.		
Disease	**Ethnic group**	**Approximate carrier frequency (%)**
Sickle cell disease	African or Afro-Caribbean	1 in 16
Thalassaemias	Mediterranean or Asian	1 in 10
Cystic fibrosis	Northern European	1 in 25
Tay–Sachs disease	Ashkenazi Jewish	1 in 25

Fig. 6.24 Examples of X-linked recessive inheritance.
Colour blindness (red–green)
Duchenne and Becker muscular dystrophies
Fragile X syndrome
Glucose-6-phosphate dehydrogenase (G6PD) deficiency
Haemophilia A and B
Hunter syndrome (mucopolysaccharidosis II)

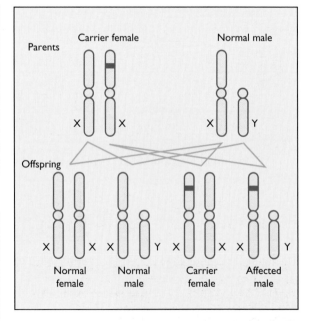

Fig. 6.25 X-linked recessive inheritance.

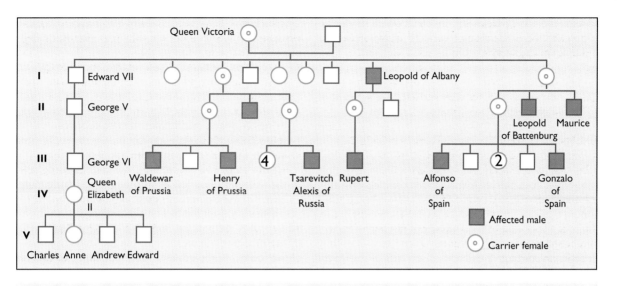

Fig. 6.26 *Typical pedigree for X-linked recessive inheritance, showing Queen Victoria, a carrier for haemophilia A, and her family. It shows affected males in several generations, related through females and that affected males do not have affected sons (contrast with autosomal dominant inheritance).*

Prader–Willi (learning difficulties, hypotonia, obesity) and Angelman (severe learning difficulties, ataxia, happy personality, characteristic facial appearance, epilepsy) syndromes. The Prader–Willi and Angelman syndrome genes are separate but both are found in the 15q11–13 region of chromosome 15 (that is, bands 11–13 on the long arm of chromosome 15). Normally, the *paternal* copy of the Prader–Willi gene and the *maternal* copy of the Angelman gene are active. Failure to inherit the particular *active* gene

will give rise to the relevant syndrome.

There are two main ways that a child can fail to inherit the active gene:

- *de novo* deletion (Fig. 6.27). Parental chromosomes are normal, and a deletion occurs as a new mutation in the child
- uniparental disomy (Fig. 6.28). This may be detected with DNA analysis. The child inherits two copies of a region of a chromosome from one parent and none

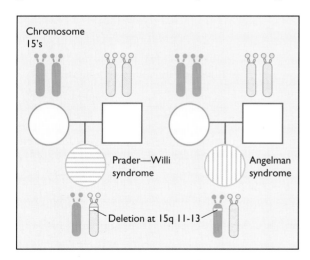

Fig. 6.27 *Imprinting resulting from a deletion. If the deletion occurs on chromosome 15 inherited from the father, the child has Prader–Willi syndrome (no active copy of the PWS gene). If the deletion occurs on chromosome 15 from the mother, the child has Angelman syndrome (no active copy of the AS gene).*

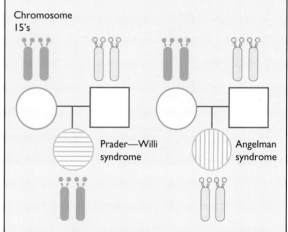

Fig. 6.28 *Imprinting resulting from uniparental disomy. A child who inherits two maternal chromosome 15s will have Prader–Willi syndrome (no active copy of the PWS gene). A child who inherits two paternal chromosome 15s will have Angelman syndrome (no active copy of the AS gene).*

from the other parent, e.g. in Prader–Willi syndrome the affected child has no paternal (but two maternal) copies of chromosome 15q 11–13.

 Imprinting is the unusual property of some genes to express only the copy derived from a parent of a given sex.

Polygenic or multifactorial inheritance

There is a spectrum in the aetiology of disease from environmental factors (e.g. trauma) at one end to purely genetic causes (e.g. Mendelian disorders) at the other. Between these two extremes are many disorders which result from the additive effect of several genes (hence the term polygenic) with or without the influence of environmental or other unknown factors (i.e. multifactorial). The two terms are often used interchangeably (Fig. 6.29).

Normal traits such as height and intelligence are also inherited in this way. These parameters show a Gaussian or normal distribution in the population. Similarly, the liability of an individual to develop a disease of multifactorial or polygenic aetiology also has a normal distribution. The condition occurs when a certain threshold level of liability is exceeded.

Relatives of an affected person show an increased liability, and so a greater proportion of them than in the general population will fall beyond the threshold and will manifest the disorder (Fig. 6.30).

The risk of recurrence of a multifactorial disorder in a family is usually low and is most significant for first-degree relatives. Empirical recurrence risk data is used for genetic counselling. It is derived from family studies which have reported the frequency at which various family members are affected. Factors which increase the risk to relatives are:

- more severe form of disorder, e.g. the risk of recurrence to sibs is greater in bilateral cleft lip and palate than in unilateral cleft lip alone
- close relationship to the affected person, e.g. overall risk to sibs is greater than to more distant relatives
- multiple affected family members, e.g. the more sibs already affected, the greater the risk of recurrence
- sex difference in prevalence, e.g. in Hirschsprung disease the male to female ratio is 3:1. An affected female must have had a greater genetic predisposition, so the risk to siblings is greater than for an affected male.

These 'rules' are in stark contrast to those in Mendelian inheritance in which the risks remain the same, regardless of the severity of the disease, number of affected sibs or sex of proband (in autosomal disorders).

It is important to note that the phenotype (clinical picture) of a disorder may have a heterogeneous (mixed) basis in different families, e.g. hyperlipidaemia leading to atherosclerosis and coronary heart disease can be due to a single gene disorder such as autosomal dominant hypercholesterolaemia, but some forms of hyperlipidaemia are polygenic and result from an interaction of the effect of genes for various lipoproteins.

In many multifactorial disorders, the 'environmental factors' remain obscure. Obvious exceptions include dietary fat intake and smoking in atherosclerosis, and viral infection in insulin-dependent diabetes mellitus. For neural tube defects, the risk of recurrence to siblings is lowered from about 3% (in low-incidence areas) to 1% or less in future pregnancies if the mother takes folate before conception and in the early weeks of pregnancy. This is a rare example of the possibility of primary prevention of a genetic disorder.

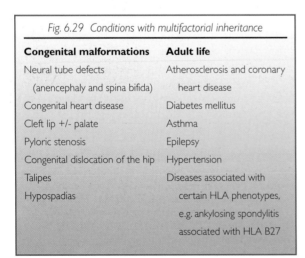

Congenital malformations	Adult life
Neural tube defects (anencephaly and spina bifida)	Atherosclerosis and coronary heart disease
Congenital heart disease	Diabetes mellitus
Cleft lip +/- palate	Asthma
Pyloric stenosis	Epilepsy
Congenital dislocation of the hip	Hypertension
Talipes	Diseases associated with
Hypospadias	certain HLA phenotypes, e.g. ankylosing spondylitis associated with HLA B27

Fig. 6.29 Conditions with multifactorial inheritance

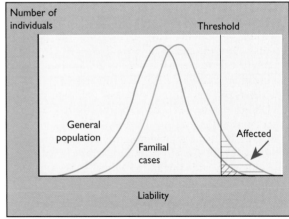

Fig. 6.30 Diagram to show the increased liability to a multifactorial disorder in relatives of an affected person.

DNA analysis

The main impact of DNA analysis for genetic counselling is:
- detection of female carriers in X-linked disorders, e.g. Duchenne and Becker muscular dystrophies, haemophilia A and B
- carrier detection in autosomal recessive disorders, e.g. cystic fibrosis
- presymptomatic diagnosis in autosomal dominant disorders, e.g. Huntington disease, myotonic dystrophy
- antenatal diagnosis of an increasing number of Mendelian conditions.

These are accomplished by means of:

1. genetic linkage
When a DNA marker is very close to or within the gene in question, use of DNA markers allows the disease gene to be 'tracked' through the family, e.g. in Duchenne muscular dystrophy it may be possible to tell if a female is a carrier by tracking the affected chromosome through the family. The family will need to be tested before any pregnancy so that useful markers can be identified for fetal sampling

2. mutation analysis
For some disorders, it is possible to detect directly the actual mutation causing the disease. Since the mutation itself is being detected this will give very accurate results. Examples are:
- deletions – DNA probes to detect these are available for α thalassaemia, some cases of β thalassaemia, haemophilia A and B, Duchenne and Becker muscular dystrophies, cystic fibrosis and many other disorders. About 78% of cystic fibrosis carriers in the UK possess the Δ F508 mutation and over 400 other mutations have been identified
- less commonly, point mutations in genes may be detectable. This is the case in sickle cell disease
- trinucleotide repeat expansion mutations. Recently, several human genetic diseases have been identified with this type of mutation. These include fragile X syndrome, myotonic dystrophy and Huntington disease. The mutation involves a repeat of a given nucleotide triplet within the gene. For example, in myotonic dystrophy (DM) the triplet is CTG. Normal individuals have from five to 40 CTG repeats in the DM gene, whereas individuals with DM have more than 40 CTG repeats. When an affected individual passes the gene to offspring, the number of repeats can expand. Greater numbers of CTG repeats are associated with increasing clinical severity of the illness. Thus the phenomenon of anticipation, which has long been recognised in DM and which refers to increasing clinical severity down the generations, now has a molecular basis (Fig. 6.31). Similarly, in fragile X syndrome, normal individuals have from 10 to 50 CGG repeats in the fragile X gene. The phenomenon of the 'normal transmitting male' (a

normal male carrier) is explained by the fact that he carries a small increase in the number of repeats (from 50 to 200). This is apparently harmless and is called a premutation. The male carrier transmits the premutation to all his daughters, who are also clinically normal. However, when they pass the gene to their children, expansion to the full mutation (200–2000 CGG repeats) can occur. All males and about 50% of females with the full mutation are affected clinically.

New techniques in DNA analysis are continually being developed which have a major impact on clinical genetics. An example is polymerase chain reaction (PCR), a technique

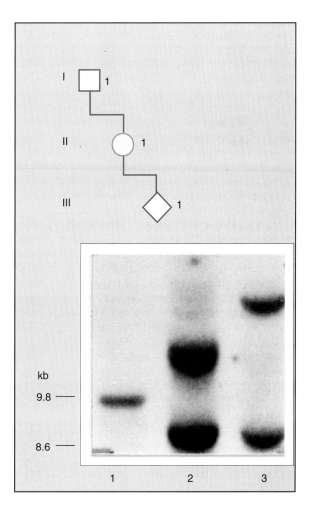

Fig. 6.31 'Anticipation', the increasing clinical severity down the generations. I1 has cataracts only, II1 has classical myotonic dystrophy and III1 is an infant with severe congenital myotonic dystrophy. The DNA results are shown below on a Southern blot. The larger a band, the higher it appears. There is increasing enlargement of the 9.8 kilobase band.

of DNA amplification. This allows:
- rapid DNA analysis. Results may be ready in 1–2 days which is particularly useful for antenatal diagnosis on chorion villus samples
- analysis of small amounts of DNA. This allows DNA analysis, e.g. for cystic fibrosis on blood spots taken for neonatal biochemical screening (Guthrie test) or even from saliva.

Anticipation is the worsening of clinical severity down the generations and can occur with trinucleotide repeat expansion mutations.

Presymptomatic testing

In many autosomal dominant disorders, clinical expression may not be evident at birth, or it may vary between mild and severe. Relatives of affected individuals may request tests to see if they are likely to develop the disorder in question. Examples include myotonic dystrophy, Huntington disease, autosomal dominant polycystic kidney disease (adult) and neurofibromatosis. Assessment may include:
- careful examination of individuals at risk, e.g. evidence of myotonia in myotonic dystrophy. In some disorders in which expression varies and may be mild, it may be impossible to determine clinically whether or not an individual carries the abnormal gene
- investigations, e.g. regular renal scans in individuals at risk of autosomal dominant polycystic kidney disease
- DNA analysis using linked markers or mutation analysis.

It is debatable whether presymptomatic tests (e.g. for myotonic dystrophy) and carrier tests (e.g. for cystic fibrosis) should be performed on children, as it removes the child's right to choose whether or not to have the information. In Huntington disease it is generally accepted that children should not be tested.

Gene therapy

Gene therapy involves the artificial introduction of genes into disease tissue in order to cure the disease.
Success requires:
- integration of the introduced gene into the chromosomal DNA of recipient cells. The simplest way is to transfer the genes into suitable cells in culture and then insert the transfected cells into the patient
- delivery to the appropriate tissue. Some tissues, such as blood, are easier to access than others, such as brain or muscle. Ways to overcome these difficulties are being developed
- the gene must be expressed appropriately.

Gene therapy has been initiated recently in adenosine deaminase deficiency (a rare recessive immune disorder), malignant melanoma and cystic fibrosis and some clinical benefit has been reported in a few patients. At present, it is generally accepted that gene therapy be limited to somatic (not germ line) cells, so that the risk of adversely affecting future generations is minimised.

Genetic counselling

The main aim of genetic counselling is to give individuals, couples and families information about hereditary disorders, so that they understand:
- what it means to have the disorder
- their risk of developing or transmitting it to offspring
- measures to treat or prevent the disorder.

The primary goal of genetic counselling is to provide information to allow for greater autonomy and choice in reproductive decisions. Prevention of genetic disease may also result from genetic counselling, but this is not the main aim. The elements of genetic counselling include:
- establishing the correct diagnosis. This includes checking hospital records and arranging to examine family members, if indicated. Special areas of diagnostic importance include making a syndrome diagnosis and perinatal deaths. It is vital to take all possible measures to establish a diagnosis in all perinatal deaths, or at least to document all details fully. Chromosome analysis, autopsy and a photograph particularly to show the face and any malformations are invaluable. X-rays are essential if a structural abnormality is suspected. A blood or tissue sample should be taken for DNA storage, if appropriate, for present or future use
- risk estimation. Even if the diagnosis is uncertain, the pedigree may allow a risk estimation to be made. Drawing a pedigree of three generations is an essential part of genetic counselling
- communication. Information should be presented in an unbiased way. For example, the impact of saying 'the risk of recurrence is 1 in 4' is different from saying 'the risk of no recurrence is 3 in 4', and so both should be presented
- discussing the options available if there appears to be a risk to offspring. These include: not having (more) children, ignoring the risk, artificial insemination by donor or ovum donation if appropriate, or antenatal diagnosis and termination of pregnancy of an affected fetus.

The counselling should be non-directive, but should also assist in the decision-making process (Fig. 6.32).
This requires:
- time and possibly several sessions
- a compassionate approach

Fig. 6.32 Influences on decisions regarding options for genetic counselling

Magnitude of risk

Severity of disorder

Availability of treatment

Person's experience of the disorder

Family size

Availability of a safe and reliable antenatal test

Parental or cultural ethical values

- awareness of psychological issues, such as denial, grief and anger which are often evoked by genetic illness
- awareness of ethnic, social, religious and educational factors
- follow-up to assess understanding and to offer support. This is an essential part of genetic counselling, particularly after a termination for fetal abnormality.

In the UK most regional health authorities have at least one clinical genetics centre where genetic counselling is carried out as a specialist service by consultants, their medical staff, specialist health visitors and others. As more disorders become amenable to antenatal diagnosis, it will be important to develop a more coordinated approach in the community which will involve:

- education of the general public and medical profession about genetic issues
- establishment of comprehensive screening programmes (e.g. for cystic fibrosis) in the community, complete with facilities not only for testing but for pre- and post-test counselling
- the non-medical genetic counsellor whose role will become increasingly important.

 Genetic counselling aims to allow parents greater autonomy and choice in reproductive decisions.

Syndrome diagnosis

Although singly most syndromes are rare, recognition of a dysmorphic syndrome may give information regarding:

- risk of recurrence
- prognosis
- likely complications which can be sought and perhaps treated successfully if detected early
- unnecessary investigations which may be avoided
- experience and information which parents can share with other affected families through self-help groups.

Dysmorphology
The study of malformations during embryogenesis.

Malformation
A primary structural defect occurring during the development of a tissue or organ, e.g. spina bifida. Isolated malformations are often multifactorial in aetiology. Multiple malformation syndromes are often associated with severe learning difficulties and may be due to:

- a single gene defect
- chromosomal defects
- exposure during pregnancy to teratogens such as alcohol, drugs (valproate, phenytoin) or viral infections
- unknown causes.

Disruption
Involves destruction of a fetal part which initially formed normally, e.g. amniotic membrane rupture may lead to amniotic bands which may cause limb reduction defects.

Deformation
Implies an abnormal physical influence in the intrauterine environment, e.g. renal agenesis in which severe oligohydramnios causes pulmonary hypoplasia and a characteristic compressed facial appearance. Oligohydramnios from any cause will result in a similar phenotype, which is referred to as Potter syndrome.

Sequence
Refers to a series of events occurring after one initiating defect. Potter syndrome is an example of a malformation sequence in which all abnormalities may be traced to one original malformation, renal agenesis.

Association
A group of malformations occurring together more often than expected by chance, e.g. the VATER association (Vertebral anomalies, Anal atresia, Tracheo-Esophageal fistula, Radial defects) and CHARGE association (Coloboma of the eye, Heart defect, Atresia choanae, Retardation of growth and development, Genital abnormalities, Ear anomalies).

The approach to diagnosis of dysmorphic syndromes includes:

- history, e.g. exposure to teratogens, fetal movements *in utero*
- examination of the child including measurements and photographs
- examination of the parents, e.g. a white forelock in the mother of a deaf child might suggest the diagnosis of Waardenburg syndrome
- investigations, such as chromosome analysis and radiology
- in some cases, the overall appearance of the child ('gestalt') will allow recognition of a syndrome. In others, checking in books containing lists of syndromes or using a computer to search for a previously described association of abnormal features may assist in diagnosing the many hundreds of rare syndromes. Despite these measures, many malformation syndromes remain unrecognised. Examples of syndromes recognisable by 'gestalt' are shown in Figures 6.33–6.35.

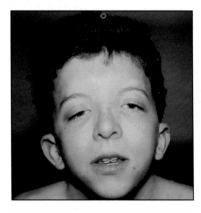

Fig. 6.33a Noonan syndrome affects males and females. There are some similarities to the phenotype in Turner syndrome, but it is caused by a faulty autosomal dominant gene and the chromosomes appear normal.

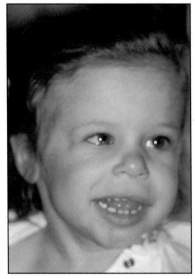

Fig. 6.34a Williams syndrome is usually sporadic.

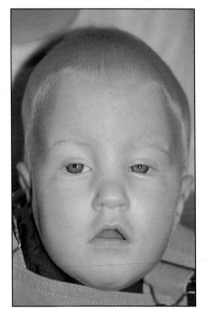

Fig. 6.35a Prader–Willi syndrome.

Fig. 6.33b

Clinical features of Noonan syndrome:

Characteristic facies

Occasional mild learning difficulties

Short webbed neck with trident hair line

Pectus excavatum

Short stature

Congenital heart disease (especially pulmonary stenosis, ASD)

Fig. 6.34b

Clinical features of Williams syndrome:

Short stature

Characteristic facies

Transient neonatal hypercalcaemia (occasionally)

Congenital heart disease (supravalvular aortic stenosis)

Mild to moderate learning difficulties

Fig. 6.35b

Clinical features of Prader–Willi syndrome:

Characteristic facies

Hypotonia

Obesity (after initial failure to thrive)

Hypogonadism

Developmental delay

FURTHER READING

Baraitser M. Winter RM. *Color Atlas of Congenital Malformation Syndromes*. Mosby–Wolfe, London 1996.

Connor JM, Ferguson-Smith MA. *Essential Medical Genetics*, 3rd ed. Blackwell Scientific Publications, Oxford, 1993. General medical genetics.

Emery AEH, Mueller RF. *Elements of Medical Genetics*. 8th ed. Churchill Livingstone, Edinburgh, 1992. General medical genetics.

Harper PS. *Practical Genetic Counselling*. 4th ed. Wright, London, 1993. Book on genetic counselling.

Jones KL. *Smith's Recognisable Patterns of Human Malformation*. 4th ed. WB Saunders, Philadephia, 1988. Diagnosing syndromes.

Kingston HM. *ABC of Clinical Genetics*. BMJ. London 1989.

McKusick VA. *Mendelian Inheritance in Man. Catalogs of autosomal dominant, autosomal recessive and X linked phenotypes*. 10th ed. Johns Hopkins University Press, Baltimore and London, 1992. A list and summary of Mendelian disorders.

Strachan T. *The Human Genome*. BIOS Scientific Publishers Ltd, Oxford, 1992. Molecular genetics.

Weatherall DJ. *The New Genetics and Clinical Practice*. 3rd ed. Oxford University Press, Oxford, 1991. Molecular genetics and its clinical applications.

CHAPTER 7

Perinatal Medicine

• *Preconceptual care* • *Antenatal diagnosis* • *Obstetric conditions affecting the fetus* • *Maternal conditions affecting the fetus* • *Maternal drugs affecting the fetus* • *Congenital infections* • *Adaptation to extrauterine life* • *Neonatal resuscitation* • *Size at birth* • *Examination of the newborn infant*

The term 'perinatal medicine' acknowledges the continuity of fetal and neonatal life. Using modern technology, such as high-resolution ultrasound and DNA analysis, detailed information about the fetus can now be obtained for a large and increasing number of conditions. There should be close cooperation between the professionals involved in the care of the pregnant mother and fetus and those caring for the newborn infant.

Preconceptual care

The better a mother's state of health and nutrition, the higher her socio-economic living standard and the quality of health care she receives, the greater is the chance of a successful outcome to her pregnancy. This is reflected in the widely varying perinatal mortality rate in different countries. In 1990, the perinatal mortality rate in Costa Rica was 16.5, in the US 8.8, in the UK 8.1 and in Japan 5.3/1000 total births.

Couples planning to have a baby often ask what they should do to optimise their chances of having a healthy child. They can be informed that for the mother:
* *smoking* reduces birthweight, which may be of critical importance if born preterm. On average, the babies of smokers weigh 170g less than non-smokers, but the reduction in birthweight is related to the number of cigarettes smoked per day. Smoking is also associated with an increased risk of miscarriage and stillbirth. The infant has a greater risk of sudden infant death syndrome (SIDS). There is some evidence that maternal smoking may adversely affect ovarian function in female children
* *medication* either prescribed or proprietary, is best avoided, unless essential, because of potential teratogenic effects
* *excess alcohol* ingestion and drug abuse may damage the fetus
* *congenital rubella* is preventable by maternal immunisation before pregnancy
* exposure to *toxoplasmosis* should be minimised by not handling cat litter, or wearing gloves if she does do so, and avoiding eating undercooked poultry
* *Listeria infection* can be acquired from eating unpasteurised dairy products, soft ripened cheeses, e.g. Brie,

Camembert and blue veined varieties, pâtés and ready-to-eat poultry unless thoroughly reheated
* *eating liver* during pregnancy is best avoided as it contains a high concentration of vitamin A
* *periconceptual folic acid* supplements reduce the risk of neural tube defects in the fetus. Low-dose folic acid supplementation is recommended for all women planning a pregnancy, with a higher dose for women with a previously affected fetus.

Any pre-existing maternal medical condition, e.g. hypertension or obstetric risk factors for complications of pregnancy or delivery, e.g. recurrent miscarriage or previous preterm delivery, should be identified and treated or monitored. Obesity increases the risk of developing gestational diabetes and pregnancy induced hypertension.

Couples at risk of inherited disorders should receive genetic counselling before pregnancy. This enables them to be fully informed, decide whether or not to proceed, and consider antenatal diagnosis if available. Pregnancies at increased risk of fetal abnormality include those in which:
* the mother is over 35 years old, when the risk of Down syndrome is greater than 1 in 380
* there is a previous abnormal child
* there is a family history of an inherited disorder
* the parents are identified as carriers of an autosomal recessive disorder, e.g. thalassaemia
* a parent carries a chromosomal rearrangement.

 Some definitions:
Stillbirth – fetal death after 24 completed weeks of pregnancy.
Perinatal mortality rate – stillbirths + deaths within the first 6 days per 1000 live and stillbirths.
Neonatal mortality rate – deaths of liveborn infants less than 28 days of age per 1000 live births.

Antenatal diagnosis

Antenatal diagnosis has become available for an increasing number of disorders. Screening tests performed on maternal blood and ultrasound of the fetus are listed in Figure 7.1. The main diagnostic techniques for antenatal diagnosis are detailed ultrasound scanning, amniocentesis, chorion villus sampling and fetal blood sampling (Fig. 7.2). Their indications are

	Fig. 7.1 Screening tests for antenatal diagnosis
Maternal blood	Blood group and antibodies for rhesus and other red cell incompatibilities
	Hepatitis B
	Syphilis
	Rubella
	HIV infection: after counselling and maternal consent, usually if at increased risk
	Testing for neural tube defects: maternal serum alphafetoprotein (MSAFP) is measured in many parts of the UK and other countries. It is raised in about 80% of open neural tube defects and more than 90% of anencephaly. These conditions are increasingly diagnosed or excluded on detailed ultrasound alone.
	Testing for Down syndrome: a risk estimate can be calculated from MSAFP (lowered), together with human chorionic gonadotrophia (HCG) and unconjugated oestriol (uE3) measurements (the 'triple' test), adjusted for maternal age. Other hormones can be measured instead, or in addition. If the risk is high, fetal chromosome analysis is offered.
Ultrasound screening	Gestational age: can be estimated reliably if performed before 20 weeks
	Multiple pregnancies: can be identified
	Structural malformations: 30–70% of major congenital malformations can be detected. If a significant abnormality is suspected, a more detailed scan by a specialist is advisable.
	Fetal growth: can be monitored by serial measurement of abdominal circumference, head circumference and femur length
	Amniotic fluid volume: oligohydramnios may result from reduced fetal urine production (from dysplastic or absent kidneys or obstructive uropathy), from prolonged rupture of the membranes or associated with severe intrauterine growth retardation. It may cause pulmonary hypoplasia and limb and facial deformities from pressure on the fetus (Potter syndrome).
	Polyhydramnios is associated with maternal diabetes and with gastrointestinal atresia in the fetus.

listed in Figure 7.3. The structural malformations and some of the other lesions which can be identified on ultrasound are listed in Figures 7.4 and 7.5.

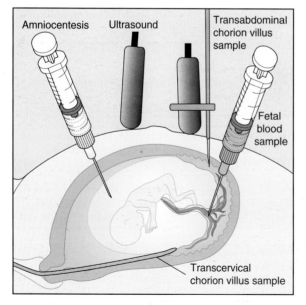

Fig. 7.2 Some of the techniques used for antenatal diagnosis.

Antenatal diagnosis may allow:
- the option of termination of pregnancy to be offered for severe disorders
- therapy to be given for a limited number of conditions
- reassurance where disorders are not detected
- optimal obstetric management of the fetus
- neonatal management to be planned in advance.

Parents require accurate medical advice and counselling to help them with these difficult decisions. Many transient or minor disorders are also detected, which may cause considerable anxiety.

> *Congenital malformations and disorders which used to be diagnosed at birth or during infancy are increasingly recognised antenatally.*

FETAL MEDICINE

The fetus can sometimes be treated by giving medication to the mother. Examples are:
- **glucocorticoid therapy** given before preterm delivery accelerates lung maturity and surfactant production, reducing the incidence and severity of respiratory distress syndrome (RDS). For optimal effect, it needs to be given at least 48 hours before delivery, but this is often not possible as delivery occurs before this time has elapsed.
- **digoxin or flecainide** can be given to the mother to treat fetal supraventricular tachycardia.

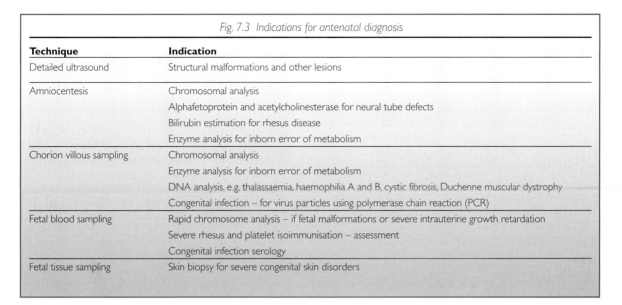

Fig. 7.3 Indications for antenatal diagnosis

Technique	Indication
Detailed ultrasound	Structural malformations and other lesions
Amniocentesis	Chromosomal analysis
	Alphafetoprotein and acetylcholinesterase for neural tube defects
	Bilirubin estimation for rhesus disease
	Enzyme analysis for inborn error of metabolism
Chorion villous sampling	Chromosomal analysis
	Enzyme analysis for inborn error of metabolism
	DNA analysis, e.g. thalassaemia, haemophilia A and B, cystic fibrosis, Duchenne muscular dystrophy
	Congenital infection – for virus particles using polymerase chain reaction (PCR)
Fetal blood sampling	Rapid chromosome analysis – if fetal malformations or severe intrauterine growth retardation
	Severe rhesus and platelet isoimmunisation – assessment
	Congenital infection serology
Fetal tissue sampling	Skin biopsy for severe congenital skin disorders

Fig. 7.4 Main structural malformations and other lesions detectable by ultrasound

Neural	Anencephaly – the unexpected birth of an affected infant is now extremely uncommon in the UK
	Spina bifida – can be difficult to recognise; associated cerebral abnormalities can be helpful
	Hydrocephalus, microcephaly
Cardiac	A four-chamber view should detect about 60% of severe malformations
Intrathoracic	Diaphragmatic hernia
Gastrointestinal	Cleft lip and palate
	Bowel obstruction – e.g. duodenal atresia; lower bowel obstruction may be difficult to detect
	Exomphalos and gastroschisis (Fig. 7.5)
Genitourinary	Dysplastic kidneys
	Obstructive disorders – readily visualised, but distinguishing mild hydronephrosis from transient, physiological pelvicalyceal dilatation is problematic
	Oligohydramnios may indicate poor renal function or outflow obstruction
Skeletal	Skeletal dysplasias, e.g. achondroplasia and limb reduction deformities
Hydrops	Oedema of the skin, pleural effusions and ascites
Chromosomal	Down syndrome – suspected from a thickened fat pad at the back of neck (nuchal translucency), duodenal atresia or an atrioventricular canal defect of the heart
	Other chromosomal disorders – suspected from identifying multiple abnormalities

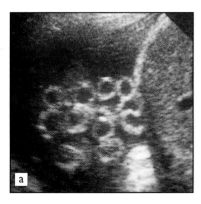

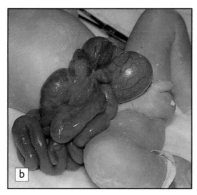

Fig. 7.5 Gastroschisis on antenatal ultrasound showing free loops of small bowel in the amniotic fluid (a) and following delivery (b). Antenatal diagnosis allowed the baby to be delivered at a paediatric surgical unit and the parents forewarned about the need for surgery. Satisfactory surgical repair was achieved. (Courtesy of Mr Karl Murphy.)

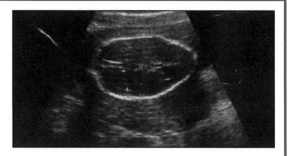
There are a few conditions where therapy can be given to the fetus directly:

- **rhesus isoimmunisation**. The incidence of rhesus incompatibility has fallen markedly since anti-D immunisation of mothers was introduced. Severely affected fetuses become anaemic and may develop hydrops fetalis, with oedema and ascites. Infants at risk are identified by maternal antibody screening. Regular ultrasound of the fetus is performed to detect oedema. Mild or moderate disease is monitored by assessing the bilirubin, measured by spectrophotometer, in the amniotic fluid obtained by amniocentesis. Severe disease is best assessed by serially measuring fetal blood haematocrit to detect anaemia. Fetal blood transfusion via the umbilical vein may be required regularly from about 20 weeks' gestation

- **perinatal isoimmune thrombocytopenia**. This condition is analogous to rhesus isoimmunisation, but involves maternal anti-platelet antibodies crossing the placenta. It is rare, affecting about 1 in 5000 births. Intracranial haemmorhage secondary to fetal thrombocytopenia occurs in up to 25%, occasionally antenatally. When the problem has been identified because of a previously affected infant, repeated intrauterine platelet transfusions can be performed.

 Maternal glucocorticoid therapy before preterm delivery markedly reduces morbidity and mortality from respiratory distress syndrome in the neonate.

FETAL SURGERY

Fetal surgery is being attempted at a number of centres in the world but the results have generally been disappointing. Procedures which have been performed include:

- **surgical correction at hysterotomy**, when the uterus is opened at 22–24 weeks' gestation to allow surgery on the fetus – has been performed for diaphragmatic hernia but may precipitate preterm delivery, and its efficacy in

preventing pulmonary hypoplasia remains uncertain

- **catheter shunts** inserted under ultrasound guidance – have been performed successfully for fetal pleural effusions, usually from a chylothorax (lymphatic fluid). One end of a looped catheter lies in the chest, the other end in the amniotic cavity

- **intrauterine shunting for obstruction to urinary outflow** – has yielded disappointing results to date

- **intrauterine shunting for hydrocephalus** – has largely been abandoned on finding an increased survival rate of severely disabled children

- **dilatation of stenotic heart valves** via a catheter inserted under ultrasound guidance into the fetal heart has been performed successfully in a few fetuses.

Careful case selection is mandatory to ensure that these novel forms of treatment are of long-term benefit.

Obstetric conditions affecting the fetus

PRETERM DELIVERY

When delivery is elective, determining its optimal time requires an evaluation of the risks to the mother and fetus of allowing the pregnancy to continue compared with the neonatal complications associated with preterm birth. Mothers with pre-eclampsia may require delivery because of the risks of eclampsia and of cerebrovascular accident. The fetus with severe growth retardation may require early delivery to prevent hypoxic damage to the gut and brain and intrauterine death.

MULTIPLE BIRTHS

Twins occur naturally in the UK in 1 in 105 deliveries, triplets 1 in 10 000 and quadruplets approximately 1 in every 500 000 deliveries. Over the last decade the number of triplets and higher multiple deliveries has more than doubled, mainly from ovarian stimulation and in-vitro fertilisation programmes.

The main problems associated with multiple births are:
- pre-eclampsia
- preterm labour. The median gestation for twins is 36 weeks, for triplets 34 weeks and for quads 32 weeks. Preterm delivery is the most important cause of the greater perinatal mortality of multiple births, especially for triplets and higher order pregnancies
- complicated deliveries, e.g. due to malpresentation of the second twin at vaginal delivery
- intrauterine growth retardation. Fetal growth, particularly of the 'second twin', may deteriorate and needs to be monitored regularly
- twin–twin blood transfusions – may cause discrepancy in growth or intrauterine death, usually of monochorionic (identical) twins
- congenital abnormalities – occur twice as frequently as in a singleton.

Finding sufficient intensive care cots for preterm multiple births can be problematic.

Maternal conditions affecting the fetus

DIABETES

Women with insulin-dependent diabetes find it difficult to maintain good diabetic control during pregnancy and have an increased insulin requirement. Poorly controlled maternal diabetes is associated with polyhydramnios and pre-eclampsia, increased rate of early fetal loss, congenital malformations and late unexplained intrauterine death. Ketoacidosis carries a high fetal mortality. With meticulous attention to diabetic control the perinatal mortality rate is now only slightly greater than in non-diabetics.

Fetal problems associated with maternal diabetes are:
- **congenital malformations**–overall, a 6% risk of congenital malformations, a threefold increase. The range of anomalies is similar to the general population, apart from an increased incidence of cardiac malformations, sacral agenesis (caudal regression syndrome) and hypoplastic left colon, although the latter two conditions are rare. Studies show that good diabetic control periconceptually reduces the risk of congenital malformations.
- **intrauterine growth retardation (IUGR)**–there is a threefold increase in growth retardation, probably because of small vessel disease in the mother.
- **macrosomia** (Fig. 7.7)–maternal hyperglycaemia causes fetal hyperglycaemia as glucose crosses the placenta. As insulin does not cross the placenta, the fetus responds

with increased secretion of insulin, which promotes growth by increasing both cell number and size. About 25% of such infants have a birthweight greater than 4 kg compared with 8% of non-diabetics. The macrosomia predisposes to cephalopelvic disproportion, shoulder dystocia and birth asphyxia and trauma.

Neonatal problems include:
- **hypoglycaemia** – transient hypoglycaemia is common during the first day of life from fetal hyperinsulinism, but can usually be prevented by early feeding. The infant's blood glucose should be closely monitored during the first 24 hours and hypoglycaemia treated
- **respiratory distress syndrome (RDS)** – is more common as lung maturation is delayed
- **hypertrophic cardiomyopathy** – hypertrophy of the cardiac septum occurs in some infants. It regresses over several weeks but may cause heart failure from reduced left ventricular function
- **polycythemia (venous haematocrit >0.65)** – makes the infant look plethoric. Treatment with partial exchange transfusion to remove blood may be required.

Gestational diabetes is when carbohydrate intolerance occurs only during pregnancy. Its definition and method of identification remain controversial. It is more common in women who are obese and in those of Afro-Caribbean and Asian ethnicity. The incidence of macrosomia and its complications is similar to that of the insulin-dependent diabetic mother, but the incidence of congenital malformations is not increased.

 Meticulous diabetic control during pregnancy markedly reduces fetal and neonatal morbidity and mortality.

HYPERTHYROIDISM

One to two per cent of newborn babies whose mothers have had Graves disease are hyperthyroid, due to circulating

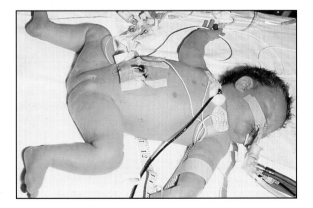

Fig. 7.7 Infant of a diabetic mother showing macrosomia and plethora. Although born at 37 weeks' gestation, she required artificial ventilation for respiratory distress syndrome.

thyroid-stimulating antibody which crosses the placenta and stimulates the fetal thyroid. Hyperthyroidism in the fetus is suggested by fetal tachycardia on a CTG trace. In the neonate it may cause irritability, weight loss, diarrhoea and exophthalmos lasting several months.

SYSTEMIC LUPUS ERYTHEMATOSUS

There is an increased rate of fetal loss in systemic lupus erythematosus (SLE), mostly during the second trimester, in mothers with high titres of antiphospholipid antibodies. Some of the infants born to mothers with antibodies to the Rho (SS-A) or La (SS-B) antigens develop neonatal lupus syndrome, in which there is a self-limiting rash and, rarely, heart block.

AUTOIMMUNE THROMBOCYTOPENIC PURPURA

In maternal autoimmune thrombocytopenia purpura (AITP) the fetus may become thrombocytopenic because maternal IgG antibodies cross the placenta and damage fetal platelets.

Severe fetal thrombocytopenia, which occurs in less than 10% of mothers with proven AITP, places the fetus at risk of intracranial haemorrhage from birth trauma. Infants with severe thrombocytopenia or petechiae at birth should be given intravenous immunoglobulin. Platelet transfusions may be required if there is acute bleeding, but the response to therapy in the neonate is poor. The platelet count continues to fall over the first few days.

MYASTHENIA GRAVIS

Transient neonatal myasthenia is seen in about 10% of infants born to mothers with myasthenia gravis and is due to anti-acetylcholine antibodies crossing the placenta. Presentation is with difficulty in feeding, muscle weakness and respiratory insufficiency for 2–3 weeks.

Maternal drugs affecting the fetus

Relatively few drugs are known definitely to damage the fetus (Fig. 7.8), but it is clearly advisable for pregnant women to avoid taking medicines unless it is essential. Whilst the teratogenicity of a drug may be recognised if it causes malformations which are severe and distinctive, as with limb shortening following thalidomide ingestion, milder and less distinctive abnormalities may go unrecognised.

The problem of establishing a link may be compounded by delay of months or years before any problems present. An example of this is diethylstilboestrol (DES), given in the past for threatened abortion, and its subsquent association with vaginal adenosis and clear-cell carcinoma of the vagina and cervix in female offspring only during adolescence or early adult life.

ALCOHOL AND SMOKING

Excessive alcohol ingestion during pregnancy is sometimes associated with the 'fetal alcohol syndrome'. Its clinical features are growth retardation, characteristic facies (Fig. 7.9), cardiac defects (up to 70%) and developmental delay. The adverse effects of less severe ingestion and binge drinking remain uncertain. The effects of smoking during pregnancy are described on page 68.

DRUG ABUSE

Drug abuse with narcotics is associated with an increased risk of prematurity and growth retardation. Many narcotic abusers take multiple drugs. During the first two weeks of life infants of mothers abusing heroin, methadone and other narcotics during pregnancy often show evidence of drug withdrawal with jitteriness, sneezing, yawning, poor feeding, vomiting, diarrhoea, weight loss and seizures. Cocaine abuse rarely causes severe withdrawal in the infant

Fig. 7.8 Maternal medication which may adversely affect the fetus	
Cytotoxic agents	Congenital malformations
Diethylstilboestrol (DES)	Clear-cell adenocarcinoma of vagina and cervix
Iodides/propythiouracil	Goitre, hypothyroidism
Lithium	Congenital heart disease
Phenytoin	Fetal hydantoin syndrome – hypoplastic nails and cranio-facial abnormalities
Progestogens (androgenic)	Masculinisation of the female fetus
Tetracycline	Enamel hypoplasia of the teeth
Thalidomide	Limb shortening (phocomelia)
Valproate/carbamazepine	Increased neural tube defects
Vitamin A	Increased spontaneous abortions, abnormal facies
Warfarin	Interferes with cartilage formation (nasal hypoplasia and epiphyseal stippling); cerebral haemorrhages and microcephaly

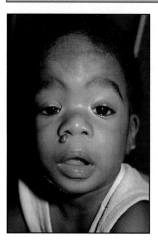

Fig. 7.9 Characteristic facies of fetal alcohol syndrome with a saddle-shaped nose, maxillary hypoplasia, absent philtrum between the nose and upper lip and a short, thin upper lip. This child also has a strawberry naevus below the right nostril.

but may result in cerebral infarction. Amphetamine abuse is also associated with gastrointestinal and cerebral infarction. The mothers and their infants are also at increased risk of hepatitis B and C and HIV infection.

Infants who develop marked features of drug withdrawal will need treatment. Morphine, methadone, phenobarbitone, diazepam and chlorpromazine are used at different centres. One of the major problems in managing these infants is that the parents' lifestyle and temperament is often not conducive to the needs of babies and young children. Close supervision or alternative care givers are often required.

 Unexplained signs in an infant – consider drug withdrawal.

DRUGS GIVEN DURING LABOUR
Potential adverse effects to the fetus of drugs given during labour are:
- opioid analgesics/anaesthetic agents – may suppress respiration at birth and result in delay in establishing normal breathing
- epidural anaesthesia – may cause maternal pyrexia during labour. It is often difficult to differentiate this from fever caused by an infection. Establishing normal feeding and behaviour during the first few days may also be delayed
- sedatives, e.g. diazepam – may cause sedation and hypotension in the newborn
- oxytocin – may cause hyperstimulation of the uterus leading to fetal hypoxia. It is also associated with a small increase in bilirubin levels in the neonate
- intravenous fluids – may cause neonatal hyponatraemia unless they contain an adequate concentration of sodium.

Congenital infections

Mothers may contract an infection during pregnancy if they do not have protective antibodies. Fortunately, few infections are known to damage the fetus. They include:
- rubella
- cytomegalovirus (CMV)
- *Toxoplasma gondii*
- varicella zoster
- parvovirus B19 (see Chapter 12)
- *Listeria monocytogenes* (see Chapter 8)
- *Treponema pallidum* (syphilis).

RUBELLA
The diagnosis of maternal infection must be confirmed serologically as clinical diagnosis is unreliable. The risk and extent of fetal damage is mainly determined by the gestational age at the onset of maternal infection. Infection before 8 weeks' gestation may cause deafness, congenital heart disease, cataracts (Fig. 7.10) and a wide range of defects (Fig. 7.11). About 30% of fetusus of mothers infected at 13–16

weeks' gestation have impaired hearing; beyond 18 weeks' gestation the risk to the fetus is minimal. Viraemia after birth continues to damage the infant. Tests used to confirm the diagnosis are shown in Figure 7.12.

Congenital rubella is preventable. In the UK, when immunisation was introduced in 1970, it was given only

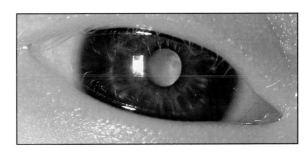

Fig. 7.10 Cataract from congenital rubella. Congenital heart disease and deafness are the other common defects.

Fig. 7.11 Clinical features of congenital rubella, CMV and toxoplasma infection

Clinical features	Rubella	CMV	Toxoplasma
Growth retardation	+++	+++	+
Anaemia	+	++	++
Petechiae, purpura	++	+++	+
Jaundice	+	+++	++
Hepatosplenomegaly	+++	+++	++
Congenital heart disease	+++	—	—
Pneumonitis	+	++	+
Eye			
Glaucoma	++	—	—
Retinopathy	+	+	+++
Cataract	++	—	+
CNS			
Encephalitis	+	++	+
Microcephaly	—	++	+
Intracranial calcification	—	+	++
Hydrocephalus	—	—	++
Bone lesions	++	—	—
Sensorineural deafness	+++	++	—

Fig. 7.12 Diagnosis of congenital rubella, CMV and toxoplasma infection

Urine	Rubella, CMV culture
Blood	Rubella-specific IgM
	CMV-specific IgM
	Toxoplasma-specific IgM and persistently raised toxoplasma IgG

to schoolgirls and susceptible adult women. However, children continued to be infected and pregnant women continued to be exposed to the virus. About 12 infants a year were born with congenital rubella syndrome. In 1988, measles/mumps/rubella (MMR) vaccine was introduced for all children. This has markedly reduced the prevalence of rubella in the community and the number of infants with congenital rubella has declined.

CYTOMEGALOVIRUS

CMV is the most common congenital infection, affecting 3–4/1000 livebirths in the UK, with higher rates reported in parts of the US. In Europe, 50% of pregnant women are susceptible to CMV. About 1% of susceptible women will have a primary infection during pregnancy and in about 40% of them the infant becomes infected. The infant may also become infected following recurrent infection in a pregnant woman who is immune, but this is much less likely to damage the fetus.

When an infant is infected:

- 90% are normal at birth and develop normally
- 5% have clinical features of infection at birth (see Fig. 7.11), most of whom will have neurodevelopmental disabilities such as sensorineural hearing loss, cerebral palsy, epilepsy and learning difficulties
- 5% develop problems later in life, mainly sensorineural hearing loss.

Infection in the pregnant woman is usually asymptomatic or causes a mild non-specific illness. Identification of infection in all pregnant women would require regular serological testing during pregnancy and might miss fetal infection following recurrence of CMV. As most infected infants develop normally, screening in pregnancy is not considered justified at present in the UK.

TOXOPLASMOSIS

Acute infection with *Toxoplasma gondii*, a protozoon parasite, may result from the consumption of raw or undercooked meat or from contact with the faeces of recently infected cats. In the UK, fewer than 20% of pregnant women have had past infection, in contrast to 80% in France and Austria.

Transplacental carriage may occur during the parasitaemia of a primary infection, and about 40% of fetuses become infected. In the UK the incidence of congenital infection is only about 0.1 per 1000 livebirths. Most infected infants are asymptomatic. About 10% have clinical manifestations, of which the most common are:

- hydrocephalus
- cerebral calcification
- retinopathy, an acute fundal chorioretinitis which sometimes interferes with vision
- other features as shown in Figure 7.11. These infants usually have long-term neurological disabilities.

Asymptomatic infants remain at risk of developing chorioretinitis into adulthood.

As the specific IgM antibody test has a low sensitivity, serial IgG antibody tests are needed to differentiate passively acquired maternal antibody from fetal infection. In some countries, e.g. France and Austria, pregnant women are screened serologically for toxoplasma infection during pregnancy. During early pregnancy, confirmation of fetal infection is obtained from cordocentesis and, if positive, termination of pregnancy or treatment with the antibiotic spiramycin can be offered. The severely affected infant may also have evidence on ultrasound of a fetal anomaly, e.g. hydrocephalus. Treatment is given to infected newborn infants (using a combination of pyrimethamine and sulphadiazine, with folinic acid, alternating with spiramycin for the first year of life). In the UK, in view of the low incidence and the lack of data on the efficacy of treatment, pregnant women are not screened.

VARICELLA ZOSTER

Fifteen per cent of pregnant women are susceptible to varicella (chickenpox). Usually, the fetus is unaffected, but is at risk if the mother develops chickenpox:

- in the first trimester, when up to 5% develop varicella embryopathy with severe scarring of the skin and possibly ocular and neurological damage
- within five days before or two days after delivery, when the fetus is unprotected by maternal antibodies and the viral load is high. About 25% develop a vesicular rash. The illness has a mortality as high as 5%. Exposed susceptible women can be protected with zoster immune globulin and treated with acyclovir. Infants born in the high-risk period should also receive zoster immune globulin. Acyclovir is often given but its efficacy when used prophylactically is unproven.

 If there is maternal chickenpox shortly before or after delivery – the infant needs protection from infection.

SYPHILIS

Congenital syphilis is now rare in the UK, though recently there has been an increase in the number of cases reported in the US, mainly among HIV-infected mothers. If mothers with syphilis identified on antenatal screening are fully treated a month or more before delivery, the infant does not require treatment and has an excellent prognosis. If there is any doubt about the adequacy of maternal treatment, the infant should be treated with penicillin.

Adaptation to extrauterine life

Fetal lungs are filled with fluid. Fetal catecholamines released during labour reduce the secretion of this lung fluid. During delivery, the thorax is squeezed and lung fluid drained. Once the infant gasps, the remaining lung fluid is absorbed via the lymphatic and pulmonary circulation.

The combination of delivery and umbilical cord occlusion results in a gasp, on average, six seconds after delivery. Lung expansion is generated by marked intrathoracic negative pressure and a functional residual capacity is established. The mean time to establishing regular breathing is 30 seconds. After an elective Caesarean section, when the mother has not been in labour and the infant's chest has not been squeezed through the birth canal, it may take up to several hours for the lung fluid to be completely absorbed.

In the fetus, oxygenated blood bypasses the lungs (Fig. 7.13). Pulmonary expansion is associated with a falling pulmonary vascular resistance and subsequent increase in pulmonary blood flow. Increased left atrial filling increases the left atrial pressure which further contributes to the closure of the foramen ovale. The flow of oxygenated blood through the ductus arteriosus causes physiological, and eventual anatomical, ductal closure.

Under experimental conditions, it is known that if a newborn animal is continuously asphyxiated by being deprived of oxygen at birth, he will initially gasp before becoming apnoeic (primary apnoea), during which time the heart rate is maintained. This is followed by irregular gasping and then a second period of apnoea (secondary apnoea), when the heart rate and blood pressure fall. At this stage, the infant will only recover if help with lung expansion is provided, for example by tracheal intubation and positive pressure ventilation (Fig. 7.14).

The human fetus rarely experiences a continuous asphyxial insult, except after severe antepartum haemorrhage or complete occlusion of umbilical blood flow in a cord prolapse. More commonly, asphyxia which occurs during labour and delivery is intermittent; only when it is severe and prolonged is an infant born whose clinical condition resembles 'secondary apnoea'. Although birth asphyxia is an important cause of failure to establish

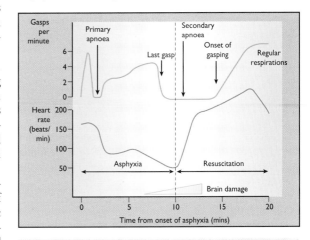

Fig. 7.14 *The changes in respiration and heart rate following continuous total asphyxia in a newborn animal. Once the infant has stopped gasping and has a marked bradycardia, resuscitation with lung expansion is required to establish regular respirations and restore the circulation. (Adapted from Dawes GS. Foetal and Neonatal Physiology. Year-Book Publishers, Chicago, 1968.)*

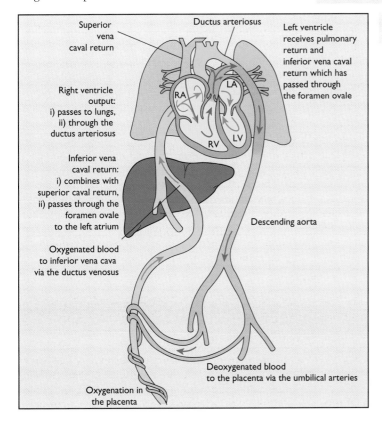

Fig. 7.13 *The fetal circulation.*

breathing at birth, there other causes, including birth trauma, maternal analgesic or anaesthetic agents, retained lung fluid, or the infant is preterm or has a congenital malformation which interferes with breathing.

The Apgar score is used to describe the neonates condition at one and five minutes after delivery (Fig. 7.15). It is also measured at five-minute intervals thereafter if the infant's condition remains poor. The most important components are the respiration and heart rate.

Neonatal resuscitation

Most infants do not require any resuscitation. Shortly after birth, the baby will gasp or cry, establish normal breathing and become pink. The baby can be handed directly to his mother, covering him with a warm towel to ensure he does not become cold.

Neonates who do not establish normal respiration quickly will need to be transferred to a resuscitation table for further assessment (Fig. 7.16). There should be an overhead radiant heater and the infant should be dried and partially covered and kept warm. The mouth and nose are gently suctioned to remove any fluid or blood. Vigorous suction of the back of the throat may provoke bradycardia from vagal stimulation and should be avoided. If the infant's breathing in the first minute of life is irregular or shallow, but the heart rate satisfactory (> 100 beats/min) additional oxygen is blown over the face and breathing encouraged with gentle tactile stimulation.

If the infant does not start to breathe, or if the heart rate drops below 100 beats per minute, basic resuscitation is initiated (Figs 7.17 and 7.18). If the baby's condition does not

Fig. 7.15 The Apgar score

	Score		
	0	**1**	**2**
Heart rate	Absent	<100 beats/min	>100 beats/min
Respiratory effort	Absent	Gasping or irregular	Regular, strong cry
Muscle tone	Flaccid	Some flexion of limbs	Well flexed, active
Reflex irritability	None	Grimace	Cry, cough
Colour	Pale/blue	Body pink, extremities blue	Pink

Fig. 7.16 Resuscitation of the newborn

All health professionals dealing with newborn infants should be proficient in basic resuscitation

Additional skilled assistance is needed if the baby does not respond rapidly and should be called without delay

A person proficient in advanced resuscitation should be available at short notice in a maternity unit at all times

The need for resuscitation can usually be anticipated and a person proficient in advanced resuscitation should be in attendance

A clock should be started at birth for accurate timing of changes in the infant's condition and Apgar scores

Babies should be prevented from becoming cold

Basic resuscitation	Mask ventilation	**Advanced resuscitation**	Tracheal intubation and ventilation
	External cardiac compression		Drug therapy (other than naloxone)
	Naloxone		VLBW infant
			Meconium aspiration

Fig. 7.17 Basic resuscitation

Mask ventilation	Mask over mouth and nose
	Neck slightly extended
	Ventilator circuit or rebreathing bag
	Rate–30–40 breaths/min
	Pressure–to match chest wall movement (in term infants 30 cm H_2O for first few breaths, up to 2 seconds inflation time, then 15–25 cm H_2O, 0.5 second inflation time)
External cardiac compression	Start if heart rate < 60 beats/min or pulse absent or poor
Naloxone	Give if mother has received narcotic analgesia within 4 h of delivery and respiration continues to be depressed after initial resuscitation
	(Naloxone 60 microg/kg im or 10 microg/kg iv, when further doses may be needed as its effect is short-lived)

improve promptly with basic resuscitation, or if the infant is clearly in very poor condition at birth, advanced resuscitation with tracheal intubation should be performed immediately (Figs 7.19 and 7.20).

MECONIUM ASPIRATION

The passage of meconium becomes increasingly common the greater the infant's gestational age. Infants who inhale thick meconium may develop meconium aspiration syndrome. Gasping may start shortly before birth. Thick meconium present at delivery should be removed from the upper airway by suction immediately after the head is delivered to try and prevent aspiration. After delivery, the cords are inspected under direct vision. If meconium is present in the trachea, a tracheal tube or large-bore suction catheter is passed below the cords and aspirated to remove as much meconium as possible. If the tube becomes blocked the procedure will need to be repeated. As much meconium as possible is removed unless the infant develops a prolonged bradycardia, when positive pressure ventilation will need to be initiated.

FAILURE TO RESPOND TO RESUSCITATION

The main reasons why infants fail to respond to resuscitation are listed in Figure 7.21. Poor response to tracheal intubation is usually because the tracheal tube is misplaced

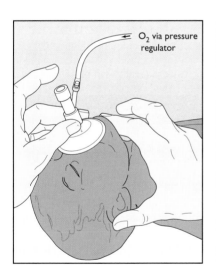

Fig. 7.18a Mask ventilation. The oxygen is given via a pressure regulator. Pressure is delivered when the T-piece is occluded. Alternatively, the mask may be attached to a rebreathing bag.

O₂ via pressure regulator

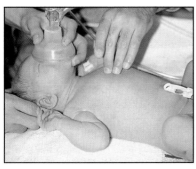

Fig. 7.18b External cardiac massage in a newborn infant.

Fig. 7.19 Advanced resuscitation

Tracheal intubation and ventilation (see Fig. 7.20)
Drug therapy – given via an umbilical venous catheter for persistent bradycardia in spite of adequate ventilation. The use of sodium bicarbonate is controversial, as it may cause further lowering of intracellular pH. Adrenaline can be delivered via the endotracheal tube and repeated as required. If the infant is shocked, colloid (20 mg/kg) should be given.

Drug	Dose
Adrenaline iv	10 microg/kg (0.1 ml/kg of 1:10 000) iv or
Adrenaline down tracheal tube	100 microg/kg (0.1 ml/kg of 1:1000)
Dextrose 10%	2ml/kg
Sodium bicarbonate (8.4% solution diluted to 4.2%)	1 mmol/kg

Flush catheter with saline after each drug

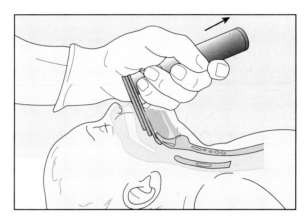

Fig. 7.20 Tracheal intubation of a newborn infant. The laryngoscope blade is advanced to lift the epiglottis, as shown, and the laryngoscope is then lifted upwards. Gentle pressure on the trachea with the fifth finger or by an assistant helps bring the vocal cords into view.

Fig. 7.21 Failure of resuscitation

Inadequate mask ventilation due to poor technique
Tracheal tube in oesophagus or down a bronchus or blocked
    with secretions or meconium
Birth asphyxia/trauma
Lung disorders
    lung immaturity/respiratory distress syndrome
    pneumothorax
    diaphragmatic hernia
    lung hypoplasia
    pleural effusion
Shock from blood loss
Upper airways obstruction
    choanal atresia

or has become blocked with secretions or meconium. Chest wall movement is a useful guide to air entry to the lungs. If there is any uncertainty about the adequacy of ventilation and resuscitation continues to be unsuccessful, it is best to replace the tracheal tube. The decision to stop resuscitation is always difficult and should be made by a senior paediatrician. Following severe birth asphyxia identified during labour, if there is no respiratory effort or cardiac output after 20 minutes of effective resuscitation, continuing is unlikely to be productive.

Size at birth

An infant's gestation and birth weight influence the nature of the medical problems likely to be encountered in the neonatal period. In the UK, 7% of babies are of low birthweight. However, they account for about 70% of neonatal deaths.

Babies with a birthweight below the tenth centile for their gestational age are called small for gestational age or small for dates (Fig. 7.22). The majority of these infants are normal but small. The incidence of neonatal problems is higher in those whose birthweight falls below the third centile (approximately two standard deviations below the mean), and some authorities restrict the term to this group of babies. An infant's birthweight may also be low because of preterm birth, or because the infant is both preterm and small for gestational age.

Small for gestational age infants may have grown normally but are small or they may be growth-retarded, when they appear thin and malnourished. Babies with a birthweight above the tenth centile may also be malnourished, e.g. a fetus

growing along the 80th centile who develops growth retardation who is born on the 20th centile for weight.

Growth retardation in both the fetus and infant has traditionally been classified as symmetrical or asymmetrical. In the more common asymmetrical growth retardation, the weight or abdominal circumference lies on a lower centile than that of the head. This occurs when the placenta fails to provide adequate nutrition late in pregnancy, but brain growth is relatively spared at the expense of liver glycogen and skin fat (Fig. 7.23). This form of growth retardation is associated with maternal pre-eclampsia, cardiac or renal disease or multiple gestation, or it may be idiopathic. These infants rapidly put on weight after birth.

In symmetrical growth retardation the head circumference is equally reduced. It suggests a prolonged period of poor intrauterine growth. This is usually due to a small but normal fetus, but may be due to a fetal chromosomal disorder or syndrome, a congenital infection or maternal smoking, drug and alcohol abuse, a chronic medical condition or malnutrition. These infants are more likely to remain small permanently.

The fetus with intrauterine growth retardation is at risk from:
• intrauterine hypoxia and death
• birth asphyxia.

After birth, these infants are liable to:
• hypothermia because of their relatively large surface area
• hypoglycaemia from poor fat and glycogen stores
• hypocalcaemia
• polycythaemia (venous haematocrit > 0.65).

The growth-retarded fetus will need to be monitored closely to determine the optimal time for delivery. This will include assessing fetal size clinically (symphysis to fundal

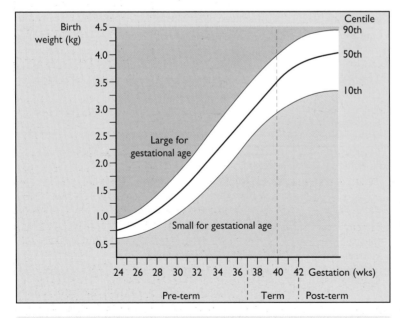

Fig. 7.22 Birthweight of small for gestational age infants is below the tenth centile for their gestation. Small for gestational age infants may be preterm, term or post-term.

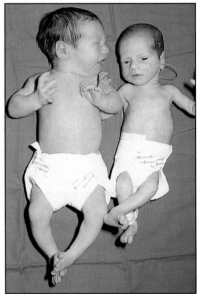

Fig. 7.23 Twins, one of whom had severe intrauterine growth retardation.

height measurement) and serial ultrasound measurements of fetal growth. Antenatal cardiotocography (CTG) to detect evidence of fetal hypoxia may be combined with an ultrasound assessment of fetal activity, breathing and amniotic fluid volume to form a biophysical profile to identify high-risk pregnancies. Doppler ultrasound is now widely used to obtain a blood flow velocity profile of the uterine artery (maternal circulation to the placental bed) and the umbilical artery (fetal circulation). Absence or reversal of blood flow velocity in diastole carries an increased risk of morbidity from hypoxic damage to the gut or brain, or of intrauterine death. The blood flow velocity in the fetal descending aorta, cerebral and other arteries may give an indication of fetal circulatory redistribution in response to hypoxia.

LARGE FOR GESTATIONAL AGE INFANTS

Large for gestational age infants are those above the 90th weight centile for their gestation. Macrosomia is a feature of infants of mothers with diabetes, either permanent or gestational. The problems associated with being large for gestational age are:

- birth asphyxia from a difficult delivery
- birth trauma, especially from shoulder dystocia at delivery
- hypoglycaemia due to hyperinsulinism
- polycythaemia.

Some definitions:
Neonate – infant ≤ 28 days old
Preterm – gestation < 37 completed weeks
Post-term – gestation ≥ 42 completed weeks
Low birthweight – < 2500 g
Very low birthweight – < 1500 g
Extremely low birthweight – < 1000 g
Small for gestational age – birthweight <10th centile for gestational age
Large for gestational age – birthweight >90th centile for gestational age

---

Fig 7.24 The routine examination of the newborn infant

Birthweight, gestational age and birthweight centile are noted
General observation of the baby's appearance, posture and movements provides valuable information about any abnormalities. The baby must be fully undressed during the examination.

The head circumference is measured with a paper tape measure and its centile noted.

The fontanelle and sutures are palpated. The fontanelle size is very variable. The sagittal suture is often separated and the coronal sutures may be overriding. A tense fontanelle, when the baby is not crying, may be due to raised intracranial pressure and cranial ultrasound should be performed to check for hydrocephalus. A tense fontanelle is also a late sign of meningitis.

The facies is observed. If abnormal, this may represent a syndrome, particularly if other anomalies are present. Down syndrome is the most common, but there are hundreds of syndromes. When the diagnosis is uncertain, a book or a computer database may be consulted and advice should be sought from a senior paediatrician or clinical geneticist.

If plethoric or pale, the haematocrit should be checked to identify polycythaemia or anaemia. Central cyanosis, which always needs urgent assessment, is best seen on the tongue.

Jaundice within 24 hours of birth requires further evaluation.

The eyes are checked for cataracts (red reflex checked with an ophthalmoscope) and other abnormalities.

The palate needs to be inspected, including posteriorly to exclude a posterior cleft palate, and palpated to detect an indentation of the posterior palate from a submucous cleft.

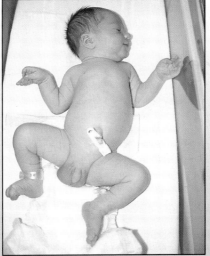

Breathing and chest wall movement are observed
On auscultating the heart, the normal rate is 110–150 beats per minute in term babies, but may drop to 85 beats per minute during sleep.

On palpating the abdomen the liver normally extends 1–2 cm below the costal margin, the spleen tip may be palpable as may the kidney on the left side. Any intra-abdominal masses, which are usually renal in origin, need further investigation.

The genitalia and anus are inspected on removing the nappy. In boys the presence of testes in the scrotum is confirmed.

The femoral pulses are palpated. Their pulse pressure is:
- reduced in coarctation of the aorta. This can be confirmed by measuring the blood pressure in the arms and legs
- increased if there is a patent ductus arteriosus.

Muscle tone is assessed by observing limb movements and on picking up the baby while supporting the head. Most babies will support their weight with their feet. On turning the baby prone, the head is lifted to the horizontal and the back straightened.

The whole of the back and spine is observed, looking for any midline defects of the skin.

The hips are checked for congenital dislocation of the hips (CDH). This is left until last as the procedure is uncomfortable.

Details of the examination, including confirmation of a normal hip examination and that the testes are palpable in the scrotum in boys, should be entered in the infant's personal child health record carried by the mother.

Examination of the newborn infant

Immediately after a baby is born, parents are naturally anxious to know if their baby is all right. To answer this the midwife, or the paediatrician or obstetrician if present, will briefly but carefully check that the baby is pink, breathing normally and has no major abnormalities. If the mother has had hydramnios, a feeding tube needs to be passed into the stomach to exclude oesophageal atresia. If a significant problem is identified, an experienced paediatrician needs to explain the situation to the parents. If the baby is markedly preterm, small for gestational age or ill, admission to a neonatal unit will be required. Should there be any uncertainty about the child's sex, it is best not to guess but to explain to the parents that further tests are necessary. In most hospitals babies are given vitamin K at birth to prevent haemorrhagic disease of the newborn.

Within 24 hours of birth every baby should have a full and thorough medical examination, the 'routine examination of the newborn infant'. Its purpose is to:
- detect congenital abnormalities not already identified at birth, e.g. congenital heart disease, congenital dislocation of the hip
- check for potential problems arising from maternal disease or familial disorders
- provide an opportunity for the parents to discuss any questions about their baby.

Before approaching the mother and baby, the obstetric and neonatal notes must be checked to identify relevant information. The examination (Fig. 7.24) should be performed with the mother or ideally both parents present. Many lesions in the newborn resolve spontaneously (Fig. 7.25). Some of the abnormalities detected at birth are shown in Figure 7.26. A serious congenital anomaly is present at birth in about 10–15/1000 live

---

Fig. 7.25a Lesions in newborn infants which resolve spontaneously

Peripheral cyanosis of the hands and feet – common in the first day
Traumatic cyanosis from a cord round the baby's neck or from a face or brow presentation – causes blue discoloration of the skin, petechiae over the head and neck or affected part but not the tongue
Swollen eyelids and distortion of shape of the head from the delivery
Subconjunctival haemorrhages – occur during delivery
Small white pearls along the midline of the palate (Epstein's pearls)
Cysts of the gums (epulis) or floor of the mouth (ranula)
Breast enlargement – may occur in newborn babies of either sex (Fig. 7.25b). A small amount of milk may be discharged.
White vaginal discharge or small withdrawal bleed in girls. There may be a

prolapse of a ring of vaginal mucosa.
Capillary haemangioma or 'stork bites' – pink macules on the upper eyelids, mid-forehead and nape of the neck are common and arise from distension of the dermal capillaries. Those on the eyelids gradually fade over the first year; those on the neck become covered with hair.
Neonatal urticaria (erythema toxicum) – a common rash appearing at 2–3 days of age, consisting of white pinpoint papules at the centre of an erythematous base. Microscopy reveals eosinophils. The lesions are concentrated on the trunk; they come and go at different sites.
Milia – white pimples on the nose and cheeks, from retention of keratin and sebaceous material in the pilaceous follicles
Mongolian blue spots – blue/black macular discoloration at the base of the spine

and on the buttocks (Fig. 7.25c) occasionally occur on the legs and other parts of the body, usually but not invariably, in Afro-Caribbean or Asian infants. They fade slowly over the first few years, and are of no significance unless misdiagnosed as bruises.
Umbilical hernia – common, particularly in Afro-Caribbean infants. No treatment is indicated, as it usually resolves within the first 2–3 years.
Positional talipes – the feet often remain in their *in-utero* position. Unlike true talipes equinovarus, the foot can be fully dorsiflexed to touch the front of the lower leg.
Harlequin colour change – when lying sideways, there is reddening down one half of the body with sharply demarcated blanching down the other side, lasting for a few minutes (Fig. 7.25d). It is thought to be due to vasomotor instability.

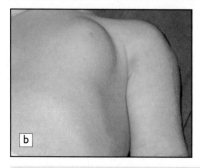
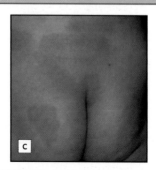
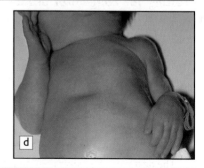

Fig. 7.25 (b) Breast enlargement in a newborn infant. (c) A Mongolian blue spot. (d) Harlequin colour change.

Fig. 7.26 Some abnormalities detected on routine examination

Port wine stain (naevus flammeus) – present from birth and usually grows with the infant (Fig. 7.26a). It is due to a vascular malformation of the capillaries in the dermis. Rarely, if along the distribution of the trigeminal nerve, it may be associated with intracranial vascular anomalies (Sturge-Weber syndrome), or severe lesions on the limbs with bone hypertrophy (Klippel-Trenaunay syndrome). Disfiguring lesions can now be improved with laser therapy.

Strawberry naevus (cavernous haemangioma) – not usually present at birth, but appears in the first month of life (Fig. 7.26b). It is more common in preterm infants. It increases in size until 3–9 months old, then gradually regresses. No treatment is indicated unless the lesion interferes with vision or the airway. Ulceration or haemorrhage may occur. Thrombocytopenia may occur with large lesions, when therapy with systemic steroids or interferon–alpha may be required.

Natal teeth consisting of the front lower incisors – may be present at birth. If loose they should be removed to avoid the risk of aspiration.

Extra digits – are usually connected by a thin skin tag and can be ligated with silk thread, but may be completely attached containing bone and should then be removed by a plastic surgeon. Skin tags anterior to the ear and accessory auricles should be removed by a plastic surgeon.

Heart murmur – poses a difficult problem, as most murmurs audible in the first few days of life resolve shortly afterwards. However, some are caused by congenital heart disease. If there are any features of a significant murmur (see Chapter 14), a chest X-ray, ECG and echocardiogram are indicated. Otherwise, a follow-up examination is arranged and the parents warned to seek medical assistance if their baby feeds poorly, develops laboured breathing or becomes cyanosed.

Midline abnormality over the spine or skull, such as a tuft of hair, swelling or naevus – requires further evaluation as it may indicate an underlying abnormality of the vertebrae, spinal cord or brain.

Palpable, large bladder – if there is urinary outflow obstruction, particularly in boys with a posterior urethral valve.

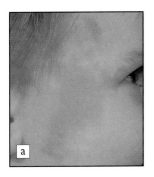
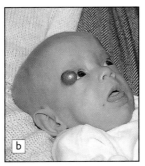

Fig. 7.26 (a) Port wine stain in an infant. (b) Strawberry naevus.

Fig. 7.27 Prevalence of serious congenital anomalies per 1000 livebirths (England & Wales 1990)

Congenital heart disease 6–8 (0.8 in the first day of life)

Congenital dislocation of the hip 1.5 (but about 6/1000 have an abnormal initial examination)

Talipes 1.5

Down syndrome 1.5

Cleft lip and palate 1.2

Urogenital (hypospadias, undescended testes) 1.2

Spina bifida/anencephaly 0.5

births (Fig. 7.27). In addition, many congenital anomalies, especially of the heart, present clinically at a later age.

PROCEDURES IN NEWBORN INFANTS
Testing for congenital dislocation of the hip (developmental dysplasia of the hip, DDH)

The infant needs to be relaxed, as kicking or crying results in tightening of the muscles around the hip and prevents satisfactory examination. The pelvis is stabilised with one hand. With the other hand, the examiner's middle finger is placed over the greater trochanter and the thumb around the distal medial femur. The hip is held flexed and adducted. The femoral head is gently pushed downwards. If the hip is dislocatable, the femoral head will be pushed posteriorly out of the acetabulum (Fig. 7.28a).

The next part of the examination is to see if the hip can be returned from its dislocated position back into the acetabulum. With the hip abducted, upward leverage is

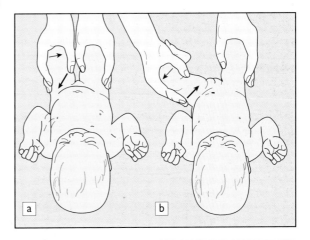

Fig. 7.28 (a) The hip is dislocated posteriorly out of the acetabulum (Barlow manoeuvre). (b) The dislocated hip is relocated back into the acetabulum (Ortolani manoeuvre).

applied (Fig. 7.28b). A dislocated hip will return with a 'clunk' into the acetabulum. Ligamentous clicks without any movement of the head of femur are of no significance. It should be possible to abduct the hips fully, but this may be restricted if the hip is dislocated. Clinical examination may not detect severe dysplasia of the hip with lack of development of the acetabular shelf.

Congenital dislocation of the hip is more common in girls (sixfold increase), if there is a positive family history (20% of affected children), if the birth is a breech presentation (30%) or if the infant has a neuromuscular disorder.

Early recognition is important as it reduces long-term morbidity. Ultrasound examination of the hip joint is performed increasingly in many hospitals, either following an abnormal examination or to screen babies at increased risk (breech presentation or positive family history). Ultrasound examination has also been performed to screen all babies, but this requires considerable resources and there are false positives. It will, however, identify some babies missed on clinical examination. Studies are in progress to ascertain the desirability of universal ultrasound screening. A specialist orthopaedic opinion should be sought in the management of this condition.

Vitamin K therapy

Vitamin K deficiency may result in haemorrhagic disease of the newborn. This can occur early, during the first week of life, or late, from one to eight weeks of age. In most affected infants the haemorrhage is mild, such as bruising, haematemesis and malaena or prolonged bleeding of the umbilical stump or after a circumcision. However, some suffer from intracranial haemorrhage, half of whom are permanently disabled or die.

Breast milk is a poor source of vitamin K, whereas infant formula milk has a much higher vitamin K content. Haemorrhagic disease of the newborn may occur in infants who are wholly breast-fed but not if fed with an infant formula. Infants of mothers taking anticonvulsants, which impair the synthesis of vitamin K-dependent clotting factors, are at increased risk of haemorrhagic disease, both during delivery and soon after birth. Infants with liver disease are also at increased risk.

The disease can be prevented by giving all newborn infants vitamin K by intramuscular injection. A recent study suggested a possible association between vitamin K given intramuscularly and the development of cancer in childhood, although this has not been confirmed in other much larger studies. The initial study has led to the recommendation that vitamin K should be given orally, but absorption via this route is variable and prophylaxis cannot be assured after a single dose. If vitamin K is given orally to breast-fed babies, several doses are needed over the first few weeks of life to achieve adequate liver storage. Mothers on anticonvulsant therapy should receive oral prophylaxis from 36 weeks' gestation and the baby be given intramuscular vitamin K.

 Vitamin K should be given to all newborn infants to prevent haemorrhagic disease of the newborn.

Biochemical screening (Guthrie Test)

Biochemical screening is performed on every baby. A blood sample, usually a heel prick, is taken when feeding has been established on day 5–9 of life. It was introduced to screen for phenylketonuria, which is rare, but is now also used to screen for hypothyroidism, which is more common. Screening for galactosaemia, maple syrup urine disease and homocystinuria is also performed. The blood spot can also be used to screen for haemoglobinopathies (mainly sickle cell and thalassaemia) and for cystic fibrosis, but this is not performed routinely throughout the UK.

 In the UK all babies are screened for congenital hypothyroidism and phenylketonuria.

FURTHER READING

James DK, Steer PJ, Weiner CP, Gonik B. *High Risk Pregnancy. Management options.* WB Saunders, London, 1994. A comprehensive textbook on perinatal medicine.

Working Party of the British Paediatric Association, College of Anaesthetists, Royal College of Midwives and Royal College of Obstetricians and Gynaecologists. *Resuscitation of the Newborn.* Royal College of Obstetricians and Gynaecologists, London, 1991. A practical manual.

CHAPTER 8

Neonatal Medicine

• *Stabilising the preterm/sick infant* • *Birth asphyxia* • *Birth injuries* • *The preterm infant* • *Jaundice* • *Respiratory distress in term infants* • *Infection* • *Neonatal seizures* • *Hypoglycaemia* • *Craniofacial disorders* • *Gastrointestinal disorders*

The dramatic reduction in neonatal mortality throughout the developed world has resulted from medical advances in the management of newborn infants together with improvements in maternal health and obstetric care. Neonatal intensive care became increasingly available in the UK from 1975, and it is since that time that the mortality of very low birthweight infants has fallen (Fig. 8.1).

About 10% of babies born in the UK require special medical and nursing care. This can be provided in special care baby units or on postnatal wards, as 'transitional care', which has the advantage that it avoids separating mothers from their babies. About 1–3% of babies require intensive care, which is undertaken in neonatal intensive care units, many of which are situated in tertiary referral centres serving a number of maternity departments. Modern technology allows even tiny preterm infants to benefit from the full range of intensive care, anaesthesia and surgery. If it is anticipated during pregnancy that the infant is likely to require long-term intensive care or surgery, it is preferable for the transfer to the tertiary centre to be made 'in-utero'. When babies need to be transferred postnatally, this transport should be done by an experienced team of doctors and nurses. Arrangements should also be made for parents to be able to be with their infant during this worrying time.

Stabilising the preterm or sick infant

Preterm infants of less than 34 weeks' gestation and newborn infants who become seriously ill require monitoring. Most of them will need respiratory and circulatory support (Fig. 8.2). If the preterm infant is allowed to develop respiratory failure, a vicious cycle of lung collapse, circulatory failure and secondary surfactant deficiency may follow. Unlike adults, the ability of preterm infants to regulate blood flow to vital organs during periods of hypo- or hypertension is impaired, and this is thought to contribute to the cerebral haemorrhages and ischaemic brain lesions to which they are susceptible during the first 72 hours of life.

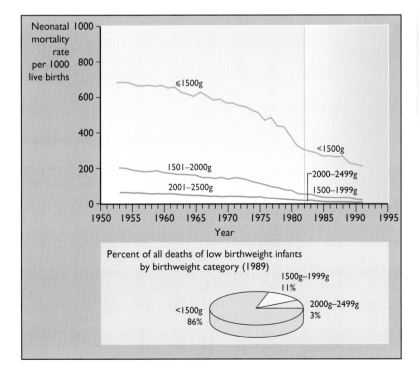

Fig. 8.1 The dramatic fall in neonatal mortality rate in England and Wales, according to birthweight. In very low birthweight infants, the marked fall in the mortality rate has been relatively recent. (Adapted from the Audit Commission. Data from OPCS.)

Stabilising the preterm or sick infant

Additional oxygen and artificial ventilation

Many infants with respiratory distress require additional inspiratory oxygen and ventilatory support. In preterm infants this is often for respiratory distress syndrome, but even in the absence of this disorder, many infants <30 weeks' gestation require artificial ventilation because of lung immaturity or to avoid recurrent apnoea.

Circulatory support

Circulatory support with colloid infusion and inotropic drugs is required to treat hypotension or if peripheral perfusion appears inadequate. Echocardiography can provide information on ventricular function.

Monitoring

The heart rate, respiratory rate and temperature are monitored continuously. Oxygenation is measured indirectly by pulse oximetry for oxygen saturation and with a transcutaneous electrode for oxygen tension. The arterial CO_2 tension can also be measured transcutaneously. Blood gas analysis is performed on arterial samples from a peripheral or umbilical artery catheter. The arterial oxygen tension is maintained at 8–12 kPa (60–90 mmHg) and the CO_2 tension at 4.5-6.5 kPa (35–50 mmHg).

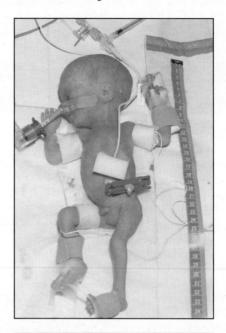

Fig. 8.2 Stabilising preterm or sick infants is important to prevent complications. This preterm infant has leads on his limbs for heart and respiratory rate, temperature and for oxygen saturation monitoring. There are arterial and intravenous cannulae and a nasotracheal tube for artificial ventilation.

A chest X-ray is required to help diagnose respiratory disorders and confirm the position of the tracheal tube and umbilical artery catheter.

Avoiding hypothermia

Hypothermia increases mortality and should be prevented by placing the baby under a radiant warmer or in an incubator.

Antibiotics

Infants requiring intensive care are often given broad-spectrum antibiotics. Infection with the Group B streptococcus and other organisms can mimic respiratory distress syndrome.

Metabolic disturbance

Blood glucose is checked regularly and iv dextrose given to prevent hypoglycaemia. Fluid requirements are very variable and must be closely monitored.

Minimal handling

All procedures, especially painful ones, adversely affect oxygenation and the circulation. Sedation and analgesia, e.g. an iv infusion of morphine, are given as required. Handling is kept to a minimum and done as rapidly and efficiently as possible.

Parents

Although medical and nursing staff are usually fully occupied stabilising the baby, time must be found for parents to allow them to see and touch their baby and to be kept fully informed.

Birth asphyxia

The incidence of this serious condition has fallen markedly in recent years to 1.5–6/1000 live births, but it remains an important cause of brain damage in children. Preventing birth asphyxia is one of the main aims of modern obstetric care.

Asphyxia, meaning suffocation, is the acute deprivation of oxygen accompanied by reduced oxygen delivery to the tissues. It has a number of different manifestations in the fetus and newborn infant. The fetal cardiotocograph (CTG) may be abnormal, but is poor at assessing the severity of asphyxia unless it is severe. However, when normal, the CTG is highly predictive of the absence of asphyxial problems in the neonate. Fetal blood sampling or cord blood analysis may identify a metabolic acidosis, but is also poor at predicting neonatal outcome unless the acidosis is very severe. Low Apgar scores at one and five minutes, reflecting delayed onset of respiration and circulatory failure at birth, are also poor at predicting outcome. If the score remains low at 15–20 minutes of age the risk of long-term disability or mortality is increased markedly. Hypoxic-

ischaemic encephalopathy is the term used to describe the clinical manifestation immediately post or up to 48 hours after asphyxia, whether antenatal, intrapartum or postnatal. Hypoxic-ischaemic encephalopathy can be graded as:

- mild – the infant is irritable, responds excessively to stimulation, may have staring of the eyes and hyperventilation and has impaired feeding
- moderate – the infant is lethargic, with reduced spontaneous movements of the limbs and seizures
- severe – there are no spontaneous movements or response to pain. Tone in the limbs may fluctuate between hypotonia and hypertonia. Seizures are prolonged and often refractory to treatment. Multi-organ failure is present.

Management

Skilled resuscitation and stabilising of sick infants will avoid or minimise asphyxia. Infants with hypoxic-ischaemic encephalopathy may need:

- respiratory support
- treatment of seizures with anticonvulsants
- prevention or reduction of cerebral oedema with fluid restriction. Infusion of mannitol, an osmotic diuretic,

is used in some centres. Hyperventilation, causing a profound reduction in CO_2 tension, is not advocated as it causes cerebral vasoconstriction and further impairs cerebral perfusion
- treatment of hypotension by colloid infusion and inotropic support
- renal support with dopamine
- monitoring and treatment of hypoglycaemia and/or hyponatraemia.

Prognosis

When hypoxic-ischaemic encephalopathy is mild, complete recovery can be expected. The prognosis is usually good if the condition is moderate, but more variable if severe. Several weeks after the insult, cystic lesions or ventricular dilatation from cerebral atrophy may be identified on cranial ultrasound, CT or MR scans. Information about cerebral metabolism from nuclear magnetic resonance (NMR) and near infrared spectroscopy is being evaluated. Infants who have recovered fully on clinical neurological examination and are feeding normally by ten days of age have an excellent prognosis. Severe hypoxic-ischaemic encephalopathy has a mortality approaching 12% and, of the survivors, 20% have neurodevelopmental disabilities, particularly cerebral palsy (Fig. 8.3).

In view of the potential medico-legal implications, it has been suggested that infants who fail to breathe at birth or develop seizures or other abnormal neurological signs should be diagnosed as having 'neonatal encephalopathy' as this does not imply that asphyxia was the cause. The diagnosis of birth asphyxia would then only be made if there is:
- evidence of severe antenatal or intrapartum hypoxia
- resuscitation needed at birth
- neurological features of encephalopathy
- evidence of hypoxic damage to other organs
- no other prenatal or postnatal cause identified.

Birth injuries

Infants may be injured at birth if they are malpositioned or too large for the pelvic outlet. Injuries may also occur during manual maneouvres or from forceps blades or at ventouse deliveries. Fortunately, now that caesarean section is available in every maternity unit, heroic attempts to achieve a vaginal delivery with resultant severe injuries to the infant have become extremely rare.

Soft tissue injuries
These include:
- caput succedaneum (Fig. 8.4) – bruising and oedema of the presenting part extending beyond the margins of the skull bones, often with overriding of the skull sutures resolves in a few days
- cephalhaematoma (Fig. 8.5) – bleeding below the periosteum, confined within the margins of the skull sutures. It usually involves the parietal bone. The centre of the

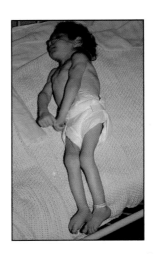

Fig. 8.3 Brain damage from severe birth asphyxia following a sudden, severe antepartum haemorrhage caused this child to become microcephalic, blind and deaf and to have spastic quadriplegia. However, less than 15% of cerebral palsy is caused by birth asphyxia.

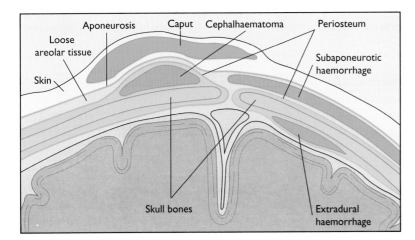

Fig. 8.4 Location of extracranial and extradural haemorrhages.

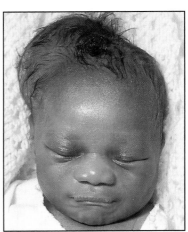

Fig. 8.5. A large cephalohaematoma.

haematoma feels soft. It resolves over several weeks. It is occasionally accompanied by a linear skull fracture

- chignon – bruising oedema from a ventouse delivery
- bruising, from even mild trauma in the delicate preterm infant, to the face after a face presentation and to the genitalia and buttocks after breech delivery
- abrasions to the skin from scalp electrodes applied during labour or from accidental scalpel incision at Caesarean section
- subaponeurotic haemorrhage (very uncommon) – may be accompanied by serious blood loss
- severe or fatal injury (very rare) from a tear of the tentorium cerebellum.

Nerve palsies

These result from traction to the cervical nerve roots. They may occur at breech deliveries or with shoulder dystocia. Upper nerve root (C5 and C6) injury results in an Erb palsy (Fig. 8.6). Less often the lower roots are injured, resulting in weakness of the wrist extensors and intrinsic muscles of the hand (Klumpke palsy). Most palsies resolve completely over a few weeks. Occasionally, following severe injury, paralysis is permanent. Surgical reconstruction of the nerves is sometimes attempted. Rarely, nerve palsies may be from damage to the cervical spine. A facial nerve palsy may result from compression of the facial nerve by forceps blades or against the mother's pelvis. It is usually transient.

Fractures

Clavicle – usually from shoulder dystocia. A snap may be heard at delivery or the infant may have reduced arm movement on the affected side or a lump from callus formation may be noticed over the clavicle at several days of age. The prognosis is excellent.

Humerus/femur – usually mid-shaft, ocurring at breech deliveries. They heal rapidly with immobilisation.

The preterm infant

The appearance, clinical problems, chances of survival and long-term prognosis depend on the infant's gestational age. Infants born at 24–26 weeks' gestation encounter many problems (Fig. 8.7), require many weeks of intensive (Fig. 8.8) and special care in hospital and have a high mortality.

At birth, they have very thin, dark red, transparent skin, no palpaple breast tissue and shapeless, soft ears. Males have no testes in the scrotum and females have widely separated labia majora and protruding labia minora. The infants lie with their arms and legs extended and have poor muscle tone. The external appearance and neurological findings can be scored to provide an estimate of an infant's gestational age (see Appendix). The number and severity of problems associated with prematurity decline markedly with increasing gestation, and with modern intensive care the prognosis is excellent after 32 weeks' gestational age. The severity of an infant's respiratory disease largely determines the neonatal course and outcome.

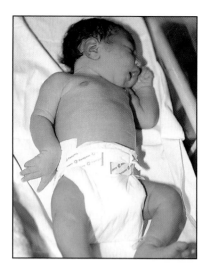

Fig. 8.6 Erb palsy. The affected arm lies straight, limp and with the hand pronated and the fingers flexed (waiter's tip position).

Fig. 8.7 Medical problems of preterm infants.

Need for resuscitation at birth
Respiratory:
    respiratory distress syndrome (RDS)
    pneumothorax
    apnoea and bradycardia
Hypotension
Patent ductus arteriosus
Temperature control
Nutrition
Metabolic
    hypoglycaemia
    hypocalcaemia
    electrolyte imbalance
    osteopenia of prematurity
Infection
Jaundice
Intracranial haemorrhage/ischaemia
Retinopathy of prematurity
Anaemia of prematurity
Iatrogenic
Bronchopulmonary dysplasia (chronic lung disease of
    prematurity)
Inguinal hernias

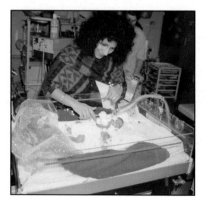

Fig. 8.8 A preterm infant receiving intensive care. Even during this period, parents need to be given the opportunity to get to know their baby.

RESPIRATORY DISTRESS SYNDROME

In respiratory distress syndrome (RDS) there is a deficiency of surfactant, the mixture of lipoproteins excreted by the alveolar epithelium which lowers surface tension. There is alveolar collapse and inadequate gas exchange. A protein-aceous exudate develops which forms a hyaline membrane seen on histology – RDS was therefore initially called hyaline membrane disease. The more preterm the infant, the higher the incidence of RDS. Whereas the majority of infants born before 28 weeks' gestation have RDS, it is uncommon in infants born at term. It is less severe in girls than boys. Surfactant deficiency may also occur secondary to hypoxia, acidosis or hypothermia.

Glucocorticoids given antenatally to the mother stimulate fetal surfactant production if there is a sufficient time interval (more than 48 hours) before birth to allow the drug to act. Surfactant production is inhibited in infants of diabetic mothers.

The recent development of exogenous surfactant therapy has been a major advance. The preparations are synthetic or derived from extracts of calf or pig lung or from human amniotic fluid. They are instilled directly into the lung via the tracheal tube. Multinational placebo controlled trials show that exogenous surfactant treatment reduces mortality from RDS by about 40%, without increasing the morbidity rate.

At delivery or within four hours of birth, babies with RDS develop clinical signs of:

- tachypnoea
- chest recession with retraction of the subcostal and intercostal muscles and diaphragm, causing indrawing of the ribs
- expiratory grunting in order to try to create positive airway pressure during expiration and maintain functional residual capacity
- cyanosis.

The characteristic chest X-ray appearance is shown in Figure 8.9.

Treatment with raised ambient oxygen is required, which may need to be supplemented with continuous positive airway pressure (delivered via nasal cannulae or face mask) or artificial ventilation via a tracheal tube. Considerable expertise is required to manage preterm babies with severe RDS. The ventilatory requirements need to be adjusted continually according to the infant's oxygenation and CO_2 tension (which are measured continuously), chest wall movements and blood gas analyses. Artificial ventilation may be synchronised as far as possible with the infant's respiration, or the infant's breathing may be partially or completely suppressed with sedatives and muscle relaxants. Whereas volume-cycled ventilators are used in adults, pressure-modulated ventilators are usually used in neonates as there is an air leak around uncuffed tracheal tubes. New modes of ventilation, such as high-frequency and oscillation, are being assessed.

 Surfactant therapy reduces the mortality of preterm infants with respiratory distress syndrome.

PNEUMOTHORAX

In respiratory distress syndrome (RDS) air from the over-distended alveoli may track into the interstitium, resulting in pulmonary interstitial emphysema (PIE) (Fig. 8.10). In up to 20% of infants ventilated for RDS, air leaks into the pleural cavity and causes a pneumothorax. When a pneumothorax occurs, the infant's oxygen requirement usually increases, the tidal volume, if monitored, is decreased and the breath sounds and chest movement on the affected side are reduced, although this can be difficult to detect clinically. A pneumothorax may be readily demonstrated by transillumination with a bright fibre-optic light source applied to the chest wall.

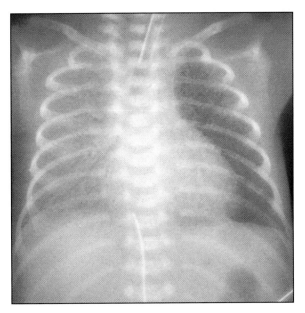

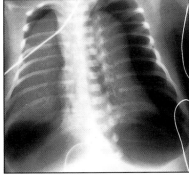

Fig. 8.9 Chest X-ray in respiratory distress syndrome showing a diffuse granular or 'ground glass' appearance of the lungs and an air bronchogram, where the larger airways are outlined. The heart border becomes indistinct or obscured completely. The diagnosis of respiratory distress syndrome is made on the basis of a characteristic chest X-ray and the clinical course.

Fig. 8.10 Chest X-ray showing right-sided pulmonary interstitial emphysema and bilateral pneumothoraces in a preterm infant with respiratory distress syndrome.

A tension pneumothorax is treated by inserting a chest drain. In order to try and prevent pneumothoraces, infants are ventilated with the lowest pressures that provide adequate chest movement and satisfactory blood gases, and ventilation is also adjusted to avoid the infant breathing against the ventilator. This is achieved by manipulating the ventilator settings, and giving sedation and muscle relaxants if necessary.

APNOEA AND BRADYCARDIA

Episodes of apnoea and bradycardia are common in very low birthweight infants until they reach about 32 weeks' gestational age. An episode of bradycardia may occur either when an infant stops breathing for sufficiently long or when the infant continues to breathe but against a closed glottis. An underlying cause for the episodes – hypoxia, infection, anaemia, metabolic disturbance, convulsions, aspiration from gastro-oesophageal reflux or heart failure – needs to be excluded. Treatment with a respiratory stimulant such as theophylline or caffeine often helps, the dosage being monitored by measuring plasma drug levels. Breathing will usually start again after gentle physical stimulation. Occasionally, continuous positive airways pressure is needed to abolish them, otherwise artificial ventilation is required.

PATENT DUCTUS ARTERIOSUS

The ductus arteriosus remains patent in many preterm infants. Shunting of blood across the ductus, from the left to the right side of the circulation, is most common in infants with respiratory distress syndrome. It may produce no symptoms or it may cause apnoea and bradycardia, increased oxygen requirement and difficulty in weaning the infant from artificial ventilation. The pulses are 'bounding' from increased blood pressure amplitude, the precordium becomes prominent and a systolic murmur may be audible. With increasing circulatory overload, signs of heart failure may develop. More accurate assessment of the infant's circulation can be obtained on echocardiography. Treatment, if necessary, is with fluid restriction, and indomethacin, a prostaglandin synthetase inhibitor. Indomethacin has widespread effects on the circulation, including reduced renal function. If these measures fail to close a symptomatic duct, surgical ligation will be required.

TEMPERATURE CONTROL

Newborn infants have a larger surface area relative to their body weight than older children. The skin of preterm infants is thin and poorly keratinised. In the first week of life it is an important source of water and heat loss. Preterm infants are unable to shiver, cannot curl up and are usually nursed naked. This adds to their difficulty in maintaining body temperature. Oxygen consumption is increased if the environment is too cold or too hot. There is a neutral temperature range in which an infant's oxygen consumption is lowest. The neutral temperature is highest in the very immature baby during the first few days of life. The temperature of these small babies is maintained using incubators (Fig. 8.11) or overhead radiant heaters.

Radiant heaters allow better access to the baby but evaporative heat loss through the skin is greater and this makes fluid balance more difficult to control. Heat loss is reduced by covering the baby with a thermal blanket or plastic shield, providing humidity and clothing the baby whenever practical. Closed incubators provide a more constant environment. Ambient humidity can be readily provided, reducing evaporative heat loss.

FLUID BALANCE

A preterm infant's fluid requirements will vary depending on gestational age, clinical condition and whether nursed in a closed or open incubator. On the first day of life, 60 ml/kg are usually required, increasing by 30 ml/kg/day to 150–180 ml/kg/day. This is adjusted according to the infant's clinical condition, plasma electrolytes and creatinine concentration, urine output and weight change.

NUTRITION

Preterm infants have a high nutritional requirement because of their rapid growth. A preterm infant born at 28 weeks gestation doubles his birthweight in six weeks and trebles it in 12 weeks, whereas a term baby doubles his weight in 4.5 months and trebles it in a year.

Infants of 35–36 weeks' gestational age are mature enough to suck and swallow milk. Less mature infants will need to be fed via an oro- or nasogastric tube. Even in very preterm infants, enteral feeds, preferably breast milk, are introduced as soon as possible. The breast milk may need to be supplemented with protein, calories and minerals. There are also special infant formulas designed to meet the increased requirements of preterm infants. In the very immature or sick infant, parenteral nutrition is often required. It is usually given through a central venous catheter, paying strict attention to aseptic technique.

In osteopenia of prematurity there is poor bone min-

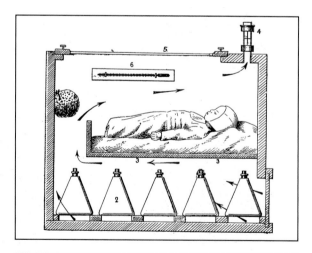

Fig. 8.11 *The importance of avoiding hypothermia in newborn infants has long been recognised. This incubator was used in the late 19th century to keep newborn infants warm.*

eralisation which can lead to rickets and bone fractures. It is common in preterm infants, but its severity can be reduced by giving sufficient phosphate in the parenteral and enteral nutrition.

Because iron is mostly transferred to the fetus during the last trimester, preterm babies have low iron stores and are at risk of iron deficiency. Iron supplements are started at 3–8 weeks of age. Blood transfusions are often required during the first few weeks of life in very immature infants to replace the blood removed for laboratory tests and to compensate for inadequate erythropoiesis. Recombinant human erythropoietin may reduce transfusion requirements and its indications and safety are currently being determined.

INFECTION

Preterm infants are at increased risk of infection, either at or shortly after birth from organisms acquired from the maternal birth canal, or at a later age when it is usually associated with indwelling catheters or artificial ventilation.

INTRACRANIAL LESIONS

Periventricular haemorrhages occur in 25% of very low birthweight infants and are readily recognised on intracranial ultrasound scans (Fig 8.12). Typically, they occur in the germinal matrix above the caudate nucleus, which supports a fragile network of blood vessels. Fortunately, the majority of haemorrhages are small and harmless, but

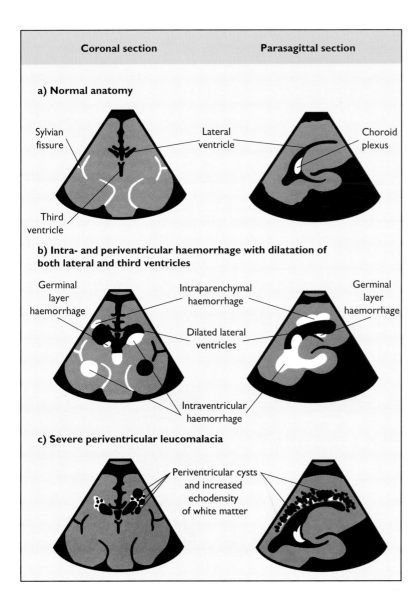

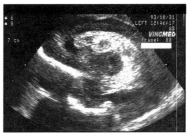

8.12a Large intraventricular haemorrhage.

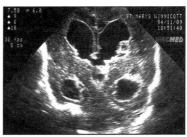

8.12b Marked ventricular dilatation. Haemorrhage is visible within the ventricles.

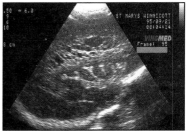

8.12c Periventricular leucomalacia following ischaemic damage.

Fig. 8.12 Intracranial ultrasound in preterm infants.

larger haemorrhages may extend into the lateral ventricles or into the brain parenchyma. This may be from extension of the haemorrhage itself or from venous infarction into an ischaemic area. Most haemorrhages occur within the first 72 hours of life. They are more common following birth asphyxia and in infants with severe respiratory distress syndrome and following a pneumothorax.

Dilatation of the ventricles is also readily detected on ultrasound. It usually follows an intraventricular bleed. The dilatation may resolve spontaneously or progress to cause hydrocephalus, when the anterior fontanelle becomes tense, the sutures separate and the head circumference increases rapidly. Convulsions or other symptoms may develop at this stage. Removal of CSF may provide symptomatic relief until a ventriculo-peritoneal shunt is inserted.

Ischaemic lesions are more difficult to detect by ultrasound. There may initially be an echodense area or 'flare' within the brain parenchyma. This may resolve, or cystic lesions may be noted some weeks later. Multiple widespread cysts, also called periventricular leucomalacia (PVL), are associated with a poor developmental outcome.

NECROTISING ENTEROCOLITIS

Necrotising enterocolitis is a serious illness mainly affecting preterm infants in the first few weeks of life. It is thought to be due to a combination of ischaemia of the bowel wall and infection from organisms colonising the bowel. The infant stops tolerating milk feeds, with milk aspirated from the stomach or vomiting, which may be bile-stained. The abdomen becomes distended (Fig. 8.13a) and the stool contains fresh blood. The infant may rapidly become shocked and require ventilatory support because of apnoeic attacks or respiratory failure. The characteristic features on an abdominal X-ray are distended loops of bowel, thickening of the bowel wall with intramural air and air in the portal tract (Fig. 8.13b). The disease may progress to bowel perforation which can be detected by X-ray or by transillumination of the abdomen (Fig. 8.13c).

Treatment is to stop oral feeding and give broad-spectrum antibiotics to cover both aerobic and anaerobic organisms. Artificial ventilation and circulatory support are often needed. Surgery is performed for bowel perforation. Total parenteral nutrition will be required. The disease has significant morbidity and a mortality of about 20%. Long-term sequelae include malabsorption if extensive bowel resection has been necessary and bowel stenosis.

RETINOPATHY OF PREMATURITY

Retinopathy of prematurity (ROP, retrolental fibroplasia) affects developing blood vessels at the junction of the vascular and non-vascularised retina. There is vascular proliferation which may progress to retinal detachment, fibrosis and blindness. It was initially recognised that the condition is caused by additional oxygen given in an uncontrolled way. Now, even with careful monitoring of the infant's oxygenation, evidence of retinopathy of prematurity is still found in about 20% of all very low birthweight infants, with a higher percentage in the very immature. It is first detected at the equivalent of 32–38 weeks' gestational age. All very low birthweight infants should have their eyes screened 6–7 weeks after birth by indirect ophthalmoscopy. The early stages of the disease are the most frequent and usually resolve completely. Cryosurgery or laser therapy may be indicated for severe disease. Severe visual impairment occurs in about 1% of low birthweight infants.

IATROGENIC DISEASE

Preterm infants, particularly those of very low birthweight or with severe lung disease, need intensive care for many days or weeks. Adverse events are inevitable when such complex techniques are used, and iatrogenic disease may result in significant morbidity and mortality unless all staff are highly skilled and pay meticulous attention to detail (Fig. 8.14).

BRONCHOPULMONARY DYSPLASIA

Infants who still require additional oxygen beyond 28 days of age are described as having bronchopulmonary dyspla-

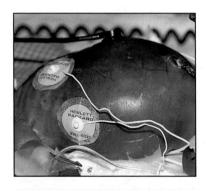

Fig. 8.13a Necrotising enterocolitis showing gross abdominal distension and tense and shiny skin over the abdomen.

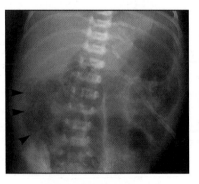

Fig. 8.13b Abdominal X-ray showing the characteristic features of distended loops of bowel and thickening of the bowel wall with intramural air (arrow).

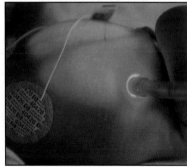

Fig. 8.13c Bowel perforation may be identified on X-ray or by transillumination.

sia (BPD) or chronic lung disease of prematurity. The lung is damaged from artificial ventilation, oxygen toxicity, infection and the accumulation of lung secretions. The chest X-ray characteristically shows widespread areas of opacification, often with cystic changes (Fig. 8.15). Some infants need artificial ventilation, but may be weaned onto continuous positive airways pressure followed by additional ambient oxygen, sometimes over several months. Corticosteroid therapy often reduces the infant's oxygen requirement and may allow earlier weaning from the ventilator. Some babies go home receiving additional oxygen for several months. Infants with severe disease may die of intercurrent infection or cor pulmonale.

PROBLEMS FOLLOWING DISCHARGE

In general, the children are shorter and thinner than full-term infants of normal birthweight. Readmission to hospital during the first year of life is increased approximately fourfold in very low birthweight infants. Those who had bronchopulmonary dysplasia are more susceptible to recurrent wheezing and chest infections. Inguinal hernias may appear in the first few months of life.

Very low birthweight infants are at risk of a wide range of neurodevelopmental problems. These include visual impairment, hearing loss, cerebral palsy and learning difficulties (Fig. 8.16). Although only 5–10% have a serious disability, they are more prone to specific learning difficulties, particularly delayed language development, poor attention span, difficulty with fine motor skills and more behavioural problems than siblings born at term. The risk of developing these problems increases markedly for those of very early gestational age. Gross abnormalities on intracranial ultrasound and abnormal neurological examination at term indicate an increased risk of long-term disability. All very low birthweight infants should have their developmental progress closely monitored to allow early detection and treatment of any problems.

Jaundice

Over 60% of all newborn infants become visibly jaundiced. This is because:

- the haemoglobin concentration falls rapidly in the first few days after birth from haemolysis (1 gram of haemoglobin yields 640 micromol (35 mg) of bilirubin) (Fig. 8.17)
- the red cell life span of newborn infants (70 days) is markedly shorter than that of adults (120 days)
- hepatic bilirubin metabolism is less efficient in the first few days of life.

Jaundice is important as:

- it may be a sign of another disorder, e.g. infection
- unconjugated bilirubin can be deposited in the brain, particularly in the basal ganglia, causing kernicterus.

Kernicterus. This is bilirubin neurotoxicity, which may occur when the level of unconjugated bilirubin exceeds the albumin-binding capacity of the blood. As this free bilirubin is fat soluble, it can cross the blood–brain barrier. The neurotoxic effects vary in severity from transient disturbance to death. Early manifestations are lethargy and poor feeding. In severe cases, there is irritability and an increase in muscle tone and the baby may lie with an arched back (opisthotonos). Infants who survive may develop choreoathetoid cerebral palsy, learning difficulties and sensorineural deafness. Kernicterus used to be an important cause of brain damage in infants with severe haemolytic disease, but has become rare since the introduction of prophylactic anti-D immunoglobulin for rhesus negative mothers.

Clinical evaluation

Babies become clinically jaundiced when the bilirubin level reaches 80–120 micromol/l. Management varies according to the infant's age at onset, bilirubin level and rate of increase, the infant's gestational age and clinical condition.

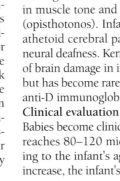

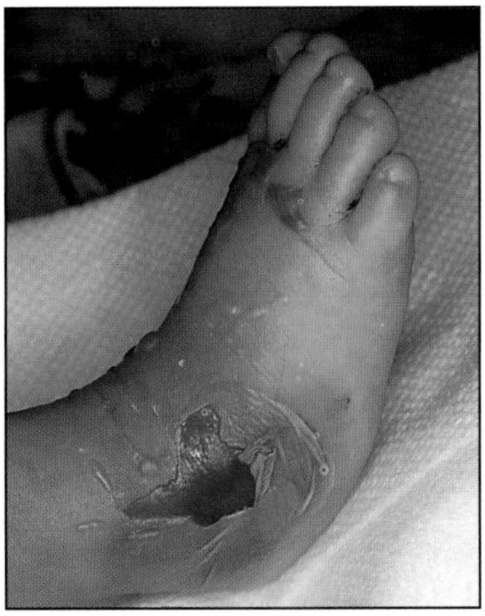

Fig. 8.14 Iatrogenic disease. Extravasation of a peripheral infusion containing calcium.

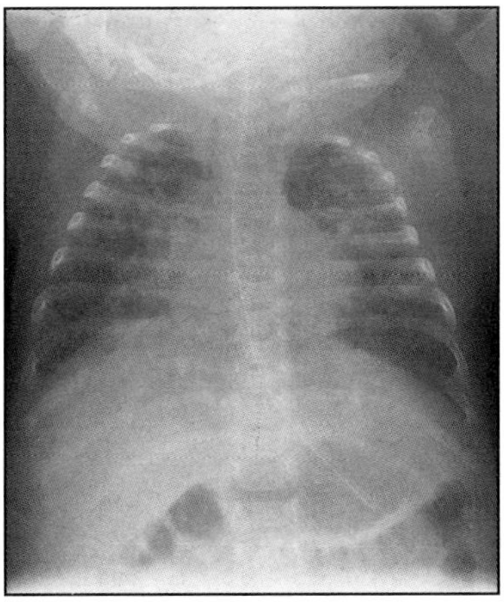

Fig. 8.15 Chest X-ray of bronchopulmonary dysplasia (BPD) showing fibrosis and lung collapse, cystic changes and over-distension of the lungs.

Fig. 8.16 Follow-up at three years of age of survivors (54%) of extremely preterm infants born at < 28 weeks' gestation admitted to a neonatal intensive care unit between 1980–1989.

Normal	72%
Lesser disabilities	9%
Moderate or severe disabilities	19%
cerebral palsy	13%
cognitive delay	10%
deafness	2%
visual impairment	6%
seizures	2%
multiple disabilities	8%

Adapted from Cooke RWI. Factors affecting survival and outcome at 3 years in extremely preterm infants. Arch Dis Ch 1994;71: F28–31.

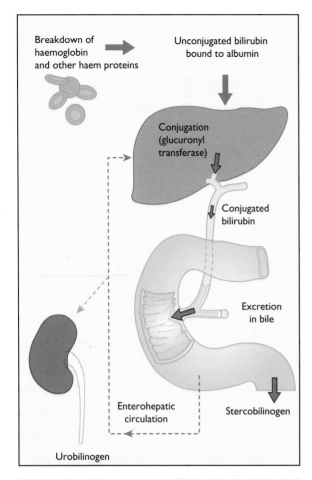

Jaundice starting at <24 hours of age	Haemolytic disorders: Rhesus incompatibility ABO incompatibility G6PD deficiency Spherocytosis, pyruvate kinase deficiency Congenital infection
Jaundice at 24 h to 2 weeks of age	Physiological jaundice Breast milk jaundice Infection, e.g. urinary tract infection Haemolysis, e.g. G6PD deficiency, ABO incompatability Bruising Polycythaemia Crigler–Najjar syndrome
Jaundice at >2 weeks of age	Unconjugated: Physiological or breast milk jaundice Infection (particularly urinary tract) Hypothyroidism Haemolytic anaemia, e.g. G6PDdeficiency High gastrointestinal obstruction Conjugated (>15% of total bilirubin): Bile duct obstruction e.g. biliary atresia Neonatal hepatitis

Fig. 8.18 Causes of neonatal jaundice.

Fig. 8.17 *The initial breakdown product of haemoglobin is unconjugated bilirubin (indirect bilirubin) which is insoluble in water but soluble in lipids. It is carried in the blood bound to albumin. It is taken up by the liver and conjugated by the enzyme glucuronyl transferase to conjugated bilirubin (direct bilirubin) which is water soluble and excreted in bile into the gut and is detectable in urine when blood levels rise. Reabsorption of bilirubin from the gut (enterohepatic circulation) is increased when milk intake is low.*

AGE AT ONSET

The age of onset is a useful guide to the likely cause of the jaundice (Fig. 8.18).

Jaundice <24 hours of age

Jaundice starting within 24 hours of birth usually results from haemolysis. This is particularly important to identify as the bilirubin is unconjugated and can rise very rapidly and reach extremely high levels.

Haemolytic disorders

Rhesus haemolytic disease. Affected infants are usually identified antenatally and given fetal therapy if necessary (see Chapter 7). The birth of a severely anaemic infant with hydrops and hepatosplenomegaly who rapidly develops severe jaundice has become rare. Antibodies may develop

to rhesus antigens other than D and also to the Kell and Duffy blood groups, but haemolysis is usually much less severe.

ABO incompatibility. This is now more common than rhesus haemolytic disease. Some group O women have an anti-A-haemolysin in the blood. This can cross the placenta, as it is an IgG immunoglobulin, and may haemolyse the red cells of a group A infant. Occasionally, group B infants are affected. Haemolysis is less severe than in rhesus disease as anti-A and anti-B haemolysins are comparatively weak and are mostly absorbed by other body tissues. The infant's haemoglobin level is usually normal or only slightly reduced and, in contrast to rhesus disease, hepatosplenomegaly is absent. The direct antibody test (Coombs test) is usually but not always weakly positive and haemolysins are usually detectable in the blood. The jaundice usually peaks in the first 12–72 hours.

G6PD deficiency. The Mediterranean and Middle and Far Eastern variants may cause neonatal jaundice (see Chapter 19). Parents of affected infants should be given a list of drugs to be avoided which may precipitate haemolysis.

Spherocytosis. Spherocytosis is considerably less common than G6PD deficiency (see Chapter 19). There is often but not always a family history. The disorder can be identified by recognising spherocytes on the blood film.

Congenital infection

Jaundice at birth can also be from congenital infection but is conjugated and the infants have other abnormal clinical signs.

Jaundice at 2 days–2 weeks of age

Physiological jaundice. Most babies who become jaundiced during this period have physiological jaundice. Other conditions need to be considered before it can be assumed that the baby's jaundice is physiological.

Breast milk jaundice. Breast milk may exacerbate jaundice in healthy infants. The hyperbilirubinaemia is unconjugated and may be prolonged. The cause is unknown. In some infants, the jaundice appears to be exacerbated if milk intake is poor from delay in establishing breast-feeding and the infant becomes dehydrated. Although the bilirubin level will fall if breast-feeding is stopped for a few days, interruption of breast-feeding for this purpose is rarely indicated.

Infection. An infected baby may develop an unconjugated hyperbilirubinaemia from poor fluid intake, haemolysis, reduced hepatic function and an increase in the enterohepatic circulation. If infection is suspected, appropriate investigations and treatment should be instigated. In particular, urinary tract infections may present in this way.

Other causes. Jaundice from haemolysis usually presents in the first day of life but may present during the next few days. Bruising and polycythaemia (venous haematocrit >0.65) will exacerbate the infant's jaundice. The very rare Crigler-Najjar syndrome, when the enzyme glucuronyl transferase is deficient or absent, may result in extremely high levels of unconjugated bilirubin.

Jaundice at >2 weeks of age (persistent neonatal jaundice)

Jaundice in babies more than two weeks old is called persistent or prolonged neonatal jaundice. In most infants the hyperbilirubinaemia will still be unconjugated, but this needs to be confirmed on laboratory testing.

In prolonged unconjugated hyperbilirubinaemia:

- 'breast milk jaundice' is the most common cause, affecting about 15% of healthy breast-fed infants. The jaundice gradually fades and disappears by 3–4 weeks of age
- infection, particularly of the urinary tract, needs to be considered
- congenital hypothyroidism needs to be excluded, as it may present with prolonged jaundice before the clinical features of coarse facies, dry skin, hypotonia and constipation become evident. While affected infants should now be identified on neonatal biochemical screening (Guthrie test), the result should be checked when there is a clinical indication.

Prolonged conjugated hyperbilirubinaemia is suggested by the baby passing dark urine and unpigmented pale stools. Its causes include neonatal hepatitis syndrome and biliary atresia. It is important to diagnose biliary atresia promptly, as delay in surgical treatment adversely affects outcome (*see* Chapter 17 for further details).

SEVERITY OF JAUNDICE

Jaundice can be observed most easily by blanching the skin with the finger. The jaundice starts on the head and face and then spreads down the trunk and limbs. A transcutaneous jaundice meter may be helpful, but if the jaundice appears clinically significant or there is any doubt about the degree of jaundice, the bilirubin should be checked on a blood sample. It is easy to under-estimate jaundice in Afro-Caribbean, Asian and preterm babies, and a low threshold should be adopted for measuring the bilirubin of these infants.

RATE OF CHANGE

The rate of rise tends to be linear until a plateau is reached, so serial measurements can be plotted on a chart and used to anticipate the need for treatment before it rises to a dangerous level.

GESTATION

Preterm infants may be damaged by a lower bilirubin level than term infants. In addition, the infant's age from birth is important, as higher bilirubin levels are tolerated with increasing age.

CLINICAL CONDITION

Infants who experience severe hypoxia, hypothermia or any serious illess may be more susceptible to damage from severe jaundice. Drugs which may displace bilirubin from albumin, eg sulphonamides and diazepam, are best avoided in newborn infants.

Management

Poor milk intake and dehydration will exacerbate jaundice, but studies have failed to show that supplementing breast-feeding with water or dextrose solution will reduce jaundice. Treatment is by phototherapy or exchange transfusion. Phototherapy. In phototherapy, light (wavelength 450 nm) from the blue band of the visible spectrum converts unconjugated bilirubin by photodegradation into a harmless water-soluble pigment. Although no long-term sequelae of phototherapy from overhead light have been reported, it is disruptive to normal nursing of the infant and should not be used indiscriminately. The infant's eyes are covered as a bright light is uncomfortable and can cause retinal damage in animals. Phototherapy can result in hypo- or hyperthermia, dehydration, a macular rash and diarrhoea.

More recently a fibre-optic blanket has been developed which can be applied directly to the skin. Both an overhead light and blanket can be used simultaneously (intensive phototherapy).

Exchange transfusion Exchange transfusion is required if the bilirubin rises to levels which are considered dangerous or continues to rise above the recommended level in spite of intensive phototherapy. Exchange transfusions have been performed traditionally via an umbilical venous catheter by alternately withdrawing 10–20 ml aliquots of the baby's blood and replacing them with donor blood. The procedure can be performed more efficiently and avoiding the complications associated with umbilical vein cannulation, by infusing the blood via a peripheral vein while extracting blood from an arterial line. Twice the infant's blood volume (80 ml/kg) is exchanged. Donor blood should be as fresh as possible and screened to exclude CMV, hepatitis B and C and HIV infection. The procedure has a low but definite morbidity and mortality.

There are no bilirubin levels which are known to be safe or which will definitely cause kernicterus. In rhesus haemolytic disease, it was found that kernicterus could be prevented if the bilirubin was kept below 340 micromol/l (20 mg/dl). As there is no consensus among paediatricians on the bilirubin levels at which phototherapy and exchange transfusion should be performed, each department should have guidelines for the management of jaundice.

Respiratory distress in term infants

Newborn infants with respiratory distress develop the following signs:
- tachypnoea
- laboured breathing, with chest wall recession and nasal flaring
- expiratory grunting
- cyanosis.

The causes in term infants are listed in Figure 8.19. Affected infants should be admitted to the neonatal unit for monitoring of heart and respiratory rates, oxygenation and circulation. A chest X-ray will be required to help iden-

tify the cause and those which need immediate treatment, e.g. pneumothorax or diaphragmatic hernia. Additional ambient oxygen, mechanical ventilation and circulatory support are given as required.

TRANSIENT TACHYPNOEA OF THE NEWBORN

By far the commonest cause of tachypnoea and respiratory distress in term infants is transient tachypnoea of the newborn caused by delay in the resorption of lung liquid. It is more common after birth by Caesarean section. The chest X-ray shows hyperinflation of the lungs and fluid in the horizontal fissure. Additional ambient oxygen may be required. The condition usually settles within the first day of life but can take several days to resolve.

MECONIUM ASPIRATION

Meconium is passed before birth by 8–20% of babies. It is rarely passed by preterm infants, and occurs increasingly commonly the greater the gestational age, affecting 20–25% of deliveries by 42 weeks. At birth these infants may inhale thick meconium into the large and small airways. Thick meconium at delivery should be aspirated from the airway (see p 77). Asphyxiated infants may start gasping and aspirate meconium before delivery. Meconium is a lung irritant and results in both mechanical obstruction and a chemical pneumonitis. It predisposes to infection. In meconium aspiration the lungs are over-inflated, accompanied by patches of collapse and consolidation. There is a high incidence of air leak leading to pneumothorax and pneumomediastinum. Artificial ventilation is often required. Infants with meconium aspiration may develop persistent pulmonary hypertension of the newborn which may make it difficult to achieve adequate oxygenation.

PNEUMONIA

Prolonged rupture of the membranes, chorioamnionitis and low birthweight predispose to pneumonia. Infants with respiratory distress will usually require investigation to identify any infection. Broad-spectrum antibiotics are started readily until the results are available.

PNEUMOTHORAX

A pneumothorax may occur spontaneously or more commonly as a complication of mechanical ventilation. Management is described on p. 87.

MILK ASPIRATION

Infants may aspirate milk. They are at increased risk if preterm, have respiratory distress or neurological damage. Babies with bronchopulmonary dysplasia often have gastro-oesophageal reflux which predisposes to aspiration. Infants with a cleft palate are prone to aspirate respiratory secretions or milk.

Fig. 8.19 Causes of respiratory distress in term infants	
Pulmonary	
Common	Transient tachypnoea of the newborn
Less common	Meconium aspiration
	Pneumonia
	Pneumothorax
	Persistent pulmonary hypertension of the newborn
	Milk aspiration
Rare	Diaphragmatic hernia
	Tracheo-oesophageal fistula (TOF)
	Respiratory distress syndrome (RDS)
	Pulmonary hypoplasia
	Airways obstruction, e.g. choanal atresia
	Pulmonary haemorrhage
Non-pulmonary	
	Congenital heart disease
	Intracranial birth trauma/asphyxia
	Severe anaemia
	Metabolic acidosis

PERSISTENT PULMONARY HYPERTENSION OF THE NEWBORN

This life-threatening condition is usually associated with birth asphyxia, meconium aspiration, septicaemia or respiratory distress syndrome. It sometimes occurs as a primary disorder. Because of the high pulmonary vascular resistance, there is right to left shunting within the lungs and at atrial and ductal levels. Cyanosis occurs soon after birth. Heart murmurs and signs of heart failure are often absent. A chest X-ray shows that the heart is of normal size and there may be pulmonary oligaemia, but this is often difficult or impossible to appreciate in the newborn period. An urgent echocardiogram is required to establish that the child does not have congenital heart disease.

Most infants require mechanical ventilation and circulatory support in order to achieve adequate oxygenation. Tolazoline, a general vasodilator, is often given but is not always beneficial. The drug may be accompanied by systemic hypotension requiring correction with colloid. Prostaglandins may also be beneficial. Recently, inhaled nitric oxide, a potent vasodilator, and new modes of artificial ventilation (using high-frequency or oscillatory ventilation) have shown promising results. Extracorporeal membrane oxygenation (ECMO), where the infant is placed on heart and lung bypass for several days, is used for severe cases.

DIAPHRAGMATIC HERNIA

This occurs in about 1 in 4000 births. If it has not been diagnosed on antenatal ultrasound, it usually presents with failure to respond to resuscitation but sometimes with increasing tachypnoea. In most cases there is a left-sided hernia through the posterolateral foramen of the diaphragm. The apex beat and heart sounds will then be displaced to the right side of the chest, and there is poor air entry in the left chest. Vigorous resuscitation may cause a pneumothorax in the normal lung, thereby aggravating the situation. The diagnosis is confirmed by X-ray of the chest and abdomen (Fig. 8.20). Once the diagnosis is suspected, a large nasogastric tube is passed and suction applied to prevent distension of the intrathoracic bowel. The diaphragmatic hernia is repaired surgically, but in most infants with this condition the main problem is pulmonary hypoplasia, where compression by the herniated viscera prevents development of the lung in the fetus. This is the cause of the high mortality (30–60%). Extracorporeal membrane oxygenation (ECMO) may be required pre- and post-operatively to provide respiratory support.

OTHER CAUSES

Other causes of respiratory distress are listed in Figure 8.21. When due to heart failure, abnormal heart sounds and/or heart murmurs may be present on auscultation. An enlarged liver from venous congestion is a helpful sign. The femoral arteries must be palpated, as coarctation of the aorta or interrupted aortic arch are important causes of heart failure in newborn infants.

Infection

Infants are exposed to a wide range of potential pathogens from the birth canal. The risk of infection is increased if there has been prolonged rupture of the membranes, especially if chorioamnionitis has developed, and if the infant is preterm.

Presentation is usually non-specific (*see* Fig. 8.21). If systemic infection is suspected, investigation and treatment must be started promptly. A septic screen will need to be performed, and antibiotics are started immediately without waiting for culture results. Intravenous, broad-spectrum antibiotics are given to cover Group B streptococci, *Listeria monocytogenes* and other Gram-positive organisms (usually penicillin or amoxycillin), combined with cover of Gram-negative organisms (an aminoglycoside or third-generation cephalosporin). The initial choice of antibiotics and length of treatment will depend on the site of infection and the pattern of pathogens in the unit. If cultures are negative and the infant has recovered clinically, antibiotics can be stopped after 48 hours.

Neonatal meningitis, though uncommon, has a mortality of 20–50%, with half of survivors having serious sequelae. Presentation is the same as for other forms of

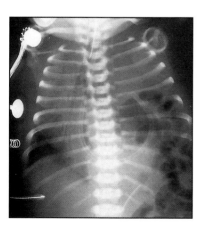

Fig. 8.20 Chest X-ray in diaphragmatic hernia showing loops of bowel in the chest and displacement of the mediastinum. There is a tracheal tube and a nasogastric tube which lies within the chest.

Fig. 8.21 Clinical features of neonatal sepsis.	
Fever or temperature instability	Apnoea and bradycardia
Poor feeding	Respiratory distress
Vomiting	Abdominal distension
Jaundice	Hypo-/hyperglycaemia
Irritability	Shock
Seizures	In meningitis:
Lethargy, drowsiness	• tense or bulging fontanelle
	• head retraction (opisthotonus)

neonatal sepsis. A bulging fontanelle and lying with the back hyperextended (opisthotonus) is a late sign of meningitis. If meningitis is thought likely, ampicillin or penicillin and a third-generation cephalosporin (e.g. cefotaxime) are given. Serial examination of the CSF and measurement of an acute phase reactant, e.g. C-reactive protein, are useful to monitor response to therapy. Complications include cerebral abscess, ventriculitis and hydrocephalus.

Nosocomially acquired infections are an inherent risk in a neonatal unit or postnatal ward. All staff must adhere strictly to effective hand washing to prevent cross infection. In intensive care, the other main sources of infection are indwelling catheters for parenteral nutrition or arterial blood gas sampling, tracheal tubes and invasive procedures which break the protective barrier of the skin. Infection of indwelling catheters usually develops after the first week of life. *Coagulase-negative staphylococcus* is the most common pathogen in this situation, but the range of organisms is very broad, and includes *Candida* and other fungal infections. Broad-spectrum antibiotics are used but are likely to include flucloxacillin or vancomycin to cover coagulase-negative staphylococcal infection.

SOME SPECIFIC INFECTIONS
Group B streptococcal infection
Up to 30% of pregnant women have faecal or vaginal carriage of Group B streptococci. Up to half of the infants born to these mothers carry the organism on their skin, but only 1% become ill. The incidence of disease varies widely between countries from 1–5 per 1000 live births. Early onset disease typically presents on day 1–3 of life with pneumonia, septicaemia and, occasionally, meningitis. Mortality is up to 20%. Transmission from mother to infant occurs during delivery or by ascending infection shortly before birth. Late onset disease, from one week to three months of age, is less common. It usually causes meningitis but may present with focal infections such as osteomyelitis or septic arthritis.

 Group B streptococcal infection may mimic respiratory distress syndrome.

Listeria monocytogenes infection
Perinatal and neonatal *Listeria* infection is uncommon but serious. It is transmitted to the mother in food, such as unpasteurised milk, soft cheeses and undercooked poultry. It can cause a mild, influenza-like illness in the mother, or there may be asymptomatic faecal and vaginal carriage. Infection in pregnancy may cause abortion, preterm delivery or fetal infection. The fetus usually acquires infection transplacentally, but also by ascending infection from the genital tract or at delivery. A characteristic feature of *Listeria* infection, even in preterm infants, is meconium staining of the liquor, which is unusual at an early gestation. There may be placental abscesses from which the organism can be cultured.

In early-onset disease, presentation is at delivery or within the first few hours of life with septicaemia and pneumonia,

a widespread rash and meningitis. The mortality is 30%. In late onset disease, presentation is at 1-8 weeks of age, most often with meningitis, and has a better prognosis.

Gram-negative infections
E. coli and other Gram-negative organisms, which are present in faeces and carried vaginally, used to be the most common cause of early-onset sepsis in the newborn. In the UK and the US, Group B streptococcal infection is now more common.

Conjunctivitis
Sticky eyes are common in the neonatal period, starting on the third or fourth day of life. Cleaning with saline or water is all that is required and the condition resolves spontaneously. A more troublesome discharge may be due to staphylococcal or streptococcal infection and can be treated with a topical antibiotic eye ointment, eg neomycin.

Purulent discharge with swelling of the eyelids within the first 48 hours of life is most likely to be due to gonococcal infection. The discharge should be Gram stained urgently as well as cultured and treatment started immediately. In countries where penicillin resistance is a problem, eg the UK and US, a third-generation cephalosporin is the antibiotic of choice. Otherwise, intravenous penicillin is used. The eye needs to be cleansed frequently.

Chlamydia trachomatis eye infection usually presents with a purulent discharge and swelling of the eyelids (Fig. 8.22) towards the end of the first week of life, but may also present shortly after birth. The organism is identified with a monoclonal antibody test on the pus. Treatment is with topical tetracycline eye ointment and oral erythromycin, both for two weeks. Both gonococcal and chlamydial eye infections need to be treated vigorously to avoid damage to the eye. The mother and partner also need to be checked and treated.

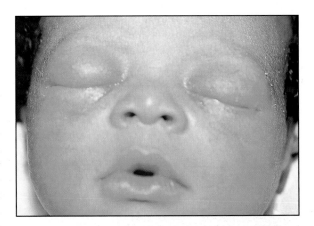

Fig. 8.22 Purulent discharge and swollen eyelids in an eight-day-old infant. This is the characteristic presentation of conjunctivitis from Chlamydia trachomatis. Neisseria gonorrhoeae *was absent.*

Umbilical infection

The umbilicus dries and separates during the first few days of life. Antibiotic powder or lotion is often applied to the area to prevent the spread of staphylococcal infection. If the skin surrounding the umbilicus becomes inflamed, systemic antibiotics are indicated. Sometimes the umbilicus continues to be sticky as it is prevented from involuting by an umbilical granuloma. This can be removed by applying silver nitrate, while protecting the surrounding skin.

Herpes simplex virus (HSV) infections

Neonatal HSV infection is uncommon, occurring in 1 in 3000 to 1 in 20 000 live births. HSV infection is usually transmitted during passage through an infected birth canal or by ascending infection. Most infections are caused by HSV-2. The risk to an infant born to a mother with a primary genital infection is high, about 40%, while the risk from recurrent maternal infection is less than 3%. In most infants who develop HSV infection, the condition is unexpected as the mother's primary infection is asymptomatic or causes a non-specific illness.

The infection is more common in preterm infants. Presentation is at any time up to four weeks of age, with localised herpetic lesions on the skin or eye, or with encephalitis or disseminated disease. Mortality of localised disease is low, but of disseminated disease is high. If the mother is recognised as having primary disease or develops genital herpetic lesions at the time of delivery, elective Caesarean section is indicated. Women with a history of recurrent genital infection can be delivered vaginally as the risk of neonatal infection is very low. Giving acyclovir prophylactically to the baby during the at risk period has been advocated but its efficacy is unproven.

Hepatitis B

Infants of mothers who are hepatitis B surface antigen (HBsAg) positive should receive hepatitis B vaccination shortly after birth to prevent vertical transmission. The vaccination course needs to be completed during infancy and antibody response checked. Babies are at highest risk of becoming chronic carriers when their mothers are 'e' antigen positive but have no 'e' antibodies. Infants of 'e' antigen positive mothers should also be given passive immunisation with hepatitis B immunoglobulin within 24 hours of birth.

 Infants of hepatitis B surface antigen (HBsAg) positive mothers should be vaccinated against hepatitis B.

Neonatal seizures

Many babies startle or are slightly jittery. It can be difficult to differentiate this from seizures. Seizure activity may be tonic, clonic or more subtle, e.g. cycling movements of the limbs or apnoea and bradycardia. About 90% of cases have a detectable cause. An EEG is helpful in identifying seizures. The causes of seizures are listed in Figure 8.23.

Whenever seizures are suspected, a low blood glucose, calcium and sodium need to be excluded immediately. An intracranial ultrasound is performed to identify haemorrhage or cerebral malformations. A septic screen, including a lumbar puncture, will be needed to exclude meningitis unless a cause has been identified. Treatment is directed at the cause whenever possible. Ongoing or repeated seizures are treated with an anticonvulsant, though their efficacy in suppressing seizures is much poorer than in older children. The prognosis depends on the underlying cause.

Hypoglycaemia

There is no agreed definition of hypoglycaemia in the newborn. Many babies tolerate low blood glucose levels in the first few days of life as they are able to utilise lactate and ketones as energy stores. Recent evidence suggests that blood glucose levels above 2.6 mmol are desirable for optimal neurodevelopmental outcome, although during the first 24 hours after birth many asymptomatic infants have a blood glucose concentration below this level. There is good evidence that prolonged, symptomatic hypoglycaemia can cause permanent neurological disability.

Hypoglycaemia is particularly likely to occur in the first 24 hours of life in babies who are growth-retarded, preterm, born to mothers with diabetes mellitus, large for dates, hypothermic, polycythaemic or ill for any reason. Growth-retarded and preterm infants have poor glycogen stores, whereas the infants of diabetic mothers have sufficient glycogen stores but hyperplasia of the islet cells in the pancreas causing high insulin levels. Symptoms are jitteriness, irritability, apnoea, lethargy, drowsiness and seizures.

Hypoglycaemia can usually be prevented by early and frequent milk feeding. In infants at increased risk of hypogly-

---

Fig. 8.23 Causes of neonatal seizures.

Hypoxic-ischaemic encephalopathy/birth trauma
Septicaemia/meningitis
Metabolic
    hypoglycaemia
    hypo-/hypernatraemia
    hypocalcaemia
    hypomagnesaemia
    inborn errors of metabolism
    pyridoxine dependency
Intracranial haemorrhage
Cerebral malformations
Drug withdrawal, e.g. maternal opiates
Congenital infection
Kernicterus

caemia, blood glucose is regularly monitored at the bedside using a reagent strip. If this suggests that the blood glucose is low, a blood sample should be checked in the laboratory for confirmation, while treatment is initiated without delay. If the infant cannot be fed or becomes symptomatic, glucose is given by intravenous infusion. The concentration of the intravenous dextrose may need to be increased from 10% to 15% or even 20%, the latter concentration given via a central venous catheter. Resolution of the hypoglycaemia should be confirmed on repeat laboratory blood glucose measurement. Intravenous infusions with a high concentration of glucose need to be monitored carefully; if there is extravasation into the tissues there is a risk of reactive hypoglycaemia and skin necrosis. If there is difficulty or delay in starting the infusion, or a satisfactory response is not achieved, glucagon can be given. Glucocorticoids or intralipid are occasionally required to treat refractory hypoglycaemia.

Craniofacial disorders

CLEFT LIP AND PALATE

A cleft lip (Fig. 8.24a) may be unilateral or bilateral. It results from failure of fusion of the fronto-nasal and maxillary processes. In bilateral cases the premaxilla is anteverted. Cleft palate results from failure of fusion of the palatine processes and the nasal septum. Cleft lip and palate affect about 1.2 per 1000 babies. Most are inherited polygenically, but they may be part of a syndrome of multiple abnormalities, e.g. chromosomal defects. Some are associated with maternal anticonvulsant therapy. They may be detected on antenatal ultrasound scanning.

Surgical repair of the lip (Fig. 8.24b) may be performed within the first week of life for cosmetic reasons, although some surgeons feel that better results are obtained if surgery is delayed. The palate is usually repaired at several months of age. A cleft palate may make

feeding more difficult but some affected infants can still be breast-fed successfully. In bottle-fed babies, if milk enters the nose and causes choking, special teats and feeding devices may be helpful. Orthodontic advice and a dental prosthesis may help with feeding. Secretory otitis media is relatively common and should be sought on follow-up. Infants are also prone to acute otitis media. Adenoidectomy is best avoided as the resultant gap between the abnormal palate and nasopharynx will exacerbate feeding problems and the nasal quality of speech. A multidisciplinary team approach is required, involving plastic and ENT surgeons, paediatrician, orthodontist, audiologist and speech therapist. Parent support groups can provide valuable support and advice for families (Cleft Lip and Palate Association, CLAPA).

PIERRE–ROBIN SYNDROME

The Pierre–Robin syndrome is an association of micrognathia (Fig. 8.25), posterior displacement of the tongue (glosoptosis) and midline cleft of the soft palate. There may be difficulty feeding and, as the tongue falls back, there is obstruction to the upper airways, which may result in cyanotic episodes. The infant may fail to thrive during the first few months. If there is upper airways obstruction, the infant may need to lie prone, allowing the tongue and small mandible to fall forward. Persistent obstruction can be treated using a nasopharyngeal tube. Eventually the mandible grows and these problems resolve. The cleft palate can then be repaired.

Gastrointestinal disorders

OESOPHAGEAL ATRESIA

Oesophageal atresia is usually associated with a tracheo-oesophageal fistula (Fig. 8. 26). It occurs in 1 in 3500 live births. It is associated with polyhydramnios during preg-

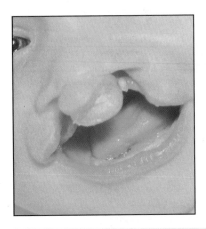
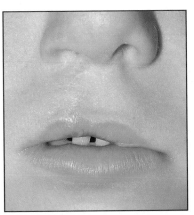
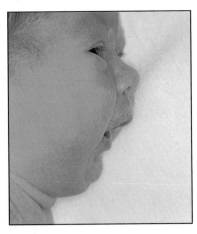

Fig. 8.24a, b Pre and post operation for cleft lip. Photographs showing the impressive results of surgery help many parents cope with the initial distress at having an affected infant. (Courtesy of Mr N Waterhouse.)

Fig. 8.25 Micrognathia in Pierre–Robin syndrome.

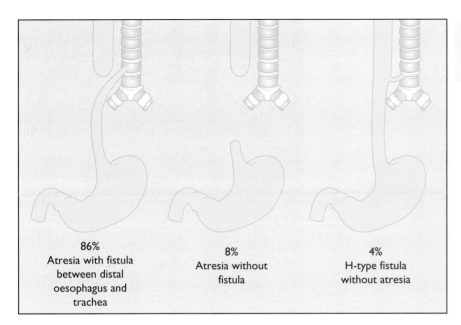

| 86%
Atresia with fistula
between distal
oesophagus and
trachea | 8%
Atresia without
fistula | 4%
H-type fistula
without atresia |

Fig. 8.26 Oesophageal atresia and tracheo-oesophageal fistula.

nancy. If there has been hydramnios during pregnancy, a wide-calibre feeding tube is passed and checked to see if it reaches the stomach. If not identified at birth, clinical presentation is with persistent salivation and drooling from the mouth after birth, associated with choking and cyanotic episodes. If the diagnosis is not made at this stage, the infant will cough, choke and vomit when fed. There will be aspiration into the lungs of saliva (or milk) from the upper airways and of acid secretions from the stomach. Almost half of the babies have other congenital malformations, e.g. as part of the VACTERL association (Vertebral, Ano-rectal, Cardiac, Tracheo-oesophageal, Renal and Radial Limb anomalies). In oesophageal atresia, a chest X-ray will confirm that a wide-calibre feeding tube fails to reach the stomach. Suction is applied to the nasogastric tube pending transfer to a neonatal surgical unit.

SMALL BOWEL OBSTRUCTION

This may be recognised antenatally on ultrasound scanning. Otherwise, small bowel obstruction presents with persistent vomiting, which is bile-stained unless the obstruction is above the ampulla of Vater. Meconium may initially be passed, but subsequently its passage is usually delayed or absent. Abdominal distension becomes increasingly prominent the more distal the bowel obstruction. High lesions will present soon after birth, but lower obstruction may not present for some days.

Small bowel obstruction may be caused by:

- atresia or stenosis of the duodenum (Fig. 8.27) – a third of such babies have Down syndrome and it is also associated with other congenital malformations
- atresia or stenosis of the jejunum or ileum – there may be multiple atretic segments of bowel
- malrotation with volvulus – a dangerous condition as it may lead to infarction of the entire mid-gut

- meconium ileus – thick inspissated meconium, of putty-like consistency, becomes packed into the lower ileum. Almost all affected neonates have cystic fibrosis
- meconium plug – a plug of inspissated meconium causes lower intestinal obstruction.

The diagnosis is made on clinical features and abdominal X-ray showing intestinal obstruction. Atresia or stenosis of the bowel and malrotation are treated surgically, after correction of fluid and electrolyte depletion. A meconium plug will usually pass spontaneously. Meconium ileus may be dislodged using gastrograffin contrast medium.

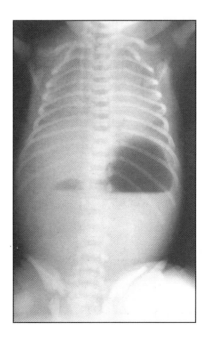

Fig. 8.27 Abdominal X-ray in duodenal atresia showing a 'double-bubble' from distension of the stomach and duodenal cap. There is absence of air distally.

LARGE BOWEL OBSTRUCTION

This may be caused by:

*   Hirschsprung disease – absence of the myenteric nerve plexus in the rectum which may extend along the colon. The baby often does not pass meconium within 48 hours of birth and subsequently the abdomen distends. About 15% present with acute enterocolitis (*see* Chapter 11)
*   rectal atresia – absence of the anus at the normal site. Lesions are high or low, depending whether the bowel ends above or below the levator ani muscle. In high lesions there is a fistula to the bladder or urethra in boys or the vagina or bladder in girls. Treatment is surgical.

  Bile-stained vomiting is from intestinal obstruction until proved otherwise.

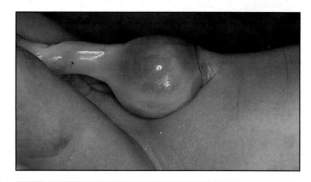

Fig. 8.28 Small exomphalos, with loops of bowel confined to the umbilicus. Care needs to be taken not to put a cord clamp across these lesions!

EXOMPHALOS/GASTROSCHISIS

These lesions are often diagnosed antenatally (see Chapter 7). In exomphalos, the abdominal contents protrude through the umbilical ring, covered with a transparent sac formed by the amniotic membrane and peritoneum (Fig. 8.28). It is often associated with other major congenital abnormalities. In gastroschisis the bowel protrudes through a defect in the anterior abdominal wall, adjacent to the umbilicus, and there is no covering sac. It is not associated with other congenital abnormalities.

At birth, the abdomen of affected infants should be wrapped in several layers of cling-film to minimise fluid and heat loss. A nasogastric tube is passed and aspirated frequently and an intravenous infusion of dextrose established. Colloid support is often required to replace protein loss into the bowel. Many lesions can be repaired by primary closure of the abdomen. With large lesions, the intestine is enclosed in a silastic sac sutured to the edges of the abdominal wall, and the contents gradually returned into the peritoneal cavity.

FURTHER READING

Klaus MH, Fanaroff AA. *Care of the High-risk Neonate*. 4th ed. Saunders, Philadelphia, 1993. Short textbook.
Roberton NRC. *Textbook of Neonatology*. 2nd ed. Churchill Livingstone, Edinburgh, 1992. Comprehensive textbook.

CHAPTER 9

Growth and Puberty

• Short stature • Tall stature • Abnormal head growth • Precocious puberty • Delayed puberty
• Disorders of sexual differentiation

Growth in children occurs in three phases.

1. Infant phase
Mainly determined by adequate nutrition, but insulin, the insulin-like growth factors (e.g. IgF II) and thyroxine are also important. Full responsiveness to growth hormone only develops in late infancy. This phase is characterised by an extremely rapid growth rate. Inadequate weight gain or growth failure in this period is usually referred to as 'failure to thrive'.

2. Childhood phase
Requires normal thyroid and growth hormone activity as well as adequate nutrition. It is the main determinant of final height as it lasts longer than other phases although the growth rate is slower.

3. Pubertal growth spurt
From the interaction of sex steroids, especially testosterone and oestradiol, and growth hormone. Growth ceases when the growth plate is eradicated by the fusion of the epiphysis and bone shaft of the long bones.

Growth parameters which should be routinely measured are:
- weight – which is readily and accurately determined with electronic scales
- height – reliable equipment must be used and attention paid to detail for accurate measurements (Fig. 9.1). In children under two years old, length is measured lying horizontally (Fig. 9.2). Accurate length measurement can be difficult to obtain as the legs need to be held straight and infants often dislike being held still. For this reason, there has been debate about the routine measurement of length in child surveillance, but it should always be performed whenever there is doubt about an infant's growth
- head circumference – the occipito-frontal circumference is measured routinely during infancy as a measure of brain growth and overall size.

Serial measurements of growth parameters should be plotted on a centile chart. In the UK, updated growth charts (see Appendix) have been published taking account of the population becoming slightly taller with time (secular trend). In addition, new lines have been added at the 0.4th and 99.6th centiles (representing 4/1000 children), as children with heights outside these centiles are more likely to have an organic cause for their short or tall stature. Puberty follows a well-defined sequence of changes (Figs 9.3a–c and 9.4). Disruption of this sequence is called dissonance.

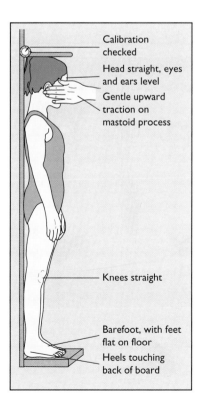

Calibration checked

Head straight, eyes and ears level

Gentle upward traction on mastoid process

Knees straight

Barefoot, with feet flat on floor

Heels touching back of board

Fig. 9.1 Measuring height accurately in children. The eyes and ears need to be level, knees straight, heels touching the back of the board and feet flat on the foot board. Gentle upward traction is applied to the mastoid process

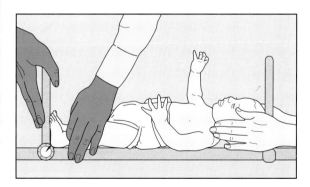

Fig. 9.2 Measuring length in infants and young children. An assistant is required to hold the legs straight and as flat as possible. The head needs to be held straight against the headboard, the feet flat against the moving footboard.

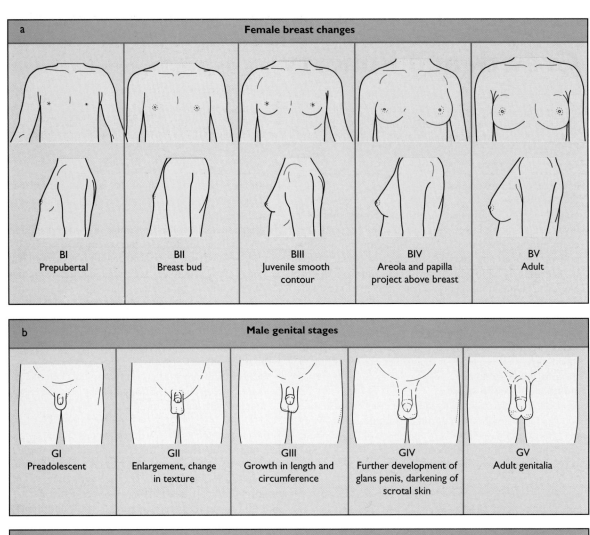

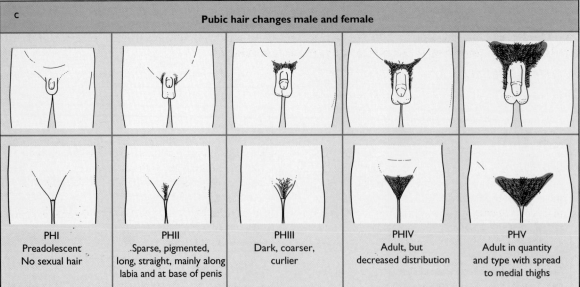

Fig. 9.3a–c Schematic drawings of male and female stages of puberty, as described by Tanner.

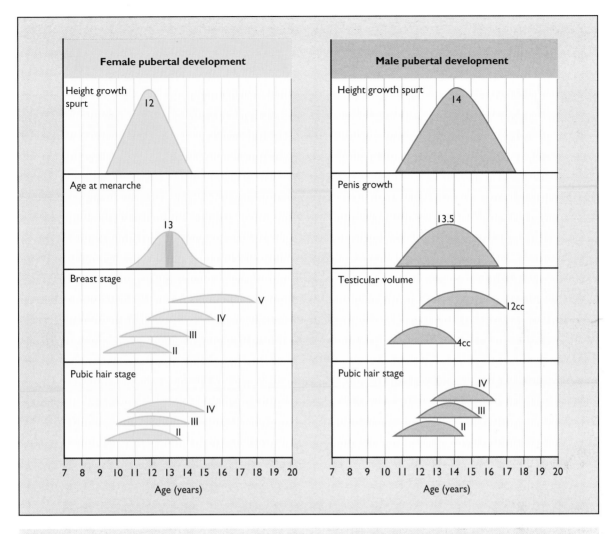

Fig. 9.4 Schematic representation of the timing of pubertal changes in males and females. Pubertal changes are shown according to the Tanner stages of puberty. (Diagrams based on Zitelli BJ, Davis HW. Atlas of Pediatric Physical Diagnosis. 2nd. ed. Lippincott, Philadelphia, 1992; and on Johnson TR, Moore WM, Jeffries JE. Children are Different; Developmental Physiology. 2nd. ed. Columbus, OH, Ross Laboratories, Division of Abbott Laboratories, 1978, pp. 26–29).

In females the features of puberty are:
- breast development, the first sign, which usually occurs between nine and 13 years, with a median of 11.5 years
- the height spurt which reaches its maximum early in puberty, before menarche
- menarche, which occurs between 11 and 15 years, with a median age of 13 years
- an increase of only about 4% of final height after menarche.

In males:
- the first sign of puberty is testicular growth, which usually starts between 10 and 15 years, with a median age of 12 years. A testicular volume greater than 4 ml indicates the onset of puberty

- the maximum height spurt is reached about two years later than in girls, at about 14 years. It occurs when the testicular volume is 12–15 ml
- the final height is greater than in females (Fig. 9.5).

When there is abnormal pubertal development this is further assessed by:
- clinical staging
- testicular volume assessment using an orchidometer in boys (Fig. 9.6)
- pelvic ultrasound to assess uterine size and endometrial thickness in girls
- bone age to determine skeletal maturation.

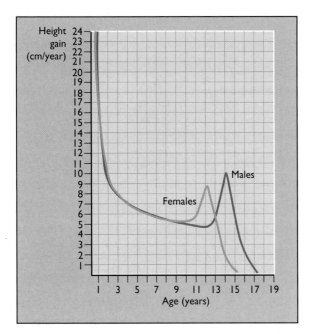

Fig. 9.5 Male and female height velocity charts (50th centile) showing that adult males are taller than females as they have a longer childhood growth phase, their peak height velocity is higher and their growth ceases later.

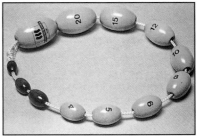

Fig. 9.6 Orchidometer to assess testicular volume (in ml).

Short stature

Short stature is usually defined as a height below the second or third centile (approximately two standard deviations below the mean). Most such children will be normal though short. The further the child is below the third

centile, the more likely there will be a pathological cause. Serial measurements are the most helpful, as they allow detection of a change in the rate of growth. Growth failure can be identified from the child's growth parameters falling across centile lines plotted on a growth chart. In this way growth failure may be identified even though the child's height is still above the second or third centile.

Measuring height velocity is a sensitive indicator of growth failure. A minimum of two accurate measurements is required, at least six months apart and preferably at a year's interval. The difference between two measurements is adjusted to cms/year (e.g. multiply by two if measured at six-monthly intervals) and plotted at the mid-point in

Familial

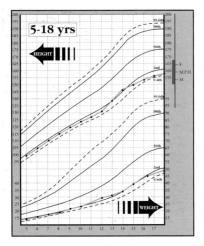

Fig. 9.7a Growth chart of familial short stature. The parent's height centiles are plotted and mid parental height (MPH) calculated.

Constitutional delay of growth and puberty

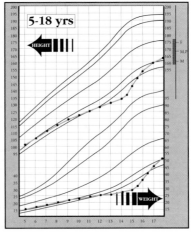

Fig. 9.7b Growth chart of constitutional delay.

Nutritional/chronic illness

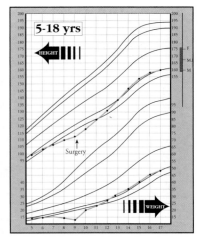

Fig. 9.7c Growth chart of nutritional short stature in a child with Crohn disease, showing catch-up growth following bowel surgery.

time. A height velocity persistently below the 25th centile is abnormal. A disadvantage of using height velocity calculations is that they are highly dependent on the accuracy of the height measurements.

Comparing height and weight in children may give useful clues towards the underlying aetiology. A discrepancy of more than two centile lines (e.g. height above 25th centile, weight below third centile) warrants further assessment. Children suffering from malnutrition or chronic illness, particularly gastrointestinal, are usually short and underweight. In contrast, hormonal causes of short stature, e.g. hypothyroidism, growth hormone deficiency or steroid excess, are often associated with the child being somewhat overweight.

Short stature may cause psychological problems. Affected children may be teased and bullied, develop poor self-esteem and are at a considerable disadvantage in competitive sport. They are also assumed by adults to be younger than their true age and are treated inappropriately. However, many short children are well adjusted psychologically to their size.

Causes (see Figs 9.7 a–f)

During infancy, when weight is the main growth parameter monitored, inadequate growth is considered as 'failure to thrive' (see Chapter 10). There are a number of causes of short stature.

Familial

This is the most common cause of short stature, though care needs to be taken that both the child and a parent do not have an inherited growth disorder. Allowance should be made for parental height. For a boy, 12.5 cm is added to his mother's height and the mean parental height calculated. For a girl, 12.5 cm is subtracted from the father's height in order to calculate the mid-parental height. The growth rate is normal.

Constitutional delay of growth and puberty

Some children are 'slow growers' and grow at a normal but slow rate. They have delayed skeletal maturity that can be demonstrated on bone age. They will also have delayed onset of puberty. Characteristically, there is a family history.

Nutritional/chronic illness

Some infants with severe intrauterine growth retardation and some very low birthweight infants remain short. Children may be underweight because they are normal but thin or from inadequate nutrition due to insufficient food, restricted diets or chronic illness, particularly of the gastrointestinal tract.

Emotional deprivation and psychological factors

Children subjected to physical and emotional deprivation may be small/underweight and show delayed puberty. It is difficult to differentiate from genetic short stature or constitutional delay of growth and puberty. Catch-up growth may be seen when placed in a nurturing environment.

Endocrine causes

Affected children have a slow growth rate.

1. Growth hormone deficiency

Causes are:

- isolated
- abnormal growth hormone secretory patterns
- pituitary deficiency – developmental or damage at breech delivery

Growth hormone deficiency

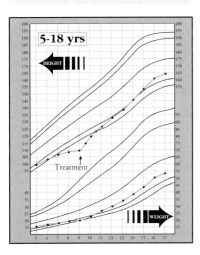

Fig. 9.7d Growth chart of a child with growth hormone deficiency, showing short stature and low height velocity.

Hypothyroidism

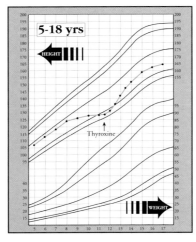

Fig. 9.7e Growth chart in hypothyroidism, showing cessation of growth until treatment is started.

Chromosomal disorders/syndromes

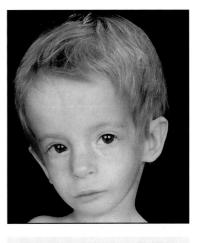

Fig. 9.7f Silver-Russell syndrome – intrauterine growth retardation, short stature, triangular facies with frontal bossing, shortened and incurved fifth fingers and hemihypertrophy of limbs.

- panhypopituitarism:
  - in association with mid-facial defects
  - secondary to a craniopharyngioma, hypothalamic tumour, cranial irradiation.

2. Hypothyroidism
Usually overweight but thyroid deficiency should be considered in any short child.

3. Cushing syndrome/steroid excess
Cushing syndrome is very unusual in childhood. Systemic corticosteroid therapy is a potent growth suppressor. This effect is greatly reduced by alternate day therapy.

Chromosomal disorders/syndromes
Many chromosomal disorders and syndromes are associated with short stature, e.g. Down, Turner and Silver–Russell syndromes. There are specific centile charts for children with the commoner syndromes.

Disproportionate short stature
Examples of disproportionate short stature are achondroplasia and other bone dysplasias and mucopolysaccharidoses.
It is confirmed by measuring:
- arm span – from tips of the fingers of one hand to the other
- sitting height – base of spine to top of head
- sub-ischial leg length – subtraction of sitting height from total height.

Investigations
Plotting present and previous heights and weights on appropriate growth charts, together with the clinical features, usually allows the cause to be identified. Bone age (Fig. 9.8) is helpful as it is markedly delayed in some endocrine disorders, e.g. hypothyroidism, and is used to estimate adult height potential.

Relatively few children will have an endocrine cause for short stature:
- thyroid function tests will identify hypothyroidism
- diagnosis of growth hormone deficiency is difficult because of the pulsatile nature of growth hormone secretion. In pituitary provocation tests, a variety of stimuli are used to provoke growth hormone release. The most common are clonidine, glucagon and insulin-induced hypoglycaemia. The hypoglycaemia induced by insulin is potentially dangerous and excessive correction with hypertonic glucose solutions can be fatal. To avoid these complications, the test should only be performed in specialist centres. Provocation tests can be misleading, with false positive and negative results. In particular, children with constitutional growth delay may not respond normally. An alternative strategy is to take regular blood samples overnight to assess spontaneous growth hormone production, but this is more complicated to perform. Urinary growth hormone measurement may also be of value.

Treatment of endocrine causes
Hypothyroidism – is treated with thyroxine replacement therapy.
Growth hormone deficiency is treated with biosynthetic

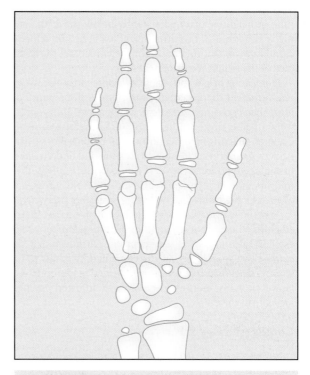

Fig. 9.8 Diagram of an X-ray of the left wrist and hand to determine bone age. It allows assessment of skeletal maturation from the time of appearance or maturity of the epiphyseal centres, using a standardised rating system. The child's height can be compared with skeletal maturation and an adult height prediction made.

growth hormone which is given by subcutaneous injection, usually daily. The best response is seen in patients with the most severe hormone deficiency. There is no longer a risk of transmission of prion diseases, e.g. Creutzfelt–Jacob disease, which unfortunately occurred in a number of instances before 1985 when cadaveric growth hormone was used. Other potential applications of growth hormone therapy under study include Turner syndrome, intrauterine growth retardation, chronic illness, e.g. chronic renal failure and catabolic states, e.g. burns.

Tall stature

Tall stature is a less frequent problem than short stature as there are social advantages in being tall. The disadvantage for younger children is that they are treated as older than they actually are. Adolescent girls may become concerned about excessive height during their pubertal growth spurt. The causes of excessive growth or tall stature are listed in Figure 9.9.

Excess growth in girls can be treated with oestrogen therapy to induce premature fusion of the epiphyses, but as it produces variable results it is seldom undertaken.

Fig. 9.9 Causes of excessive growth or tall stature	
Familial	Most common cause
Hormonal	Excess adrenal androgen steroids (congenital adrenal hyperplasia)
	Excess sex steroids (precocious puberty)
	Excess growth hormone from a pituitary secretory adenoma (very rare).
	Hyperthyroidism
Syndrome:	Marfan syndrome, homocystinuria
	Klinefelter syndrome (47 XXY)
	Sotos syndrome – cerebral gigantism associated with large hands and feet, facial features and mild learning difficulties
	Beckwith syndrome.

ASYMMETRIC HEADS

Skull asymmetry may result from an imbalance of the growth rate at the coronal, sagittal or lambdoid sutures although the head circumference increases normally. Plagiocephaly, a parallelogram-shaped head, may be seen in infants from asymmetric posture. It improves with time as the child becomes more mobile. Plagiocephaly is also seen in infants with neuromuscular disorders. Preterm infants may develop long, flat heads (Fig. 9.11).

CRANIOSYNOSTOSIS

The sutures of the skull bones do not finally fuse until about 12 years of age. Premature fusion of a suture (craniosynostosis) may lead to distortion of the head shape (Fig. 9.12). The fused suture may be felt or seen as a palpable ridge and confirmed on skull X-ray or cranial CT scan. If necessary, the condition can be treated surgically because of raised intracranial pressure or for cosmetic reasons. Such operations are performed in specialist centres for craniofacial reconstructive surgery (Fig. 9.13).

Abnormal head growth

Head growth in childhood largely reflects brain growth, but head size may be familial and is affected by the thickness of the skull. 80% of adult head size is achieved before the age of five years. The anterior fontanelle varies considerably in size at birth and is usually closed by 12–18 months of age.

MICROCEPHALY

Microcephaly, a head circumference below the third centile with abnormally slow head growth may be:
- familial, when it is not associated with developmental delay
- an autosomal recessive condition, where it is associated with severe learning difficulties
- caused by a congenital infection
- caused by an insult to the brain, e.g. perinatal hypoxia or neonatal meningitis resulting in loss of brain tissue from infarction. In these circumstances, microcephaly is often accompanied by cerebral palsy, seizures and visual impairment.

MACROCEPHALY

Macrocephaly is a head circumference above the 97th centile and excessive head growth. The head circumference may rapidly cross centile lines in infants experiencing catch up growth in the first few months of life, especially those born preterm or small for gestational age.

The causes of a large head are listed in Figure 9.10. Most are normal, tall children. Progressive hydrocephalus must be identified as quickly as possible in order to initiate treatment. It is suggested by the head circumference crossing centile lines or deviating upwards from the 97th centile. There may be a bulging fontanelle, but this may be absent initially or if the hydrocephalus has arrested. When the anterior fontanelle is still open, cranial ultrasound allows assessment of ventricular size, otherwise a cranial CT or MR scan is needed.

Fig. 9.10 Causes of a large head
Tall stature
Familial macrocephaly
Hydrocephalus – progressive or arrested
Chronic subdural haematomas
Macrocephaly with severe learning difficulties and cerebral gigantism (Sotos syndrome)
Neurofibromatosis
Cerebral tumour
CNS storage disorders, e.g. mucopolysaccharidoses (Hurler syndrome)

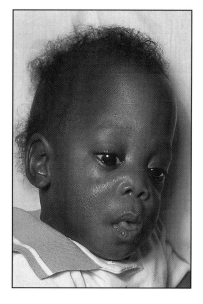

Fig. 9.11 Long flat head of a preterm infant. This can be avoided by lying preterm infants on a soft surface and regularly changing their head position.

Fig. 9.12 Forms of craniosynostosis	
Localised	Coronal suture only – asymmetrical skull
	Sagittal suture only – a long narrow skull
Generalised	Multiple sutures resulting in microcephaly and developmental delay
	Genetic syndromes,
	e.g. with syndactyly in Apert syndrome,
	with exophthalmos in Crouzon syndrome

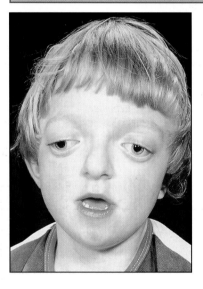

Fig. 9.13 Crouzon syndrome showing the typical shallow orbits and exophthalmos. Craniofacial reconstructive surgery is required to prevent visual loss and cerebral damage from raised intracranial pressure.

Precocious puberty

The development of secondary sexual characteristics before eight years in females and nine years in males is outside the normal range. It may be due to:
- precocious puberty, when it is accompanied by a growth spurt
- premature breast development (thelarche)
- premature pubic hair development (adrenarche).

Precocious puberty may be categorised according to the levels of the pituitary-derived gonadotrophins, follicle stimulating hormone (FSH) and luteinizing hormone (LH), as:
- gonadotrophin dependent (central, true) from premature activation of the hypothalamic–pituitary–gonadal axis
- gonadotrophin independent (pseudo, false) from excess sex steroids.

Precocious puberty in females
This is usually idiopathic or familial and follows the normal sequence of puberty. Organic causes (Fig. 9.14) are rare and are associated with:
- dissonance, e.g. isolated pubic hair with virilisation of

the genitalia suggesting excess androgens either from congenital adrenal hyperplasia or an androgen secreting tumour
- rapid onset
- neurological symptoms and signs, e.g. neurofibromatosis.

McCune–Albright syndrome is a rare cause of precocious puberty, usually in females, where there is a mutation in a protein subunit controlling cyclic AMP in cells. There is:
- skin hyperpigmentation, with cafe-au-lait patches
- fibrous dysplasia of bone, identified as radiolucent long bones. Affected children may present with pathological bone fractures
- endocrine overactivity involving the ovary, thyroid, adrenal and pituitary.

Ultrasound examination of the ovaries and uterus is helpful in establishing the cause of precocious puberty. In the premature onset of normal puberty, multicystic ovaries and an enlarging uterus will be identified.

 Precocious puberty in females is usually due to the premature onset of normal puberty.

Precocious puberty in males
This is uncommon and usually has an organic cause, particularly intracranial tumours. Examination of the testes may be helpful:
- bilateral enlargement suggests gonadotrophin release, usually from an intracranial lesion
- prepubertal testes suggests an adrenal cause (e.g. a tumour or adrenal hyperplasia)
- a unilateral enlarged testis suggests a gonadal tumour.

Tumours in the hypothalamic region are best investigated by cranial MR scan.

 Precocious puberty in males usually results from a brain tumour.

Fig. 9.14 Causes of precocious puberty
Gonadotrophin dependent (↑FSH, ↑LH)
Idiopathic/familial
CNS abnormalities
Congenital anomalies, e.g. hydrocephalus
Acquired, e.g. post irradiation, infection, surgery
Tumours, e.g. microscopic hamartomas
Hypothyroidism
Gonadotrophin independent (↓FSH, ↓LH, rare)
McCune-Albright syndrome
Adrenal disorders – tumours, congenital adrenal hyperplasia
Ovarian – tumour (granulosa cell)
Testicular – tumour (Leydig cell)
Exogenous sex steroids

Management

The management of precocious puberty is directed towards:

- detection and treatment of any underlying pathology, e.g. intracranial tumour in males
- reducing the rate of skeletal maturation if necessary. Skeletal maturation is assessed by bone age. An early growth spurt may result in early cessation of growth and a reduction in adult height
- addressing psychological/behaviour difficulties associated with early progression through puberty.

Deciding whether to treat a girl who is simply going through puberty early needs consideration of all these factors. If treatment is required for gonadotrophin dependent disease, gonadotrophin releasing hormone (GnRH) analogues are the treatment of choice. In gonadotrophin independent cases, the source of excess sex steroids needs to be identified. Inhibitors of androgen or oestrogen production or action may be used.

PREMATURE BREAST DEVELOPMENT (THELARCHE)

This is relatively common and usually affects females between six months and two years of age (Fig. 9.15). The breast enlargement may be asymmetrical. It is differentiated from precocious puberty by the absence of axillary and pubic hair and of a growth spurt. It is self-limiting and investigations are not usually required.

PREMATURE ADRENARCHE

This occurs when pubic hair develops before eight years of age in females and before nine years in males but with no other signs of sexual development. It is more common in Asian and Afro-Caribbean children. There may be a slight increase in growth rate. It is usually self-limiting but an adrenal tumour may need to be excluded.

Delayed puberty

Delayed puberty is often defined as the absence of pubertal development by 14 years of age in females and 15 years in males. The causes of delayed puberty are listed in Figure 9.16. In contrast to precocious puberty, the problem is more common in males, in whom it is mostly due to constitutional delay. Affected males are short during childhood and have delayed skeletal maturity on bone age. There is often a family history of delayed puberty in a parent. Eventually, puberty will occur and a near predicted height attained as growth will continue for longer than his peers. The boys may suffer from teasing, poor self-esteem and do badly in competitive sports. Assessment includes:

- pubertal staging
- identification of chronic systemic disorders
- karyotype if indicated
- gonadotrophin, sex steroid and thyroid hormone levels if required. These investigations will identify if the gonadotrophin levels are high or low.

The aims of management are to:

- identify and treat any underlying cause
- ensure normal psychological adaptation to puberty and adulthood
- accelerate growth and promote entry into puberty if necessary.

Fig. 9.16 Causes of delayed puberty	
Low gonadotrophin secretion	
Constitutional	Familial
	Sporadic
Systemic disease	Cystic fibrosis, severe asthma, Crohn disease, organ failure, anorexia nervosa, starvation, excess physical training
Hypothalamo-pituitary disorders	Acquired hypothyroidism
	Panhypopituitarism
	Isolated gonadotrophin or growth hormone deficiency
	Intracranial tumours (including craniopharyngioma)
	Kallmann syndrome (GnRH deficiency and inability to smell)
High gonadotrophin secretion	
Chromosomal abnormalities	Klinefelter syndrome (47, XXY)
Gonadal dysgenesis/agenesis	Turner syndrome (45, XO)
Steroid hormone enzyme deficiencies	
Acquired gonadal disease	Post surgery, chemotherapy, radiotherapy, trauma, torsionof the testis, autoimmune disorder

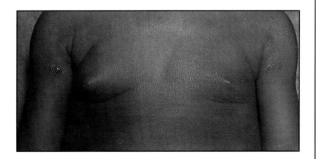

Fig. 9.15 Premature breast development in a 14-month-old girl. The absence of a growth spurt and axillary and pubic hair differentiates it from precocious puberty. It often resolves.

Following reassurance that puberty will occur, treatment is often not required. Should treatment be wanted, oral oxandrolone can be used in males. This weakly androgenic anabolic steroid will induce a growth spurt but not secondary sexual characteristics. Low-dose testosterone will accelerate growth as well as inducing secondary sexual characteristics. Females may be treated with ethinyloestradiol or oxandrolone.

Disorders of sexual differentiation

The fetal gonad is initially undifferentiated (Fig. 9.17). In the male, there is a testis determining gene on the Y chromosome (SRY antigen) which is responsible for differentiation of the gonad into a testis. In its absence the gonads become ovaries and the genitalia female. Testosterone produces development of male internal genitalia and its metabolite, dihydrotestosterone, the external genitalia. When an error occurs in this process there may be uncertainty about the sex of a newborn infant (hermaphroditism) and ambiguous external genitalia. The genitalia may range from those of an inadequately developed male to a virilised female.

The most common cause of ambiguous genitalia is congenital adrenal hyperplasia leading to a virilised female. The condition needs to be promptly identified as it may result in adrenal failure in the neonatal period.

Inadequate virilisation of the male can rarely arise from an inability to convert testosterone to dihydrotestosterone (5-alpha-reductase deficiency) or from androgen receptor defects. There are a number of syndromes in which the genitalia are poorly virilised in the male, e.g. Prader–Willi syndrome.

When the genitalia are ambiguous a definite sex cannot and should not be ascribed immediately. The cause of the intersex needs to be identified, the genitalia carefully assessed regarding future development and potential child-rearing and the family given counselling.

Chromosomal analysis, ultrasound imaging of the internal genitalia and adrenal glands and adrenal steroid measurements are undertaken. While the karyotype is vital for diagnosis it does not necessarily indicate the sex of rearing.

In many intersex conditions it is preferable to raise the child as a female, as it is possible to fashion female external genitalia, whereas it is not possible to create surgically an adequately functioning penis.

 The most common cause of ambiguous genitalia in newborn infants is congenital adrenal hyperplasia leading to female virilisation.

CONGENITAL ADRENAL HYPERPLASIA

Congenital adrenal hyperplasia is a group of autosomal recessive disorders of adrenal steroid biosynthesis. Its incidence is about 1 in 10 000 births. Over 90% have a deficiency of the enzyme 21-hydroxylase which is needed for cortisol and aldosterone biosynthesis (Fig. 9.18). In the fetus the resulting cortisol deficiency stimulates the pituitary to produce ACTH. This also stimulates production of the adrenal androgens which are converted to testosterone. In female infants, this will result in virilisation of the external genitalia. Presentation is with:

- virilisation of the female external genitalia, with clitoral hypertrophy and variable fusion of the labia
- in the male, the penis may be enlarged and the scrotum pigmented, but these changes are difficult to detect
- salt losing adrenal crisis, at 1–3 weeks of age, with vomiting and weight loss, floppiness and circulatory collapse. About two-thirds of affected children are salt-losers
- neonatal death if the condition has not been recognised and treated
- tall stature in the first few years of life
- precocious puberty.

Whereas most females with congenital adrenal hyperplasia are recognised and treated at birth, male infants often present with a salt-losing crisis or may not be identified.

Diagnosis

This is made by finding markedly raised levels of the metabolic precursor, 17-hydroxyprogesterone, in the blood. In salt-losers, the biochemical abnormalities are:

- low plasma sodium
- high plasma potassium
- metabolic acidosis
- hypoglycaemia in a salt-losing crisis.

Management

Although females with congenital adrenal hyperplasia may present with intersex, their internal genitalia are female and they should be reared as girls and are able to have children.

In a salt-losing crisis, the initial treatment is with intravenous saline and dextrose and intravenous hydrocortisone.

Long-term management is with:

- surgery during infancy to reduce clitoral size and reconstruct the vagina if abnormal
- steroid replacement for life. Glucocorticoid is given as hydrocortisone, usually three times daily (25 mg/m²/day), or prednisolone or dexamethasone in older children. Mineralocorticoid is given as fludrocortisone (0.05–0.1mg daily) if there is salt loss, and additional sodium chloride may be needed in infants
- monitoring growth, skeletal maturity and plasma androgens and 17-hydroxyprogesterone. Insufficient hormone replacement results in increased ACTH secretion and

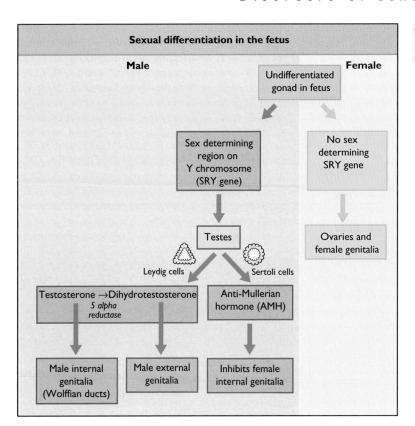

Fig. 9.17 Sexual differentiation in the fetus.

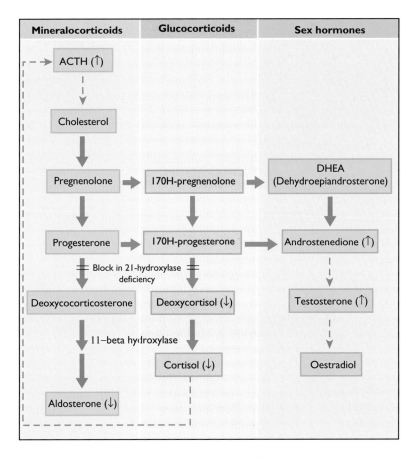

Fig. 9.18 Abnormal adrenal steroid biosynthesis in congenital adrenal hyperplasia.

androgen excess, which will cause rapid initial growth and skeletal maturation, at the expense of final height. Excessive hormonal replacement will result in skeletal delay and slow growth

- additional hormone replacement during illness or surgery.

Antenatal diagnosis and treatment are possible when a couple have had a previously affected child. If the affected fetus is female, dexamethasone may be given to the mother to reduce fetal ACTH drive and reduce the virilisation of affected females.

Other variants

The next most common variant of congenital adrenal hyperplasia is 11-betahydroxylase deficiency, which causes virilisation, salt retention and hypertension. Other variants mainly present with ambiguous genitalia.

 Salt-losing adrenal crisis needs urgent treatment with glucose and saline given intravenously.

Case History

AMBIGUOUS GENITALIA AT BIRTH

The appearance of this newborn infant's genitalia is shown in Figure 9.19.
Investigation revealed:

- a normal female karyotype, 46XX
- the presence of a uterus on ultrasound examination
- a markedly raised plasma 17-hydroxyprogesterone concentration, obtained some days later, confirming congenital adrenal hyperplasia.

After detailed explanation with her parents, she was started on oral hydrocortisone replacement therapy. Plasma electrolytes were checked every few days for the first four weeks to check for salt loss, which was absent. Surgery was performed to reduce clitoral size and separate the labia.

 Severe hypospadias and bilateral undescended testes – a male or virilised female? The karyotype is required.

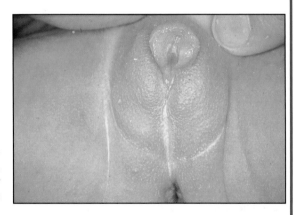

Fig. 9.19 *Ambiguous genitalia at birth. Investigation established that this was a female infant with congenital adrenal hyperplasia causing clitoral hypertrophy with fusion of the labia.*

FURTHER READING

Brook CGD. *A Guide to the Practice of Paediatric Endocrinology*. Cambridge University Press, Cambridge, 1993. A short textbook.
Buckler JMH. *Growth Disorders in Children*. BMJ Publications, London, 1995. Short book.

Nutrition

Children need an adequate quantity and balance of food for optimal growth and development. If their nutritional intake is inadequate they will fail to gain or lose weight and will subsequently fail to grow in height. Prolonged or severe nutritional deficiency will result in malnutrition.

The nutritional vulnerability of infants and children

Infants and children are more vulnerable to under-nutrition than adults. There are a number of reasons for this.

1. Low nutritional stores
Newborn infants, particularly those born preterm, have poor stores of fat and protein (Fig. 10.1). The smaller the child, the smaller the calorie reserve and the shorter the period he is able to withstand starvation.

2. High nutritional demands for growth
The nourishment children require is greatest, per unit body size, in infancy (Fig. 10.2), because of their rapid growth during this period. At four months of age, 30% of an infant's energy intake is used for growth, but by one year of age this falls to 5% and by three years to 2%. Infants during the first six months of life are therefore at greater risk of growth failure from restricted energy intake than in later childhood. Even regular small deficits in early childhood will lead to a cumulative deficit in weight and height.

3. Rapid neuronal development
The brain grows rapidly during the last trimester of pregnancy and throughout the first two years of life. The complexity of interneuronal connections also increases substantially during this time, and the process appears to be sensitive to under-nutrition. Even modest energy deprivation during periods of rapid brain growth and differentiation is thought to lead to an adverse neurodevelopmental outcome. This is not surprising when one considers that, at birth, the brain accounts for approximately two-thirds of basal metabolic rate, and for about 50% at one year of age (Fig. 10.3). Many studies have drawn attention to the delayed development seen in children suffering from protein energy malnutrition due to inadequate food intake, although inadequate psychosocial stimulation may also contribute.

A child's nutrition may be compromised following an acute illness or surgery. After a brief anabolic phase, when catecholamine secretion is increased, the metabolic rate is increased and urinary nitrogen losses may be so great that it is impossible to achieve a positive nitrogen balance. Weight is lost, and the patient's energy requirements are considerably increased. After uncomplicated surgery this phase may

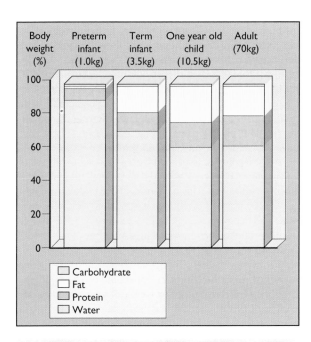

Fig. 10.1 Body composition of preterm and term infants, children and adults. Newborn infants, particularly the preterm, have poor stores of fat and protein.

Fig. 10.2 Reference values for energy and protein requirements		
Age	**Energy (kcal/kg/d)**	**Protein (g/kg/day)**
0–6 months	115	2.2
6–12 months	95	2.0
1–3 years	95	1.8
4–6 years	90	1.5
7–10 years	75	1.2
Adolescence		
11–14 years (males/females)	65/55	1.0
15–18 years	60/40	0.8

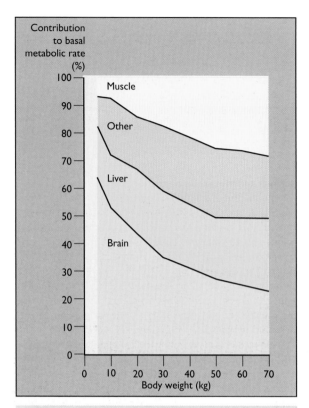

Fig. 10.3 *The relative contribution to basal metabolic rate derived from brain, liver and muscle changes with growth. Whereas the brain accounts for two-thirds of the basal metabolic rate at birth, this falls to 25% in adults. (Adapted from Halliday et al 1971)*

last for a week, but can last several weeks following extensive burns, complicated surgery or severe sepsis. Thereafter, previously lost tissue is replaced and positive energy and nitrogen balance can be obtained. However, infants may not show catch-up growth unless their energy intake is more than 150 kcal/kg/day and up to 200 kcal/kg/day.

Long-term outcome of early nutritional deficiency
Linear growth of populations
Growth and nutrition are closely related, such that the mean height of a population reflects nutritional status. Thus in the developed world people are getting taller. Height is adversely affected by lower socio-economic status and increasing numbers of children in families. Children's size increases among populations emigrating from poor to more affluent countries.

Disease in adult life
An association has been described between restricted growth during critical periods of development in fetal life and infancy with an increase in cardiovascular and obstructive lung disease in later life. For example, chronic obstructive lung disease in men is more common in those of low weight at one year of age. The same is true for ischaemic heart disease and its risk factors, such as blood pressure and plasma fibrinogen. Similarly, glucose tolerance is impaired in those adults who were of low birthweight and whose weight was low at one year of age.

Infant feeding

BREAST-FEEDING
There can be no doubt that breast milk is the best diet for babies, although the popularity of breast-feeding has frequently reflected the whim of fashion.
Advantages (Fig. 10.4)
In developing countries, where the environment is often highly contaminated, breast-feeding dramatically improves survival during infancy as a result of reduced gastrointestinal infection. Consequently, breast-feeding is one of the four most important World Health Organisation strategies for improving infant and child survival. While human milk is undoubtedly the preferred food for term infants, the superiority of breast milk over modern adapted cow's milk formulas has been difficult to prove in developed countries, despite exaggerated claims to the contrary. This is partly because it is impossible to conduct randomised studies and partly because of confounders such as social class, education and smoking.

There is convincing evidence that gastrointestinal infection is less common in breast-fed infants even in developed countries. There is also evidence that human milk feeds reduce the incidence of necrotising enterocolitis in preterm infants.

Many mothers who breast-feed find that it helps them establish an intimate, loving relationship with their baby. However, establishing breast-feeding is not always straightforward, and many mothers need help and encouragement.

Breast-feeding may confer an advantage in long-term neurological development in preterm infants, although the problem of allowing for other variables is considerable. The probable nutrients in breast milk for conferring this advantage are long chain polyunsaturated fatty acids. These have now been added to some formula feeds.

Breast-feeding is associated with a reduced incidence of inflammatory bowel disease and diabetes mellitus in children when they grow up. The incidence of breast cancer in mothers who breast-feed is reduced. Claims have not been substantiated that breast-feeding reduces the incidence of allergic disorders and sudden infant death syndrome.
Disadvantages (Fig. 10.5)
As one cannot readily tell how much milk a baby is taking from the breast, the baby's weight should be checked regularly, every few days in the first couple of weeks, then weekly until feeding is well established. Successful breast-feeding of twins can be achieved, but is more difficult (Fig. 10.6). It is rarely possible to breast-feed triplets and higher-order births totally. Preterm infants can be breast-fed, but the milk will need to be expressed from the breast until the infant can suck. Maintaining the supply of milk can be a problem for

Fig. 10.4 Why breast is best – the advantages of breast milk

Anti-infective properties
Humoral

Secretory IgA	Comprises 90% of immunoglobulin in human milk. Mucosal protection, but of uncertain benefit
Bifidus factor	Promotes growth of *Lactobacillus bifidus*, which metabolises lactose to lactic and acetic acids. The resulting low pH may inhibit growth of gastrointestinal pathogens
Lysozyme	Bacteriolytic enzyme
Lactoferrin	Iron-binding protein. Inhibits growth of *E. coli*
Interferon	Antiviral agent

Cellular

Macrophages	Phagocytic. Synthesise lysozyme, lactoferrin, C3, C4
Lymphocytes	T cells may transfer delayed hypersensitivity responses to infant. B cells synthesise IgA

Nutritional properties

Protein quality	More easily digested curd (60:40 whey/casein ratio)
Hypoallergenic	May reduce subsequent atopic disease. Conflicting evidence
Lipid quality	Rich in oleic acid (with palmitate in C-2 position). Improved digestibility and fat absorption
Breast milk lipase	Enhanced lipolysis
Calcium/phosphorus ratio of 2 : 1	Prevents hypocalcaemic tetany and improves calcium absorption
Low renal solute load	
Iron content	Bioavailable (40–50% absorption)
Long chain polyunsaturated fatty acids	Structural lipids, important in retinal development

Other advantages

Emotional	If successful, promotes close attachment between mother and baby
Contraceptive effects	Not a reliable contraceptive, but overall increases the time interval between children. Important in reducing birth rate in developing countries
Reduction in breast cancer	

Fig. 10.5 Disadvantages of breast-feeding

Unknown intake	Volume of milk intake not known
Transmission of infection	CMV, hepatitis and HIV from infected mother identified in breast milk and increase the risk of transmission to the baby
Breast milk jaundice	Mild, self-limiting, unconjugated hyperbilirubinaemia and not a contraindication
Transmission of drugs	Antithyroid drugs, cathartics, antimetabolites
Nutrient inadequacies	Prolonged breast-feeding without introduction of appropriate solids may lead to poor weight gain and rickets
Vitamin K deficiency	There is insufficient vitamin K in breast milk to prevent haemorrhagic disease of the newborn
Potential transmission of environmental contaminants	Nicotine, alcohol, caffeine etc
Less flexible	Other family members cannot help or take part. More difficult in public places
Emotional upset if unsuccessful	Breast-feeding can be problematic to establish. Difficulties or lack of success can be upsetting if determined to breast feed

mothers of preterm babies.

While two-thirds of mothers in the UK initially breast-feed, this proportion rapidly declines during the first few months (Fig. 10.7). Nearly 90% of social class I mothers start breast-feeding, but less than half of mothers from social class 5. Breast-feeding is restrictive for the mother as others cannot take charge of her baby for any length of time. This is particularly important if she goes to work.

Facilities for breast-feeding in public places are still limited. Although breast-feeding avoids the preparation needed for infant formulas, it is not necessarily cheaper for the family if it delays a mother returning to work.

 Exclusive breast-feeding in early infancy is life-saving in developing countries.

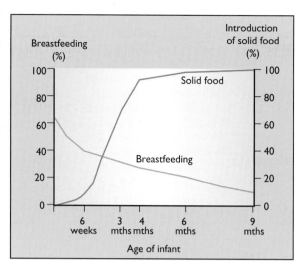

Fig. 10.7 Prevalence of breast-feeding and proportion of infants given solid feeds during the first nine month of life in the UK (1990).

Fig. 10.6 Successful breast-feeding of preterm twins.

Establishing breast-feeding

Colostrum, rather than milk, is produced for the first few days. Colostrum differs from mature milk in that the content of protein and immunoglobulin is much higher. Volumes are low but water or formula supplements are not required while the supply of breast milk is becoming established.

The first breast-feed should take place as soon as possible after birth. Subsequently, frequent suckling is beneficial as it enhances the secretion of the hormones initiating and promoting lactation.

Primates probably do not breast-feed instinctively. Monkeys bred in captivity in zoos have to be taught how to breast-feed by their keepers. It is therefore important that breast-feeding should have as high a profile as possible. Women who have never seen an infant being breast-fed are less likely to want to breast-feed themselves. Education in schools and during pregnancy about the advantages of breast-feeding is important. Advice and support from other women who have breast-fed may be important in dealing with early problems such as engorgement or cracked nipples.

'Bonding', a critical period shortly after birth in establishing a maternal–infant relationship is seen in many animals. In humans, there is no evidence for a similar critical period, and there is considerable flexibility in the timing and manner in which this close relationship develops.

FORMULA FEEDING

Infants who are not breast-fed require a formula feed based on cow's milk. Unmodified cow's milk is unsuitable for feeding in infancy, as it contains too much protein and electrolyte and inadequate iron and vitamins. Even after considerable modification, differences remain between formula feeds and breast milk (Fig. 10.8).

Most modern cow's milk-based formulas may be divided into two types, depending upon whether or not the casein to non-casein ratio has been modified by the addition of demineralised whey (soluble protein). A whey/casein ratio of 60 to 40 forms a smaller curd and provides an amino acid profile more like breast milk than a higher casein milk.

All milks currently available in the UK have been modified to make their mineral content and renal solute load comparable with that of mature human milk. Since these changes were introduced in the UK (in the 1970s), there has been an impressive reduction in the incidence of hypernatraemic dehydration in infants with gastroenteritis. There is no evidence that any of the many brands is superior to any other.

INTRODUCTION OF WHOLE PASTEURISED COW'S MILK

Breast or formula feeding is recommended until the age of six months, and there are advantages in continuing to 12 months of age. Pasteurised cow's milk is deficient in vitamins A, C and D and in iron, and if introduced in the first year will require supplements unless the infant is having a good diet of mixed solids. Alternatively, 'follow-on' formulas can be used from six months of age. They contain more protein and sodium than infant formulas and, in contrast to cow's milk, are fortified with iron and vitamins.

SOYA FORMULAS

Soya formulas have been widely used instead of cow's milk formulas in the belief that they may help prevent atopic

	Breast milk at term	Cow's milk	Infant formula (modified cow's milk)
Energy (kcal)	70	67	65–60
Protein (g)	1.3	3.5	1.5–1.9
Carbohydrate (g)	7.0	4.9	7.0–8.6
Casein : whey	40:60	63:37	40:60–63:37
Fat (g)	4.2	3.6	2.6–3.8
Sodium (mmol)	0.65	2.3	0.65–1.1
Calcium (mmol)	0.88	3.0	0.88–2.1
Phosphorus (mmol)	0.46	3.2	0.9–1.8
Iron (micromol)	1.36	0.9	8–12.5

Fig. 10.8 A comparison of human milk, cow's milk and infant formula (per 100 ml)

manifestations such as eczema or asthma, but there is no compelling evidence that their use leads to a reduced risk of these disorders. Although modern soya protein formulas are nutritionally adequate and support normal growth, there are a number of disadvantages associated with their use and they cannot be regarded as a satisfactory, routine alternative to cow's milk formulas. Approximately 20–30% of infants with cow's milk protein intolerance who are fed on a soya milk will subsequently develop clinical soya intolerance. Soya formulas contain a higher aluminium content, and the infants have lower serum immunoglobulin levels and a poorer response to vaccinations than those fed cow's milk formula.

WEANING

Solid foods are usually introduced between the ages of three and six months (see Fig. 10.7). Although human milk may be nutritionally adequate until six months of age, many babies will exhibit behavioural changes from three months, such as increased crying and poor sleeping, which may represent hunger and a need for solid food. After six months of age, breast milk becomes increasingly nutritionally inadequate, leading to deficiencies in energy, vitamins and iron.

Early weaning foods such as pureed cereals, fruit and vegetables tend to be high in energy, vitamins and minerals. Once babies can chew (at about six months), more lumpy foods and a variety of tastes and textures should be introduced. Added sugar and salt are best avoided in weaning foods because early exposure may produce bad dietary habits in later childhood and adult life.

Breast- or formula-fed infants obtain about half their energy from fat. After one year of age, whole cow's milk still provides a major contribution to the diet of most children. Some nutritionists have suggested that dietary fat intake should be reduced to supply less than 35% of energy requirements and fibre intake increased. The later introduction of solids, more breast-feeding and the fact that many weaning foods are gluten-free may be responsible for the reduction in the incidence of coeliac disease in infancy. Less gastroenteritis may also be a factor.

Failure to thrive

The term 'failure to thrive' is used to describe sub-optimal weight gain or growth in infants and toddlers. Recognition of the entity depends upon demonstration of inadequate weight gain when plotted on a centile chart, showing a consistent fall across two major centile lines (Fig. 10.9a,b). Changes in weight are compared with changes in head circumference in infants and/or in length. Repeated observations are therefore essential in making the diagnosis; a single observation is difficult to interpret unless it is well below the third centile or markedly discrepant from the head circumference or length. Weighing infants is of

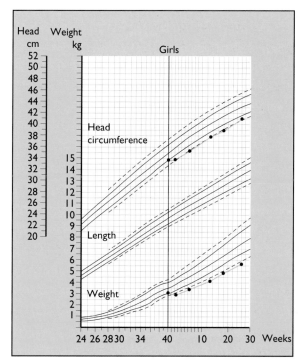

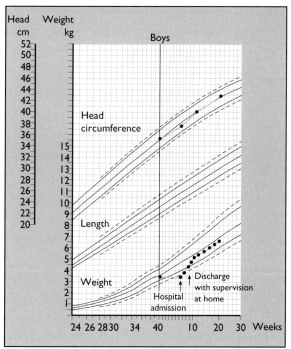

Fig. 10.9 Growth charts in failure to thrive. (a) Normal weight gain and growth in a constitutionally small child. The further below the third centile, the more likely there will be an organic cause. (b) This infant was referred by the health visitor as he was just below his birthweight at six weeks of age. His mother was 17 years old, single and unsupported, and developed postnatal depression. He gained weight in hospital on standard feeding.

relatively little value unless the weights are accurate and plotted on a centile chart.

Differentiating the infant who is failing to thrive from a normal but small or thin baby is often a problem. Normal but short infants have no symptoms, are alert, responsive and happy, and their development is satisfactory. The parents may be short (low mid-parental height) or the infant may have been extremely preterm or growth-retarded at birth. Any intercurrent illness will be accompanied by a temporary failure to gain weight. An additional diagnostic problem is 'catch-down' (as opposed to 'catch-up') weight. This is when an infant's weight falls from the birth centile, which is a product of the intrauterine environment, to a lower, genetically determined growth centile. These infants need only close monitoring of their growth over a few months.

It has been traditional to divide the causes of failure

Fig. 10.10 Some causes of failure to thrive

Organic

1. Inadequate intake of food

Primary undernutrition

    Breast-feeding – insufficient milk or poor technique (the infant may appear content)

    Bottle-feeding – too dilute (poverty may predispose to this)

    Food not available – incorrect feeding, not offered or famine

    Inability to feed – mechanical problem, e.g. cleft palate, lack of coordination in sucking and swallowing e.g. cerebral palsy

    Iatrogenic, e.g. exclusion diets, dietary fads

    Vomiting – gastro-oesophageal reflux, pyloric stenosis

Chronic illness causing anorexia

    Gastrointestinal – malabsorption, diarrhoea or vomiting

    Respiratory – cystic fibrosis

    Cardiac – congenital heart disease

    Renal – urinary tract infection, chronic renal failure, Renal tubular acidosis

2. Diminished absorption of food

Pancreatic disease – cystic fibrosis, Schwachman syndrome (pancreatic insufficiency, neutropenia and bony abnormalities)

Small intestinal disease – coeliac disease

Short gut (postoperative)

Protracted diarrhoea

3. Increased losses of protein from the gut (protein-losing enteropathy)

Intestinal lymphangiectasia

Milk protein intolerance

4. Increased energy requirements

Malignancy, cystic fibrosis

Severe burns/trauma

5. Metabolic

Hypothyroidism, congenital adrenal hyperplasia, amino acid and organic acid disorders

6. Miscellaneous

Chromosomal disorders, syndromes, congenital infection

Non-organic

Environmental deprivation:

    Maternal psychiatric illness

    Parental learning difficulties

    Parental low income, poor education, poor social support

---

to thrive into organic and non-organic (Fig. 10.10). Non-organic failure to thrive can be associated with a broad spectrum of psychosocial and environmental deprivation and is often accompanied by a delay in those aspects of development which rely on environmental stimulation, e.g. speech. It seems likely that under-nutrition is the final common pathway for poor weight gain in non-organic failure to thrive, usually from a combination of inadequate or inappropriate feeding as well as psychosocial factors. The mother may be depressed or have poor understanding of her baby's needs. This may even be part of the spectrum of child abuse. It is often accompanied by poor housing, poverty, inadequate social support and lack of an extended family which make good child care even more difficult. Some of the mothers may have eating disorders themselves.

Failure to thrive is a common reason for referral to a paediatrician. A careful history and examination is the key to its evaluation. Most can be managed without admission to hospital. While it is essential not to miss organic disease, it is equally important to make the diagnosis of non-organic failure to thrive on positive grounds, rather than exposing the infant to unnecessary investigations. Further information about the child and family from the health visitor, general practitioner or other professionals involved with the family can be particularly helpful. Hospital admission may occasionally be required for a period of assessment and observation of the child and family or when detailed investigations are required.

 Failure to thrive is a description and not a diagnosis.

Malnutrition

Worldwide, malnutrition is common and is responsible directly or indirectly for about half of all deaths of children under five years of age. Primary malnutrition also continues to occur in developed countries, as a result of poverty, parental neglect or poor education. Specific nutritional deficiencies, particularly of iron, also remain common. Restrictive diets may be iatrogenic or from parental food fads or self-inflicted.

Malnutrition is far from rare in hospital, affecting 20–40% of patients in a children's hospital. The chronically ill are at particular risk, especially preterm infants and those children with congenital heart disease or chronic gut or respiratory disorders. In these children, malnutrition may result from a combination of anorexia, malabsorption and increased requirements because of infection or inflammation. Anorexia nervosa and other feeding disorders cause malnutrition in older children and adolescents. The diencephalic syndrome, which is extremely rare, comprises severe protein-energy malnutrition in association with a cerebral tumour, usually of the hypothalamus. Food intake is often high, suggesting a possible defect in energy metabolism.

Assessment of nutritional status

Malnutrition must be recognised and accurately defined for rational decisions to be made about refeeding. Evaluation is divided into assessment of past and present dietary intake, anthropometry and laboratory assessments (Fig. 10.11).

Dietary assessment

Parents are asked to record as best they can all the food the child eats during several days. This gives a reasonably accurate assessment of habitual food intake. Children under 12 years are likely to give unreliable information if questioned directly.

Anthropometry

Regular growth measurements are valuable, as a fall off is one of the earliest indicators of incipient malnutrition. Height, weight, triceps skinfold thickness and mid-arm circumference are basic measures which permit a reasonably accurate assessment of nutritional status. The World Health Organisation recommends that nutritional status is expressed as:

- weight for height, a measure of wasting and an index of acute malnutrition (Fig. 10.12)
- height for age, a measure of stunting and an index of chronic malnutrition.

Subcutaneous fat stores can be assessed by measuring skinfold thickness, while upper arm circumference in conjunction with triceps skinfold thickness is an indication of skeletal muscle mass. However, it is difficult to measure skinfold thicknesses accurately in young children, so this reduces its use in reflecting short-term changes in body composition.

Laboratory investigations

These are useful in the detection of early physiological adaptation to malnutrition, but a clinical history, examination and anthropometry are of greater value than any single biochemical or immunological measurement.

Consequences of malnutrition

Malnutrition is a multi-system disorder. When severe, immunity is impaired, wound healing is delayed and operative morbidity and mortality increased. Malnutrition worsens the outcome of illness, e.g. respiratory muscle dysfunction may delay a child being weaned from mechanical ventilation. Malnourished children are less active, less exploratory and more apathetic. These behavioural abnormalities are rapidly reversed with proper feeding. Prolonged and profound malnutrition probably causes some permanent delay in intellectual development.

The role of intensive nutritional support

Malnutrition from many childhood disorders is due to inadequate nutrient intake and responds to tube feeding nasogastrically or by gastrostomy. Thus, malnourished children with cystic fibrosis, malignancy, inflammatory bowel disease, advanced liver disease, congenital heart disease, cerebral palsy and chronic renal failure will all grow if given supplementary enteral feeds. Other than in Crohn disease, whether such nutritional support alters prognosis or quality of life remains uncertain.

Assessment of nutritional status

Anthropometry
- Weight
- Height
- Mid-arm circumference
- Skinfold thickness

Laboratory
- Low plasma albumin
- Low concentration of specific minerals and vitamins

Food intake
- Dietary recall
- Dietary diary

Immunodeficiency
- Low lymphocyte count
- Impaired cell-mediated immunity

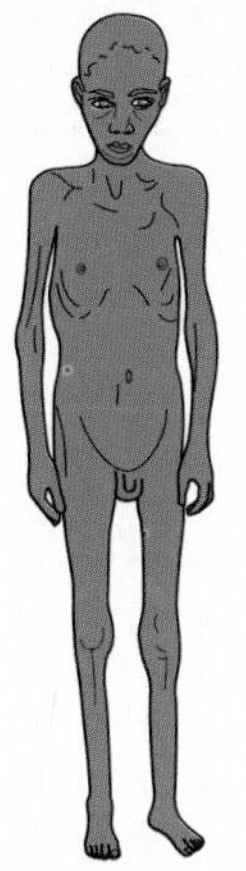

Fig. 10.11 Assessment of nutritional status. This cannot be determined by a single measurement, but is a composite of a number of variables.

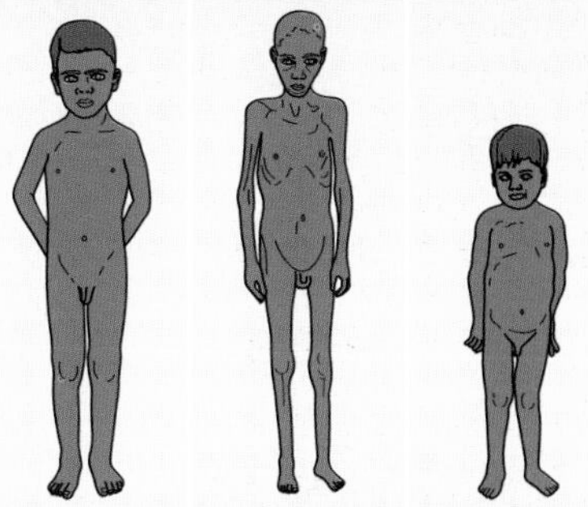

	Normal	Wasted	Stunted
Weight/age %	100	70	70
Weight/height%	100	70	100
Height/age %	100	100	84

Fig. 10.12 Comparison of a normal, wasted and stunted child at one year. Low weight for height reveals a child of normal height, but who is thin and wasted, whereas low height for age reveals a short, non-wasted child. (% is of expected value).

MARASMUS AND KWASHIORKOR

Severe protein-energy malnutrition in children usually leads to marasmus, with a weight less than 60% of the mean for age, and a wasted, wizened appearance (Fig. 10.13). Oedema is not present. Skin fold thickness and mid-arm circumference are markedly reduced and affected children are often withdrawn and apathetic.

Kwashiorkor is another manifestation of severe protein malnutrition (Fig. 10.14), in which body weight is 60–80% of expected and oedema is present. In addition, there may be:

- a 'flaky-paint' skin rash with hyperkeratosis and desquamation
- a distended abdomen and enlarged liver
- angular stomatitis
- hair which is sparse and depigmented
- diarrhoea, hypothermia, bradycardia and hypotension
- low plasma albumin, potassium, glucose and magnesium.

It is unclear why some children with protein energy malnutrition develop kwashiorkor and others develop marasmus. Kwashiorkor is a feature of children reared in traditional, polygamous societies, where infants are not weaned from the breast until about 12 months of age. The subsequent diet tends to be relatively high in starch. Kwashiorkor often develops after an acute intercurrent infection, such as measles or gastroenteritis. There is some evidence that kwashiorkor is a manifestation of primary protein deficiency with energy intake relatively well maintained, or alternatively that it results from excess generation of free radicals.

Management

Urgent treatment for severe malnutrition involves correcting dehydration, acid–base disturbance, hypocalcaemia and treating infection. Hypothermia is common and children require careful wrapping, particularly at night. Children with severe malnutrition are deficient in potassium and magnesium, and these should be supplemented. Diarrhoea is a frequent complication of refeeding, but parenteral nutrition is not usually required. Overzealous treatment with fluids may lead to

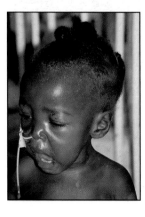

Fig. 10.13 Marasmus in a three-month-old baby from a developing country who was unable to establish breast-feeding because of a cleft palate.

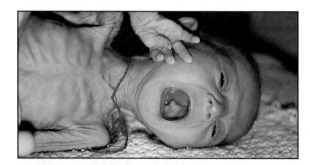

Fig. 10.14 Kwashiorkor, a particular manifestation of severe protein-energy malnutrition in some developing countries where infants are weaned late from the breast and the young child's diet is high in starch. There is hyperkeratosis and depigmentation of the skin and redness of the hair. (Courtesy of Dr Sharon Taylor.)

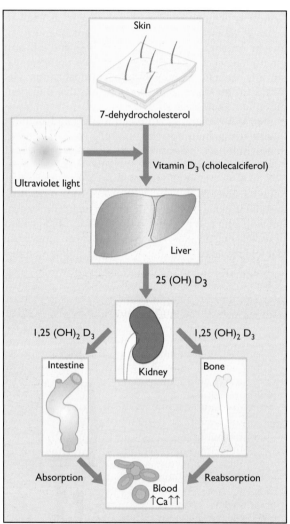

Fig. 10.15 Vitamin D metabolism. In most countries, sunlight is the most important source of vitamin D. Vitamin D is not abundant naturally in foods except in fish liver oils, fatty fish and egg yolk. Vitamin D_2 (ergocalciferol) is the form used to fortify foods such as margarine. Vitamin D_3 is hydroxylated in the liver and again in the kidney to produce 1-25 dihydroxy vitamin D ($1,25 (OH)_2D_3$), the most active form of the vitamin. It is produced following parathormone secretion in response to a low plasma calcium.

cardiac failure. In kwashiorkor, severe hypoglycaemia is frequently associated with coma, hypothermia and infection and carries a high mortality. Feeding 2–4 hourly, including during the night, has reduced the frequency of hypoglycaemia and the mortality. The overall mortality of severe malnutrition among children treated in hospital is about 30%.

Fig. 10.16 Causes of rickets

Nutritional (primary) rickets

Risk factors

 Living in northern latitudes

 Decreased exposure to sunlight, e.g. in some Asian children
  living in the UK

 Diets low in calcium, phosphorus and vitamin D,
  e.g. exclusive breast-feeding into late infancy or, rarely,
  toddlers on unsupervised 'dairy-free' diets

 Prolonged parenteral nutrition in infancy with an inadequate
  supply of parenteral calcium and phosphate

Intestinal malabsorption

Defective production of $25(OH)D_3$
 Liver disease

Increased metabolism of $25(OH)D_3$
 Enzyme induction by anticonvulsants

Defective production of $1,25(OH)_2D_3$
 Hereditary Type I vitamin D-dependent rickets
  (defective synthesis of renal hydroxylase)
 Familial (X-linked) hypophosphataemic rickets
  renal tubular defect in phosphate transport)
 Chronic renal disease
 Fanconi syndrome (renal loss of phosphate)

Target organ resistance to $1,25 (OH)_2D_3$
 Vitamin D-dependent rickets (Type II)

RICKETS

Rickets, derived from the old English word 'wrickken' meaning to twist, is used to describe the clinical syndrome arising from an excess of undermineralised bone matrix in growing bone. It usually results from deficient intake or defective metabolism of vitamin D (Figs 10.15–10.16). It can also occur from a nutritional deficiency of calcium, particularly in developing countries, or from a deficiency of phosphate in breast milk or unsupplemented cow's milk formulas in preterm infants.

Mineralisation of osteoid is impaired, and the epiphyseal growth area becomes disorganised and hypertrophic. The clinical features are listed in Figure 10.17. Bones are soft and the long bones easily deformed. Skull bones can be indented easily by finger pressure (craniotabes), and expansion of the costochondral junctions produces a 'rickety rosary'. Indrawing of the softened ribs along the attachment of the diaphragm produces a hollowing called Harrison sulcus (Fig 10.18).

Diagnosis

Serum calcium is low or normal, phosphorus is low, and plasma alkaline phosphatase activity is greatly increased. X-ray of the wrist joints shows cupping and fraying of the metaphyses and a widened epiphyseal plate (Fig 10.19).

Treatment

Nutritional rickets is treated with oral supplements of vitamin D_2 (calciferol) and correction of the predisposing risk factors. Response is monitored biochemically and radiographically. The disorder can be prevented by health education about a balanced diet, exposure to sunlight and vitamin D supplementation when indicated..

VITAMIN A (RETINOL)

In developed countries, biochemical vitamin A deficiency is seen as a complication of fat malabsorption, when

Fig. 10.17 Clinical features of rickets

Misery

Failure to thrive/short stature

Frontal bossing

Craniotabes

Delayed closure of anterior fontanelle

Delayed dentition

Rickety rosary

Harrison sulcus

Expansion of metaphyses (especially wrist)

Bowing of weight-bearing bones

Hypotonia

Seizures (late)

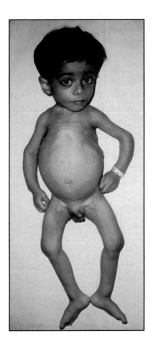

Fig. 10.18 Rickets in a three-year-old boy secondary to coeliac disease. He has frontal bossing, a Harrison sulcus, expansion of the metaphyses and bowing of the legs.

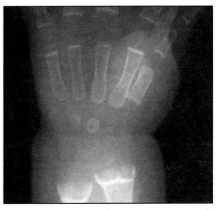

Fig. 10.19 An X-ray of the wrist showing rickets. The ends of the radius and ulna are expanded, rarefied and cup-shaped and the bones are poorly mineralised. This infant was exclusively breast-fed until 12 months of age, when he presented with a hypocalcaemic seizure.

supplementation has been inadequate. Clinical manifestations in these circumstances are rare, except for impaired dark adaptation. Vitamin A deficiency is common in many developing countries, where it causes eye damage from corneal scarring and acceleration of malnutrition from impairment of mucosal function and immunity. A number of community-based trials of supplementation have shown a marked reduction in mortality by reducing the incidence of infection.

Obesity

This is difficult to define and to measure. A commonly accepted definition is more than 120% weight for height, and examining the undressed child rarely leaves doubt about the diagnosis. At least 2–3% of UK school children are obese, more in adolescence. Obesity may result from genetic factors, a high carbohydrate diet, eating large infrequent meals or reduced activity.

In obesity:

- babies who are obese at six months are more likely to be obese school children, over three-quarters of whom will remain obese in adult life
- overnutrition accelerates growth and the onset of puberty. Most obese children are above the 50th centile for height. This makes the differentiation from hypothyroidism or Cushing syndrome easier, as these conditions lead to short stature from a decline in growth velocity
- a syndome, e.g. Prader-Willi, in which it is a clinical feature, needs to be considered
- emotional disturbances are seen in some affected children and unhappiness may lead to further excessive eating
- the child or teenager may be teased and develop a poor self-image, adversely affecting self-confidence, particularly in establishing relationships with the opposite sex. Psychological support may be required
- if severe, it may lead to hypoventilation and hypercapnia, somnolence and heart failure (Pickwickian syndrome).

Management

The aim is for energy intake to be less than expenditure. The child and parents need to be highly motivated, as obesity in the child is often a reflection of parental obesity and eating habits. A reduced-energy diet designed to lose 1 kg per week is reasonable, coupled with a programme of increased exercise. Some families will need psychiatric assessment. Unfortunately, compliance is poor and many who start a weight reduction programme continue with it only for a short period and do not reach a normal weight. Some prefer to join a group of others with the same problem. The more frequent the follow-up the more likely are children to adhere to the regimen.

Long-term consequences

The link between obesity in adults and risk factors for cardiovascular disease is well recognised. Maturity onset diabetes, hypertension, hypertriglyceridaemia, lower HDL-cholesterol and high LDL-cholesterol are all more common. It is uncertain whether the tracking of these risk factors is inevitable, but it seems likely that weight reduction and exercise reduce the level of risk.

Dental caries

Dental destruction occurs as a result of exposure to organic acids produced by bacterial fermentation of carbohydrate. Prevention involves:

- a reduction in cariogenic plaque bacteria (brushing and flossing)
- less frequent ingestion of carbohydrates
- regular inspection by a dentist
- an optimal intake of fluoride up to puberty to improve the resistance of the tooth to damage.

Incorporation of fluoride in enamel by ionic substitution leads to replacement of calcium hydroxyapatite by calcium fluorapatite, which is less soluble in organic acids. In areas where drinking water contains a low concentration of fluoride, supplementation with fluoride drops or tablets is needed. Additionally, topical fluoride in toothpaste or mouthwashes is also advisable. Excess fluoride administration before enamel has formed may lead to mottled enamel (dental fluorosis).

Infants and children who are put to bed with a bottle containing fermentable liquid (milk or a sucrose-containing fruit juice) are at particular risk of developing severe dental caries. Characteristically, fluid collects around the upper anterior and posterior teeth, which become extensively damaged. Because of reduced salivation and swallowing during sleep, clearance and neutralisation of organic acids is also reduced. So called 'prop feeding' should therefore be energetically discouraged.

FURTHER READING

Barker DJ. *Fetal and infant origins of adult disease.* BMJ 1992. Book based on original papers.

Department of Health. *Dietary reference values for food energy and nutrients in the United Kingdom.* London, HMSO, 1991. Reference manual.

Garrow JS, James WPT, (eds.) *Human Nutrition and Dietetics.* Churchill Livingstone, Edinburgh, 1993. Textbook.

McLaren DS, Burman D, Belton NR, Wiliams AF. *Textbook of Paediatric Nutrition,* 3rd ed. Churchill Livingstone, Edinburgh, 1991. Brief textbook.

Tanner JM. *Foetus in Man,* 2nd ed. Castlemead, 1989. Brief book.

Waterlow JC. *Protein energy malnutrition.* Edward Arnold, Sevenoaks, Kent, 1992. Brief book.

CHAPTER 11

Gastroenterology

• Vomiting • Crying • Acute abdominal pain • Recurrent abdominal pain • Gastroenteritis • Malabsorption
• Toddler diarrhoea • Inflammatory bowel disease • Constipation

Few children reach adulthood without experiencing gastrointestinal disorders such as gastroenteritis, recurrent abdominal pain or constipation. This is evident from their high frequency of consultations in both general practice and paediatric outpatient clinics. In spite of the enormous reserve capacity of the gut, which ensures adequate digestion and absorption in the face of substantial disease, chronic gastrointestinal disorders are a potent cause of weight loss and poor growth.

Vomiting

Posseting and regurgitation are terms used to describe the non-forceful return of milk, but differ in degree. Posseting describes the small amounts of milk which often accompany the return of swallowed air ('wind'), whereas regurgitation is used to described larger, more frequent losses. Posseting occurs in nearly all babies from time to time, whereas regurgitation usually indicates the presence of gastro-oesophageal reflux.

Vomiting implies the forceful ejection of gastric contents and when prolonged is likely to imply more serious pathology. It is a common problem in infancy and childhood (Figs 11.1 and 11.2). It is usually benign and is caused by feeding disorders or mild gastro-oesophageal reflux or gastroenteritis, but potentially serious disorders need to be excluded. In infants, vomiting may be associated with infection outside the gastrointestinal tract, especially urinary tract and central nervous system infections. In intestinal obstruction, the more proximal the obstruction, the more prominent the vomiting. As the obstruction becomes more distal, the abdomen will become distended.

GASTRO-OESOPHAGEAL REFLUX

Physiological, asymptomatic reflux may occur in any adult or child, but is infrequent. Measurement of lower oesophageal pH shows that normally there is reflux for only 4% of a 24-hour period. Reflux occurring more frequently than this and giving rise to symptoms is common in the first year of life. It results from functional immaturity of the lower oesophageal sphincter leading to episodes of inappropriate relaxation. A short intra-abdominal length of oesophagus-

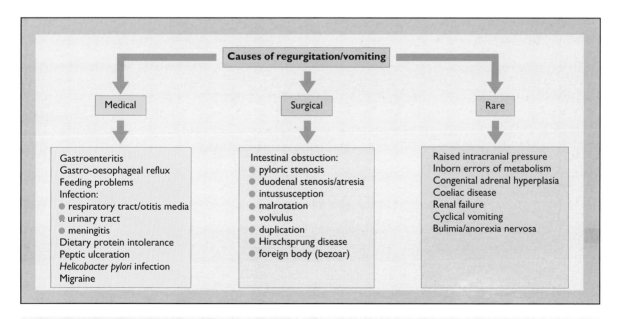

Fig. 11.1 Causes of regurgitation/vomiting.

Fig. 11.2 Diagnostic clues in a vomiting infant
Bile stained vomit – intestinal obstruction must be excluded
Blood in the vomit – suggests oesophagitis or peptic ulcer
Projectile vomiting in the first few weeks of life – is it pyloric stenosis?
Are there symptoms to suggest urinary tract, central nervous system or gastrointestinal infection?
Is the infant dehydrated?
Abdominal distension – is there lower intestinal obstruction?

Fig. 11.3 Complications of gastro-oesophageal reflux
Failure to thrive
Feeding problems
Pulmonary aspiration leading to 'bronchitis' or pneumonia
Oesophagitis – pain, bleeding, iron deficiency
Peptic stricture – associated with oesophagitis
Dystonic movements of head and neck (Sandifer syndrome)
Apnoea in preterm infants
Sudden infant death syndrome (SIDS) – controversial

probably also contributes. By 12 months of age, nearly all symptomatic reflux will have resolved spontaneously, presumably due to a combination of maturation of the lower oesophageal sphincter, assumption of an upright posture and more solids in the diet. A sliding hiatus hernia occurs in some symptomatic infants but is not invariable. Also, many children with a hiatus hernia are symptom-free.

Severe reflux is uncommon, but may be associated with potentially serious complications (Fig. 11.3). Reflux often occurs in children with cerebral palsy and its energetic management, surgically if necessary, may transform the child's quality of life. Reflux is also common in neonates who develop bronchopulmonary dysplasia (BPD).

Case History

GASTRO-OESOPHAGEAL REFLUX

This infant had a history of frequent regurgitation from the first few days of life. He developed two chest infections. Some of the vomits started to contain altered blood. A 24-hour oesophageal pH study showed severe gastro-oesophageal reflux (Fig. 11.4a–c). Endoscopy showed oesophagitis. He had probably had episodes of aspiration pneumonia. Symptoms resolved on treatment with feed thickeners, cisapride and cimetidine. His parents also commented on how much better he slept at night. Treatment was withdrawn at 15 months of age and symptoms did not recur.

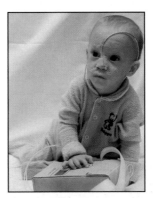

Fig. 11.4a The pH study in progress.

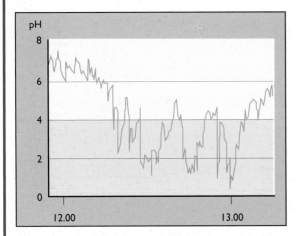

Fig. 11.4b Part of his 24-hour oesophageal pH study showing severe reflux, with frequent drops in pH below 4.

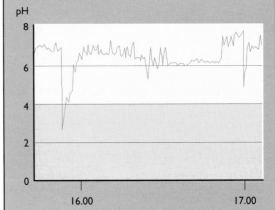

Fig. 11.4c Part of a normal oesophageal pH study. The lower oesophageal pH is above 4 for most of the time.

Management

Patients with mild, uncomplicated reflux can be diagnosed clinically and treated without further investigation. However, when the history is not typical or when complications are present, further investigation is indicated. The best diagnostic test is 24-hour ambulatory oesophageal pH monitoring. Barium studies are performed in patients with severe reflux in order to exclude underlying anatomical abnormalities in the oesophagus, stomach and duodenum, as is endoscopy in patients with suspected oesophagitis.

It is worthwhile treating all infants with symptomatic reflux; repeated regurgitation is smelly and unpopular with the family. Mild reflux responds well to the addition of inert carob-based thickening agents to feeds, and positioning in a 30° head-up prone position after feeds. Drugs which enhance gastric emptying and increase lower oesophageal sphincter pressure (e.g. cisapride) are useful in more severe forms of reflux. If there is associated failure to thrive, a period of continuous nasogastric feeding for 2–3 weeks may occasionally be needed to reduce the reflux sufficiently to allow control by other measures. Surgery, called fundoplication, in which the fundus of the stomach is wrapped around the intra-abdominal oesophagus, is reserved for those patients with complications failing to respond to intensive medical treatment, with oesophageal stricture or severe pulmonary aspiration.

PYLORIC STENOSIS

This disorder is four times more common in males than in females. Firstborns are more commonly affected. It affects 5–10% of the infants of parents who had pyloric stenosis, especially if it was the mother. Unexplained hypertrophy of the circular muscles of the pylorus develops in early infancy. Gastric peristalsis is visible, moving across the epigastrium following a feed (Fig. 11.5). There is:

- non bile-stained vomiting beginning between the second and fourth weeks of life, in both term and preterm infants
- vomiting which is projectile
- vomiting within 30 minutes of a feed and an infant who is hungry afterwards
- constipation and dehydration
- a hypochloraemic alkalosis from vomiting acid stomach contents
- a mild, unconjugated hyperbilirubinaemia in many infants.

Management

The diagnosis is made by palpation of the enlarged hard pylorus deep in the right upper quadrant during a test feed or immediately after a vomit. Ultrasound examination is used increasingly to confirm the diagnosis (Fig. 11.6). A barium meal is now used very infrequently, only when the diagnosis remains in doubt. Initial management is to correct any fluid and electrolyte disturbance with intravenous fluids. Treatment is with Ramstedt pyloromyotomy, when an incision is made in the pyloric canal to divide the hypertrophied muscles fibres down to but not through the pyloric mucosa.

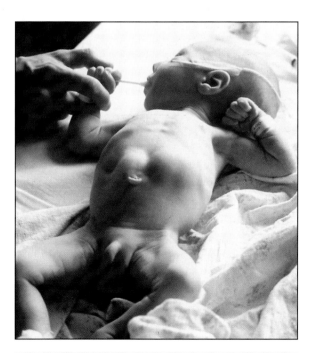

Fig. 11.5 Visible gastric peristalsis in an infant with pyloric stenosis.

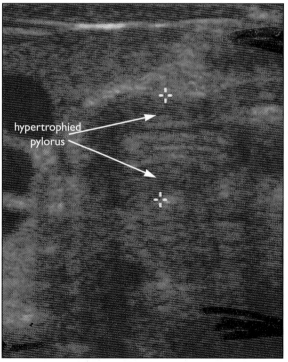

hypertrophied pylorus

Fig. 11.6 Ultrasound examination showing pyloric stenosis.

Crying

Excessive crying in infants is distressing for all concerned. Advice on appropriate feeding and wrapping, and reassurance will usually suffice. The emotional climate within a home is readily transmitted to a baby and tense, anxious or irritable care givers are likely to have similar babies. Practical help and emotional support to replace the missing extended family are often important. Organic causes must not be overlooked. Crying of sudden onset may point to a urinary tract infection, meningeal or middle ear infection, pain from an unrecognised fracture, oesophagitis or torsion of the testis. Severe nappy rash, constipation or coeliac disease may produce a miserable, crying infant. The complaint that a baby is 'always crying' may be an important pointer to potential or actual non-accidental injury. On the basis of countless reports of parents, there seems little doubt that the eruption of teeth is painful in some infants. However, teething does not cause convulsions, vomiting, diarrhoea or high fever.

INFANT 'COLIC'

This term is used to describe a common symptom complex which occurs in infants during the first few months of life. Paroxysmal, inconsolable crying or screaming accompanied by drawing up of the knees takes place several times a day, particularly in the evening. There is no firm evidence that the cause is intestinal, biliary or renal colic. Cow's milk protein intolerance or gastro-oesophageal reflux may be responsible in the occasional baby. Sympathetic counselling is helpful. The condition is essentially benign although it may precipitate non-accidental injury in infants already at risk. In severe, persistent cases an empirical two-week trial of a cow's milk-free diet followed by a trial of anti-reflux treatment may be worthwhile.

Acute abdominal pain

Managing acute abdominal pain in children requires considerable skill. In nearly half the children admitted to hospital, the pain resolves undiagnosed. In young children it is essential not to delay the diagnosis and treatment of acute appendicitis, as progression to perforation can be very rapid. It is easy to belittle the clinical signs of abdominal tenderness in young children. Of the surgical causes, appendicitis is by far the most common. It needs to be differentiated from mesenteric adenitis and the other surgical and medical conditions listed in Figure 11.7. The testes, hernial orifices and hip joints must always be checked.

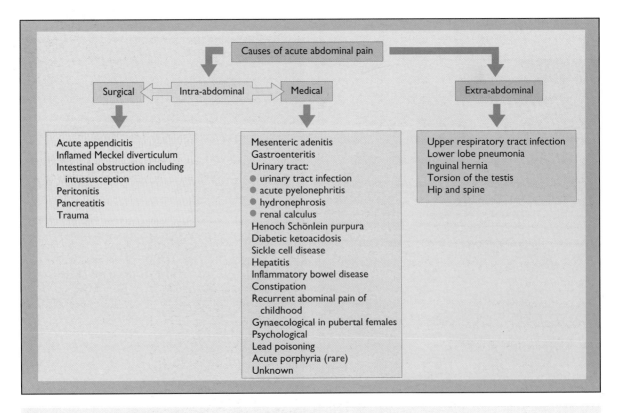

Fig. 11.7 Causes of acute abdominal pain.

It is notewothy that:
- lower lobe pneumonia may cause pain referred to the abdomen
- primary peritonitis is seen in patients with ascites from nephrotic syndrome or liver disease
- diabetic ketoacidosis may cause severe abdominal pain
- urinary tract infection, including acute pyelonephritis, is a relatively uncommon cause of acute abdominal pain, but a diagnosis that should not be missed. It is clearly important to test a urine sample in order to identify not only diabetes mellitus but conditions affecting the liver and urinary tract
- the role of laparoscopy is being assessed.

ACUTE APPENDICITIS

This important cause of acute abdominal pain may present at any age, with one-fifth of children being under three years old. Classically, it presents with a history of:
- central abdominal pain moving to the right iliac fossa
- pain aggravated by movement
- pain of increasing severity
- minimal early vomiting
- a low-grade fever.

Abdominal examination reveals:
- localised tenderness and guarding at McBurney point in the right iliac fossa
- the child wishes to lie still as the pain is worse on moving
- in young children poorly localised tenderness and absence of guarding.

Sometimes, with a retrocaecal appendix, there is no localised rigidity or rebound tenderness and in a pelvic appendix there may be few abdominal signs. In general, the younger the child the more difficult it is to make the diagnosis and the more likely it is to be delayed.

No routine or laboratory investigation is consistently helpful in making the diagnosis. In particular, a routine blood count is rarely indicated.

Appendicectomy is simple in early appendicitis, but the time between onset and perforation may be only a few hours in a pre-school child. Following perforation, correction of fluid and electrolyte loss and administration of broad-spectrum antibiotics are important. 'Active observation' with repeated reassessment in hospital reduces the number of non-inflamed appendices removed at unnecessary operations. In the young child it is vital that this period of observation is confined to a few hours.

 In young children with appendicitis, it is easy to underestimate their abdominal signs.

MESENTERIC ADENITIS

This is a poorly defined symptom complex of central abdominal pain, often in association with an upper respiratory tract infection and systemic illness. It is thought that inflammation of mesenteric lymph nodes leads to a peritoneal reaction, though pathological evidence for this tends to be lacking. Tenderness, often moving in location, is present. Careful observation with reassessment every couple of hours in hospital may be required to differentiate mesenteric adenitis from acute appendicitis. Management is conservative, but persisting local tenderness lasting more than a 3–6 hours warrants surgical exploration.

INTUSSUSCEPTION

Idiopathic intussusception describes the invagination of one segment of bowel into an adjacent lower segment. The blood supply to the bowel is shown in Figure 11.8 and shows why relief of this form of obstruction is urgent. It most commonly begins proximal to the ileocaecal valve. It is the most common cause of intestinal obstruction in infants after the neonatal period, usually occuring between six and nine months of age.

Presentation is with:
- paroxysmal, colicky pain and pallor. During episodes of screaming the baby becomes pale and draws up his legs
- vomiting and diarrhoea
- abdominal distension and dehydration
- a sausage-shaped mass in the abdomen (Fig. 11.9), with its curve and position following the surface markings of the colon

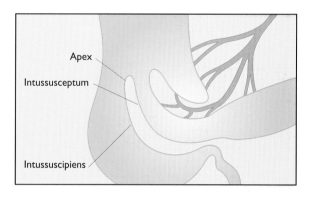

Apex

Intussusceptum

Intussuscipiens

Fig. 11.8 Intussusception, showing why the blood supply to the gut rapidly becomes compromised, making relief of this form of obstruction urgent.

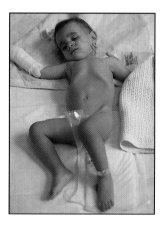

Fig. 11.9 A child with an intussusception. The mass can be seen in the upper abdomen. The child has become shocked.

- passage of a characteristic 'red-currant jelly' stool comprising blood-stained mucus. This may be first seen following rectal examination, an essential part of the assessment.

Usually no underlying intestinal cause for the intussusception is found, although there is some evidence that viral infection leads to enlargement of Peyer's patches, which may form the lead point of the intussusception. An identifiable lead point such as a Meckel diverticulum or polyp or rarely a lymphoma is more likely to be present in children over two years old. Intravenous fluid replacement with plasma volume expansion is particularly important in intussusception as there is often pooling of fluid in the gut and danger of circulatory failure.

An X-ray of the abdomen may show small bowel obstruction and paucity of gas in the right iliac fossa. Sometimes the outline of the intussusception itself can be visualised. Unless there are signs of peritonitis, reduction of the intussusception with barium, or now more often by air insufflation, is usually attempted initially (Fig. 11.10). The success rate of this procedure is 75%, although attempted reduction should be brief in the presence of radiological obstruction, bleeding or clinical deterioration during the procedure. The remaining 25% are treated surgically. Recurrence of the intussusception occurs in less than 5% but is more frequent after hydrostatic reduction.

 Shock is an important complication of intussusception.

MECKEL DIVERTICULUM

Two per cent of individuals have an ileal remnant of the vitellointestinal duct, in the form of a Meckel diverticulum which contains ectopic gastric mucosa or pancreatic tissue. Most are asymptomatic. Presentation is usually with severe rectal bleeding which is neither bright red nor true melaena. Alternative presentation is as an intussusception, a volvulus or diverticulitis which mimics appendicitis. A technetium scan will demonstrate increased uptake by ectopic gastric mucosa in 70% of cases (Fig. 11.11).

MALROTATION

Malrotation of the intestine is related to the abnormal movement of the intestine around the superior mesenteric artery during embryological development.

Failure to complete normal rotation and fixation (incomplete rotation) is the most common abnormality (Fig. 11.12). The caecum remains high and near the

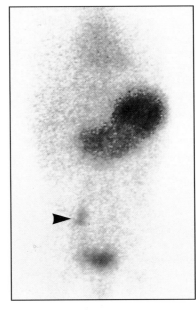

Fig. 11.11 A technetium scan showing uptake by ectopic gastric mucosa in a Meckel diverticulum in the right iliac fossa.

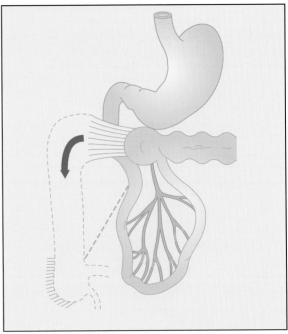

Fig. 11.12 The most common form of malrotation, with the caecum remaining high and fixed to the posterior abdominal wall, obstructing the duodenum.

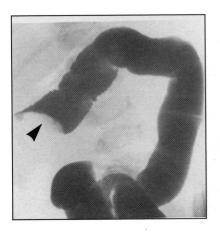

Fig. 11.10 An abdominal X-ray demonstrating an intussusception (see arrow), taken during reduction by air insufflated per rectum.

midline. As it fixes to the posterior abdominal wall the duodenum may be extrinsically obstructed. The midgut loop is also suspended from a narrow stalk containing superior mesenteric vessels instead of the normal broad base. The midgut loop is therefore prone to volvulus. Other forms of malrotation occur, such as reversed rotation, with the colon passing behind the duodenum. They are all much less common. Malrotation is a constant feature of exomphalos and congenital diaphragmatic hernia and is commonly associated with intrinsic duodenal atresias.

Bile-stained vomiting as a result of high intestinal obstruction in the newborn period is the most common presentation. Urgent surgery is required to avoid possible strangulation.

Older children may present with recurrent abdominal pain, abdominal distension and vomiting, a symptom complex which requires radiological investigation. Malrotation found by chance in an asymptomatic patient should probably be treated surgically in order to avoid midgut volvulus at a future date.

Recurrent abdominal pain

Recurrent pain, sufficient to interrupt normal activities and lasting episodically for at least three months, occurs in 10% of school-age children. Less than 10% of affected children will have a definable organic cause. The widely held belief that the remainder have psychogenic pain is without foundation.

A number of studies have failed to show psychosocial differences between such children and their families and controls. However, in some individual children it may be a manifestation of stress (see Chapter 20) or becomes part of a vicious cycle of anxiety and escalating pain leading to family distress and demands for increasingly invasive investigations. There is evidence that this anxiety leads to increased intestinal motility which may be perceived by the child as pain.

The pain is characteristically:
- peri-umbilical
- often worse on waking
- associated with a family history of cranial migraine, irritable bowel syndrome or travel sickness
- not accompanied by any other features of ill health.

The list of possible causes of organic pain is extensive and exclusion by investigation is therefore impossible and inappropriate.

The history and examination are therefore of paramount importance in deciding whom to investigate and how (Fig. 11.3). Urinary tract infection may cause abdominal pain in the absence of any clinical pointers. Urine microscopy and culture is therefore the only routine investigation in all these children.

Management

In the management of non-organic pain, it is important that a full history and examination is seen to be done. Moreover, reassurance is never acceptable to parents and to children without adequate explanation, and in this context it is often helpful to explain the pain in terms of 'the intestine becoming so sensitive from time to time that it is as if the child can feel food going round the bends'. Recent manometric evidence suggests that this explanation is remarkably accurate; children with recurrent 'non-organic' pain often have abnormalities in small bowel motility in association with pain.

The prognosis of non-organic abdominal pain is:
- about one-half of children have a rapid, spontaneous resolution of their symptoms following referral to a paediatrician
- one-quarter have a delayed resolution
- one-quarter will continue to have abdominal pain which often becomes recognisable as irritable bowel syndrome by the time adulthood is reached.

 No organic cause is identified in most children with recurrent abdominal pain, but this does not mean that it is psychogenic.

GASTRITIS AND PEPTIC ULCERATION

The greater use of endoscopy in children and the recent identification of a Gram-negative organism, *Helicobacter pylori*, in association with antral gastritis, has focused attention on it as a potential cause of abdominal pain in children.

Fig. 11.13 Pointers towards an organic basis of recurrent abdominal pain

History

Asymmetrical, non-central or referred pain

Nocturnal pain and/or a family history of peptic ulcer
   – suggests peptic ulceration

Pain worse before or relieved by defaecation
   – suggests colonic origin

Associated vomiting and distension – malrotation

Diarrhoea – possible inflammatory bowel disease

Blood in the stool – colitis

Loin pain – pelviureteric obstruction or renal stones

Urinary symptoms

Worse after milk – lactose intolerance

Related to menstruation

Examination

The presence of growth failure or of anal fissures or skin tags
   – Crohn disease

Hypertension – a catecholamine-secreting tumour

Jaundice – liver disease

Testicular mass – tumour

The relationship between *H. pylori* and duodenal ulceration in adults is becoming clearer, and there is now substantial evidence that *H. pylori* is a strong predisposing factor to duodenal ulcers. This association in children is much less clear. Duodenal ulcers are relatively uncommon in children, but should always be sought in children with night pain, particularly if it wakes them, or when there is a history of peptic ulceration in a first-degree relative.

H. pylori causes a nodular antral gastritis but in the absence of a duodenal ulcer is seldom associated with abdominal pain. It is usually identified in gastric antral biopsies, but may also be present on micro-aerophilic culture. The organism produces urease which forms the basis for a laboratory test on biopsies, and the ^{13}C breath test following the administration of ^{13}C-labelled urea by mouth. Serological tests are generally unreliable in children. Treatment comprises triple therapy (with omeprazole, clarithromycin and tinidazole).

Gastroenteritis

In the developing world gastroenteritis claims the lives of 5 million children under the age of five each year. Infective diarrhoea and vomiting also remains an important problem in developed countries, although mortality has decreased substantially over the past forty years.

The most common cause of gastroenteritis in developed countries is rotavirus infection, which accounts for up to 60% of cases in children less than two years of age, particularly during the winter months. Other viruses, particularly adenovirus, calicivirus, corona and astroviruses have been implicated in outbreaks but are numerically much less common and their role as pathogens is less clear.

Bacterial causes are less common in developed countries. *Campylobacter jejunii* infection, usually the most common of the bacterial infections in developed countries, is often associated with severe abdominal pain and blood in the stools. *Shigella* and some salmonellae produce a dysenteric type of infection with blood and pus in the stool, pain and tenesmus. *Shigella* may be accompanied by high fever causing a febrile convulsion. Cholera and enterotoxigenic *E. coli* infection are associated with profuse, rapidly dehydrating diarrhoea. However, clinical features are a poor guide to the pathogen.

A number of disorders may masquerade as gastroenteritis (Fig. 11.14) and in cases of diagnostic doubt hospital referral is essential. Dehydration and its complications are the usual cause of death in gastroenteritis, and its correction is the fundamental aim of treatment. Infants are at high risk. Accurate clinical assessment of dehydration is required but is difficult (Fig. 11.15).

Electrolyte disturbances

Infants are at greater risk of dehydration because of their:
- higher basal fluid requirements (100–120 ml/kg/day)
- inability to gain access to fluids when thirsty
- higher surface area to weight ratio, leading to greater insensible water losses (300 ml/m²/ day, equivalent in infants to 15–17 ml/kg/day)
- immature renal tubular reabsorption.

Fig. 11.14 Differential diagnosis of gastroenteritis	
Systemic infection	Septicaemia, meningitis
Local infections	Respiratory tract, otitis media, hepatitis A, urinary tract infection
Surgical disorders	Pyloric stenosis, intussusception, acute appendicitis, necrotising enterocolitis, Hirschsprung disease
Metabolic disorder	Diabetic ketoacidosis,
Renal disorder	Haemolytic uraemic syndrome
Other	Coeliac disease, cow's milk protein intolerance, adrenal insufficiency, Reye syndrome

 The cause of death in gastroenteritis is dehydration. Its correction is the mainstay of treatment.

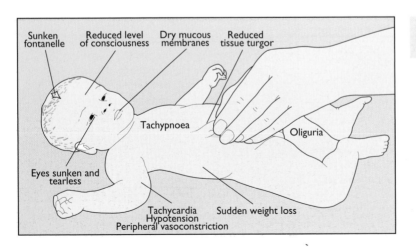

Fig. 11.15 *Clinical features of dehydration in an infant.*

Sunken fontanelle — Reduced level of consciousness — Dry mucous membranes — Reduced tissue turgor — Tachypnoea — Oliguria — Eyes sunken and tearless — Tachycardia — Hypotension — Peripheral vasoconstriction — Sudden weight loss

Isonatraemic and hyponatraemic dehydration

In dehydration, there is a total body deficit of sodium and water. In most instances the losses of sodium and water are proportional and plasma sodium remains within the normal range (isonatraemic dehydration). When sodium losses exceed those of water, plasma sodium falls (hyponatraemic dehydration) and this is associated with a shift of water from extra- to intracellular compartments. The increase in intracellular volume leads to an increase in brain volume, sometimes resulting in convulsions, whereas the marked extracellular depletion leads to a greater degree of shock per unit of water loss. This form of dehydration is more common in poorly nourished infants in developing countries.

Hypernatraemic dehydration

Infrequently, water loss exceeds the relative sodium loss, and plasma sodium concentration increases (hypernatraemic dehydration). This usually results from high insensible water losses (high fever or hot, dry environment) or from profuse, low-sodium diarrhoea. The extra cellular fluid becomes hypertonic with respect to the intracellular fluid and there is a shift of water into the extracellular space from the intracellular compartment. Signs of extracellular fluid depletion are therefore less per unit of fluid loss; depression of the fontanelle, reduced tissue elasticity and sunken eyes are late signs. Therefore, this form of dehydration is more difficult to recognise clinically, particularly in an obese infant. It is a particularly dangerous form of dehydration as water is drawn out of the brain and cerebral shrinkage within a rigid skull may lead to multiple small cerebral haemorrhages and convulsions. Transient hyperglycaemia occurs in some patients with hypernatraemic dehydration; it is self-correcting and does not require insulin.

Management

Mild dehydration (<5% body weight loss)

In most cases of gastroenteritis in infants and toddlers in developed countries, dehydration is mild with less than 5% loss of body weight and there are few, if any, clinical signs of dehydration. It can usually be managed by substitution of normal feeds with a maintenance type of glucose–electrolyte solution (Fig. 11.16). The glucose or sucrose is present in oral rehydration solutions to enhance sodium and water absorption, not as a calorie source. Rehydration solutions may be rice-based. The solution is given until vomiting and profuse diarrhoea subside. This usually lasts less than 24 hours and a normal diet can then be introduced immediately. There is no need to re-introduce milk gradually or to avoid milk or milk-containing foods.

Moderate dehydration (5–10% body weight loss)

These children have clinical signs of dehydration. (Fig. 11.17). There is a role for a six-hour trial of oral rehydration, aiming to give 100 ml/kg over this period (orally or by nasogastric tube). If there is no improvement in the child's symptoms and state of hydration, intravenous rehydration should be given.

Severe dehydration

Intravenous rehydration is always indicated. Patients who are shocked require immediate resuscitation with plasma volume expansion with 20–30 ml/kg, or more as indicated, of normal sodium chloride solution (0.9 g NaCl/100ml)

Fig. 11.16 Composition (mmol/l) of oral rehydration solutions		
	Standard solution	**WHO/UNICEF**
Sodium	60	90
Potassium	20	20
Chloride	50	80
Citrate	10	10
Glucose	75–110	110

The WHO/UNICEF solution is designed principally for use in developing countries in children with moderate to severe dehydration. The sodium concentration is too high for routine use in developed countries.

Throughout the world, oral rehydration solution saves the lives of millions of children each year.

Fig. 11.17 Clinical assessment of dehydration		
	Moderate	**Severe**
Body weight loss	5–10%	>10%
General appearance	Thirsty, restless or lethargic	Drowsy, cold, sweating
Tears	Reduced/absent	Absent
Tissue elasticity	Reduced/absent	Absent
Mucous membranes	Dry	Very dry
Capillary return	Normal/prolonged	Prolonged (>4 sec)
Blood pressure	Normal or low	Low or unrecordable
Urine output	Reduced	Marked oliguria
Pulse	Rapid	Rapid, weak, may be impalpable
Eyes	Sunken	Grossly sunken
Anterior fontanelle	Sunken	Very sunken

or plasma (Fig. 11.18). Rehydration is corrected to replace the fluid deficit, maintenance fluids and continuing fluid losses (Figs 11.19 a and b). The child's fluid balance needs to be closely monitored by clinical reassessment and measurement of plasma electrolytes.

Potassium chloride is added to the intravenous infusion once the child is passing urine. Acute renal failure may rarely complicate severe dehydration. Failure to recognise continuing oliguria leads to overhydration and pulmonary oedema.

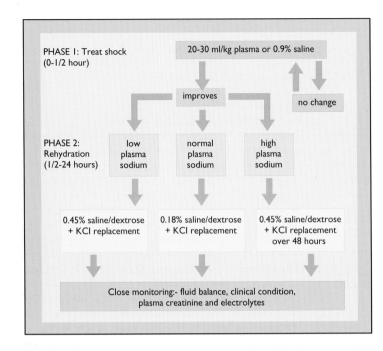

Fig. 11.18 Initial intravenous fluid management of severe dehydration.

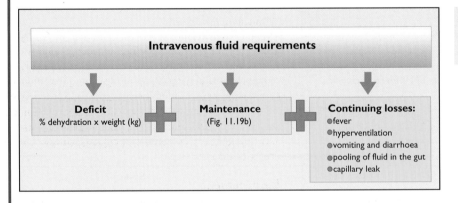

Fig. 11.19a Intravenous fluid requirements in severe dehydration.

Fig. 11.19b Maintenance intravenous fluid and electrolyte requirements per 24h

Body weight	Fluid (ml/kg)	Sodium (mmol/kg)	Potassium (mmol/kg)
<10 kg	100–120	2.5–3.5	1.5–2.5
10–30 kg	60–90	1.0–2.5	2.0–2.5
>30 kg	40–90	1.5–2.0	1.5–2.0

Too rapid correction of hypernatraemic dehydration may result in convulsions and cerebral damage.

Hypernatraemic dehydration

The management of hypernatraemic dehydration is particularly difficult. Once circulation has been restored, a too rapid reduction in plasma sodium concentration and osmolality will lead to a shift of water into cerebral cells resulting in cerebral oedema and possible convulsions. The reduction in plasma sodium should therefore be slow, over 48 hours, in order not to exceed a reduction in plasma sodium of 10 mmol/l/24 h.

Antidiarrhoea drugs (e.g. loperamide, Lomotil) and anti-emetics

There is no place for medications for the vomiting or diarrhoea of gastroenteritis as they are:

- ineffective
- may prolong the excretion of bacteria in stools
- can be associated with side-effects
- add unnecessarily to cost
- focus attention away from oral rehydration.

Antibiotics are indicated only rarely, for specific bacterial or protozoal infections (e.g. cholera, shigellosis, giardiasis).

POST-GASTROENTERITIS SYNDROME

Infrequently, following an episode of gastroenteritis, the introduction of a normal diet results in a return of watery diarrhoea. Lactose intolerance may be prominent, with non-absorbed sugar in the stools, giving a positive Clinitest result. In such circumstances, a return to an oral rehydration solution for 24 hours, followed by a further introduction of a normal diet is usually successful. The precise aetiology of this disorder is uncertain but it may result from the interaction within the small intestinal mucosa of an infecting organism with an acquired dietary protein intolerance. Multiple dietary intolerances may result, such that specialist dietary management is essential, in the implementation of a diet which excludes cow's milk, disaccharides and gluten. In severe cases a period of parenteral nutrition is required to enable the injured small intestinal mucosa to recover sufficiently to absorb luminal nutrients.

Malabsorption

Disorders affecting the digestion or absorption of nutrients manifest as:

- abnormal stools
- failure to thrive or poor growth in most but not in all cases
- specific nutrient deficiencies, either singly or in combination.

In general, parents know when their child's stools have become abnormal. The truly offensive stool is difficult to flush down the toilet and has an odour which pervades the whole house. In general, colour is a poor guide to abnormality. Reliable dietetic assessment is important. It is inappropriate to investigate children for malabsorption as a cause of their failure to thrive when dietary energy intake is demonstrably low and other symptoms are absent. Some disorders affecting the small intestinal mucosa or pancreas may lead to the malabsorption of many nutrients (panmalabsorption), whereas others are highly specific, for example, zinc malabsorption in acrodermatitis enteropathica.

COELIAC DISEASE

Coeliac disease is an enteropathy in which the gliadin fraction of gluten provokes a damaging immunological response in the proximal small intestinal mucosa. As a result, the rate of migration of absorptive cells moving up the villi (enterocytes) from the crypts is massively increased but is insufficient to compensate for increased cell loss from the villous tips. Villi become progressively shorter, and then absent, leaving a flat mucosa.

Overall, the incidence of coeliac disease varies between 1 in 500 and 1 in 3000. It has been particularly frequent in the West of Ireland, but in common with some parts of Europe, including the UK, the frequency in early childhood is falling. In contrast, the frequency in other European countries, e.g. Sweden, has recently increased. These changes appear to be related to the amount and timing of the introduction of gluten in the diet in the first year of life. The picture in the UK is unclear. It seems likely that a lower rate in infancy will be reflected in a higher rate in later childhood, i.e. manipulating dietary gluten in infancy postpones rather than prevents the disease.

Children normally present in the first two years of life with failure to thrive following the introduction of gluten in cereals. General irritability, abnormal stools, abdominal distension and buttock wasting are the usual symptoms. Occasionally, children present in later childhood with anaemia (iron and/or folate deficiency) or growth failure, with little or no gastrointestinal symptoms.

Diagnosis

The diagnosis depends upon the demonstration of a flat mucosa on jejunal biopsy followed by the resolution of symptoms and catch-up growth upon gluten withdrawal. There is no place for the empirical use of a gluten-free diet as a diagnostic test for coeliac disease in the absence of a jejunal biopsy. Serological tests such as anti-gliadin and anti-endomysial antibodies are not sufficiently sensitive and specific to replace jejunal biopsy in diagnosis, but are useful as screening tests.

Management

All products containing wheat, rye and barley are removed from the diet and this results in resolution of symptoms. Supervision by a dietician is essential. In children in whom the initial biopsy or the response to gluten withdrawal is doubtful or when the disease presents before the age of two, a gluten challenge is required in later childhood to demonstrate continuing susceptibility of the jejunal mucosa to damage by gluten. The gluten free diet should be adhered to for life. The incidence of small bowel malignancy in adulthood is increased in coeliac disease although a gluten-free diet probably reduces the risk to normal.

Case history

COELIAC DISEASE (FIG. 11 20a–d)

This two year old had a history of poor growth from 12 months of age. His parents had noticed that he tended to be crotchety and had three or four foul-smelling stools a day. A jejunal biopsy performed at two years of age showed sub-total villous atrophy and he was started on a gluten-free diet. Within a few days his parents commented that his mood had improved and within a month he was a 'different child'. He subsequently exhibited good catch-up growth.

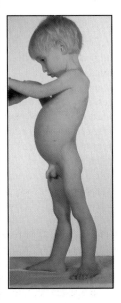

Fig. 11.20a Coeliac disease causing wasting of the buttocks and distended abdomen.

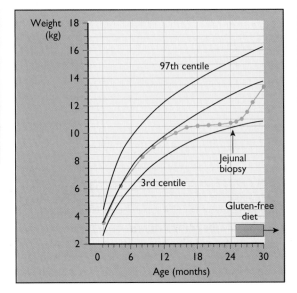

Fig. 11.20d Growth chart showing failure to thrive and response to a gluten-free diet.

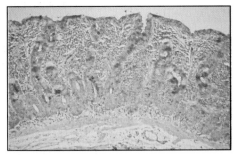

Fig. 11.20b Histology of his jejunal biopsy showing lymphocytic infiltration and villous atrophy confirming coeliac disease.

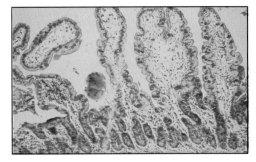

Fig. 11.20c Normal jejunal histology is shown for comparison.

TRANSIENT DIETARY PROTEIN INTOLERANCES

In contrast to coeliac disease, which requires lifelong gluten withdrawal, there are a number of transient intolerances to dietary proteins. These usually manifest as:

- diarrhoea and/or vomiting with failure to thrive
- eczema
- acute colitis
- migraine
- occasionally as an acute anaphylactic reaction with urticaria, stridor, bronchospasm and shock.

Cow's milk protein is the most commonly incriminated antigen but intolerance to soya and less frequently to wheat, fish, egg, chicken and rice are also described. When an acute reaction occurs immediately after ingestion, the diagnosis can be readily established. When the reaction is delayed, diagnosis is more problematic. Intolerances occur more commonly in those infants with IgA deficiency or with a strong family history of atopy. Although no single laboratory test is diagnostic, affected children may have:

- eosinophilia in the peripheral blood
- positive antibody tests to specific food proteins
- a high IgE concentration in plasma.

Those children who present with failure to thrive and protracted diarrhoea may require a jejunal biopsy to establish the diagnosis, in particular to differentiate it from coeliac disease. In cow's milk protein intolerance there is a patchy enteropathy in the jejunal mucosa, usually with prominent eosinophils in the lamina propria. Elimination of the offending antigen results in rapid resolution of symptoms, and this together with their return upon challenge is the only diagnostic test. The advice of an experienced dietician is essential in the supervision of all exclusion diets in infancy and childhood, not only to assure complete antigen exclusion but also to maintain a nutritionally adequate diet.

In the case of cow's milk protein intolerance, a casein hydrolysate-based formula is preferred to a soya-based feed as up to 20% of infants will also be or become intolerant to soya. Most children have outgrown their intolerance by the age of two years, which is therefore an appropriate time to conduct a challenge. Although infrequent, anaphylaxis may occur, so the challenge should be conducted in hospital, beginning with a skin test followed by the ingestion of an increasing quantity of antigens orally.

OTHER CAUSES OF NUTRIENT MALABSORPTION

Abnormal nutrient absorption occurs in blind loops from *small intestinal bacterial contamination*, when there is colonisation of the small intestine by Gram-negative organisms or anaerobes normally found in the colon. *Bile salt deficiency*, from cholestatic disorders or following resection of the distal ileum, leads to substantial malabsorption of fat and fat-soluble vitamins.

Impaired fat transport may occur in the rare disorders of intestinal lymphangiectasia, in which there are abnormal lymphatics, and in a-betalipoproteinaemia, in which there is a failure to make chylomicrons. The latter disorder presents in childhood with steatorrhoea, acanthocytosis of red blood cells, retinal degeneration and fat soluble vitamin malabsorption, particularly vitamin E which causes severe neuronal degeneration in later childhood and adolescence. Large oral doses of vitamin E from early childhood are preventive.

CONGENITAL ENZYME DEFECTS

Congenital sucrase–isomaltase deficiency is rare and has very variable clinical expression. It leads to diarrhoea following sucrose, and to a lesser degree, starch ingestion. Some children present with florid symptoms in infancy, usually after the introduction of solids, whereas others present in later childhood with a picture very similar to toddler diarrhoea.

In contrast to transient lactose intolerance following diarrhoea, *primary congenital lactase deficiency* is very rare indeed. A third sort of lactose deficiency – hereditary *late-onset lactase deficiency* – is very common and is the norm in most of the world's population. Lactase is no longer expressed in the small intestine after early childhood in non-Caucasians. Symptoms vary considerably and are not present before the age of two or three years. Northern Europeans and North Americans are unusual in continuing to express lactase throughout life.

SPECIFIC TRANSPORT DEFECTS

There are many such defects, each limited to a specific carrier protein. They are all rare. *Glucose–galactose malabsorption* results in severe, life-threatening diarrhoea from the introduction of milk feeds, and affected children are only able to tolerate fructose as their dietary carbohydrate.

Acrodermatitis enteropathica results from a congenital defect in zinc transport in the small intestine. Affected children present in infancy with a symmetrical erythematous rash mainly affecting mucocutaneous junctions. Plasma zinc is very low, as are the activities of zinc-dependant enzymes such as alkaline phosphatase in plasma.

Toddler diarrhoea

This condition, also called chronic non-specific diarrhoea, is the most common cause of persistent loose stools in preschool children. Characteristically, the stools are of varying consistency, sometimes well formed, sometimes explosive and loose. The presence of undigested vegetables in the stools is common, giving rise to the alternative title of 'peas and carrots syndrome'. Affected children are well and thriving and there are no precipitating dietary factors.

The uncommon disorder, sucrose-isomaltase deficiency should be excluded, as it may be clinically indistinguishable from toddler diarrhoea. This is done by an oral sucrose challenge and testing the stool for sucrose. Toddler diarrhoea probably results from an underlying maturational delay in intestinal motility. Most children have grown out of their symptoms by five years of age.

No treatment is usually required. Loperamide used cautiously is often helpful in children with socially disruptive symptoms.

Inflammatory bowel disease

CROHN DISEASE

From the 1950s, there has been a marked increase in the incidence of Crohn disease in all age groups. It becomes progressively more common throughout childhood. In Northern Europe and North America, the overall incidence is about 4 per 100 000. About one-quarter of patients with Crohn disease present in childhood or adolescence.

Crohn disease is a transmural, focal, sub-acute or chronic inflammatory disease. It affects any part of the gastrointestinal tract from the mouth to the anus, but most commonly the distal ileum and proximal colon. The affected intestine is thickened and adhesions between affected loops are common. Perianal skin tags, fissures and fistulae are also common. The histological hallmark is the presence of non-caseating epithelioid cell granulomata.

Abdominal pain, diarrhoea and growth failure with pubertal delay are the most common presenting features. There may be oral and perianal ulcers. The disease may be insidious in onset, and extra-intestinal symptoms such as growth failure, intermittent fever, arthritis, uveitis and erythema nodosum may be present, with few or no pointers towards gastrointestinal disease. Some adolescents may present with a clinical picture virtually indistinguishable from anorexia nervosa.

Diagnosis rests upon the demonstration of characteristic abnormalities on barium follow-through (narrowing, fissuring, mucosal irregularities and mural thickening), and at colonoscopy and on histology of a biopsy. Acute phase reactants, e.g. C-reactive protein and ESR, are usually raised and can be useful in monitoring disease severity.

The aims of treatment are to induce remission by suppressing inflammation by treatment with steroids or by using an elemental diet for about six weeks. Recurrence is common and, with the exception of azathioprine in Crohn colitis, no medical regimen has been shown to maintain remission. Overnight enteral feeding may be helpful in correcting growth failure. Surgery is necessary for complications of Crohn disease – obstruction, fistulae, failed medical treatment, growth failure or abscess formation. In general, the long-term prognosis for Crohn disease beginning in childhood is good and most patients lead normal lives despite occasional recurrent disease.

 In Crohn disease, up to one-third of children will experience growth failure and delayed puberty.

ULCERATIVE COLITIS

Ulcerative colitis is a recurrent, inflammatory and ulcerating disease involving the mucous membrane of the colon. Characteristically, the disease presents with rectal bleeding, diarrhoea, colicky pain and weight loss.

The diagnosis is made by identification of the characteristic macroscopic and histological appearances at colonoscopy, following exclusion of infective causes of colitis. Extra-intestinal complications include erythema nodosum, pyoderma gangrenosum, arthritis and spondylitis. There is an increased incidence of adenocarcinoma of the colon in adults (1 in 200 risk for each year of disease between ten and 20 years).

Mild attacks are managed by topical steroids when the disease is confined to the rectum and sigmoid colon, or sulphasalazine for more extensive disease. More severe disease requires systemic steroids. Severe fulminating disease is a medical emergency and requires treatment with broad-spectrum antibiotics and intravenous fluids and steroids. One-third of patients require colectomy during the course of their disease. It is required for chronic poorly controlled disease, prevention of malignancy in long-standing disease, or severe fulminating disease sometimes complicated by toxic megacolon which fails to respond promptly to intensive medical treatment.

Constipation

In healthy infants there is a wide range in bowel frequency. Breast-fed infants may not pass stools for several days. In young children, constipation, which is the painful passage of hard, infrequent stools, is common. It often follows an acute febrile illness. A transient superficial anal tear may be an important precipitating factor. Most such cases resolve with mild laxatives and extra fluids. Occasionally, following such an event, or perhaps in association with forceful potty training, the use of strange, uncomfortable lavatories on holiday or at school or psychological stress in the family, more protracted constipation results. Children may withhold passage of stool for fear of the associated pain. The rectum becomes full and over distended and the sensation of needing to defaecate is lost. Involuntary soiling usually follows as the full rectum overflows. Children of school age are frequently teased as a result and secondary behavioural problems are common. At this stage, the use of stimulant laxatives without first emptying the rectum completely is likely to make soiling worse.

Examination often reveals an abdominal mass and on rectal examination stool is present down to the anal margin. Organic causes of constipation are uncommon, but hypothyroidism, hypercalcaemia, a urinary concentrating defect or Hirschsprung disease should be considered.

It needs to be explained to the child and his parents that soiling is involuntary and that recovery of normal rectal sensation often takes a long time.

The first aim of management is to empty the rectum and colon completely. Following 1–2 weeks of stool softeners (lactulose or docusate), large doses of powerful oral laxatives (sodium picosulphate and senna) are given daily for 2–3 days until the stools are liquid. This is followed immediately by daily evening doses of a stimulant laxative (e.g. senna) to prevent reaccumulation of stool and encourage a daily bowel action.

Treatment with senna is often needed for several months before the dose is gradually tailed off. Laxative treatment is combined with regular post-prandial visits to the lavatory and a star chart is introduced to record and reward progress.

Encouragement by family and doctor is essential, as relapse is common particularly in children from socially disadvantaged backgrounds. Occasionally, the degree of faecal retention is so severe that evacuation is only possible by using enemas or surgical disempaction under an anaesthetic. Great care must be used to avoid distress if the rectal route is used (see Chapter 20).

HIRSCHSPRUNG DISEASE

The absence of ganglion cells from the myenteric and sub-mucosal plexuses of part of the large bowel results in a narrow, contracted segment, ending proximally in a normally innervated, dilated colon. In 75% of cases the lesion is confined to the rectosigmoid, but in 5% the entire colon is involved. Presentation is usually in the neonatal period with intestinal obstruction, heralded by failure to pass meconium within the first 24 hours of life. Abdominal distension and later bile-stained vomiting develop (Fig. 11.21). Rectal examination may reveal a narrowed segment; withdrawal of the examining finger often releases a gush of liquid stool and flatus. There may be a temporary improvement in the obstruction following the dilatation, caused by the rectal examination, which can lead to a delay in diagnosis. Occasionally infants present with severe, life-threatening Hirschsprung enterocolitis during the first few weeks of life, probably due to *Clostridium difficile* infection. In later childhood presentation is with chronic constipation, usually profound, and associated with abdominal distension but usually without soiling. Growth failure may also be present.

Diagnosis is made by demonstrating the absence of ganglion cells together with the presence of large, acetyl cholinesterase-positive nerve trunks on a suction rectal biopsy. Anorectal manometry or barium studies may be useful in giving the surgeon an idea of the length of the aganglionic segment but are unreliable for diagnostic purposes. Management is surgical and usually involves an initial colostomy followed by an operation to bypass the aganglionic segment by anastomosing normally innervated bowel to the anus.

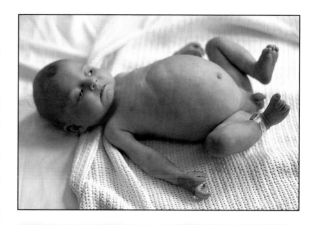

Fig. 11.21 Abdominal distension in Hirschprung disease.

FURTHER READING

Booth IW. Silent gastro-oesophageal reflux: how much do we miss? *Arch Dis Ch* 1992;**67**:1325–1327. Review article.

Booth IW. Chronic inflammatory bowel disease. *Arch Dis Ch* 1991;**66**:742–744. Review article.

Booth IW. Dietary management of acute diarrhoea in childhood. *Lancet* 1993;**341**:996–997. Review article.

Navarro J, Schmitz J, eds. *Paediatric Gastroenterology*. Oxford University Press, Oxford, 1992. Short textbook.

Nixon H, O'Donnell B, eds. *Essentials of Paediatric Surgery*. 4th ed. Butterworth/Heinemann, Oxford, 1992. Short textbook.

Walker WA, Durie PR, Hamilton JR, Walker-Smith JA, Watkins JBBC, eds. *Pediatric Gastrointestinal Disease*. Decker, Ontario, 2nd edn 1995. Comprehensive textbook.

CHAPTER 12

Infection and Immunity

• *Common childhood infections* • *Staphylococcal and streptococcal infections* • *Kawasaki disease*
• *Tuberculosis* • *Lyme disease* • *Tropical infections* • *Immunodeficiency disorders* • *Immunisation*

Infections are the most common cause of acute illness in children. Worldwide, acute respiratory infections, gastroenteritis, measles and malaria, often accompanied by malnutrition, are major causes of death. It has been estimated that they are responsible for about 14 million children under five years old dying each year.

In developed countries, with improved nutrition, living conditions, sanitation, immunisation, antibiotic therapy and modern medical care, morbidity from infections has declined dramatically, and deaths from infectious diseases are uncommon. However, some infections remain a major problem, e.g. meningococcal disease and some have re-emerged, e.g. TB and diptheria. There are also new infections, e.g. HIV and Lyme disease.There has also been an increase in the number of immunocompromised children who are vulnerable to unusual or opportunist pathogens and in the incidence of antibiotic-resistant bacteria.

At birth, infants possess all the essential components of the immune system. However, their circulating immunoglobulins, derived from their mother (Fig. 12.1) decrease during the first few months of life, leaving them susceptible to the common infections.

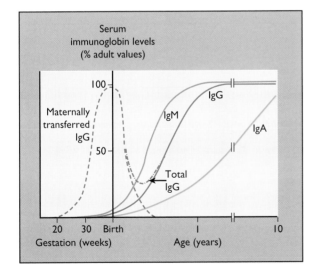

Fig. 12.1 *Serum immunoglobulin levels in the fetus and infant.When maternal immunoglobulin levels decline, infants become susceptible to infections.*

Common childhood infections

MEASLES
Since the introduction of an effective vaccine in 1968, the incidence of measles in England and Wales has declined dramatically, from a peak of 800 000 per year in the early 1960s to just under 10 000 in 1993. This has been accompanied by a decline in its complications. However, the mean age of infection has increased, so that a significant proportion are now over ten years old, in whom the disease is often more severe.

Clinical features
These are shown in Figures 12.2, 12.2a and 12.2b. There are a number of serious complications. In previously healthy children, serious neurological complications are rare. They are:

- **encephalitis** – occurs in only 1 in 5000, about eight days after the onset of the illness. Initial symptoms are headache, lethargy and irritability, proceeding to convulsions and ultimately coma. Mortality is 15%. Serious long-term sequelae include seizures, deafness, hemiplegia and severe learning difficulties affecting up to 40% of survivors

- **subacute sclerosing panencephalitis (SSPE)** – a rare but devastating illness which presents on average seven years after infection with measles, in about 1 in 100 000 cases. The disorder presents with motor incoordination, visual impairment, speech abnormalities, behaviour disturbances and seizures, progressing over several years to dementia, stupor and finally decorticate rigidity and death. The diagnosis is essentially clinical, supported by finding high levels of measles antibody in both blood and CSF and by characteristic EEG abnormalities. Even more rarely, SSPE may follow measles immunisation, but since the introduction of measles immunisation in the US in 1963, there has been a hundredfold decrease in its incidence.

In developing countries, where malnutrition and particularly vitamin A deficiency lead to impaired cell-mediated immunity, measles often follows a protracted course with severe complications. The rash may progress to a dark red/violet colour followed by desquamation and depigmentation, which may last weeks or months. Pre-existing malnutrition is further exacerbated by oral infections and diarrhoea.

In immunocompromised patients measles is a dangerous

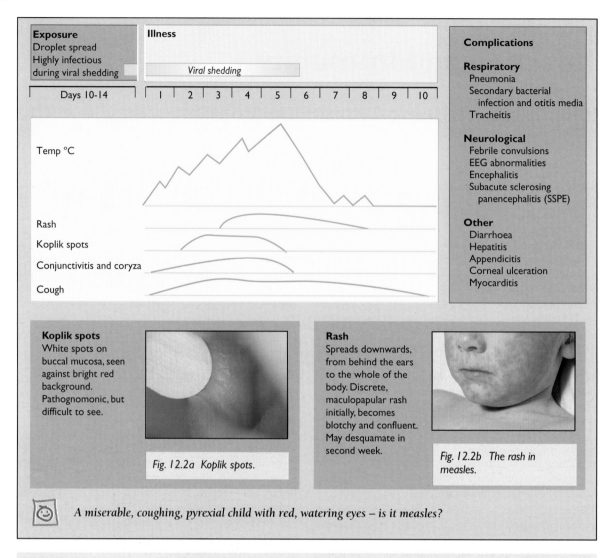

Exposure
Droplet spread
Highly infectious
during viral shedding

Illness

Viral shedding

Days 10-14

| 1 | 2 | 3 | 4 | 5 | 6 | 7 | 8 | 9 | 10 |

Temp °C

Rash

Koplik spots

Conjunctivitis and coryza

Cough

Complications

Respiratory
  Pneumonia
  Secondary bacterial
    infection and otitis media
  Tracheitis

Neurological
  Febrile convulsions
  EEG abnormalities
  Encephalitis
  Subacute sclerosing
    panencephalitis (SSPE)

Other
  Diarrhoea
  Hepatitis
  Appendicitis
  Corneal ulceration
  Myocarditis

Koplik spots
White spots on
buccal mucosa, seen
against bright red
background.
Pathognomonic, but
difficult to see.

Fig. 12.2a Koplik spots.

Rash
Spreads downwards,
from behind the ears
to the whole of the
body. Discrete,
maculopapular rash
initially, becomes
blotchy and confluent.
May desquamate in
second week.

Fig. 12.2b The rash in
measles.

A miserable, coughing, pyrexial child with red, watering eyes – is it measles?

Fig. 12.2 Clinical features and complications of measles.

illness. Giant cell pneumonia is an important cause of death in children with malignant disease, even when in remission. These children are also susceptible to a measles encephalopathy.

Treatment and prevention

As there is currently no treatment for measles, management is symptomatic. In immunocompromised patients, the antiviral drug, ribavirin is currently under evaluation. Vitamin A, which may modulate the immune response, should be given in developing countries and to susceptible children in developed countries. Children with measles should be kept away from school for seven days after the emergence of the rash. Those who are admitted to hospital should be isolated.

Prevention by immunisation is the most successful strategy for reducing the morbidity and mortality of measles. In the UK, there was concern that up to 40% of school age children were susceptible to measles due to poor immu-

nisation coverage in the past and a vaccine failure rate of up to 10%. The combination of higher uptake rates since the change from measles vaccine alone to MMR, and the immunisation campaign of school age children in 1994 has markedly reduced the number of susceptible children.

MUMPS

Mumps occurs worldwide, but its incidence has been reduced dramatically with the introduction of the MMR vaccine. Mumps usually occurs in the winter and spring months. It is spread by droplet infection to the respiratory tract, where the virus replicates within epithelial cells. The virus gains access to the parotid glands before further dissemination to other tissues.

Clinical features

The incubation period is 14–21 days. Onset of the illness is with fever, malaise and parotitis. Only one side may be swollen initially but bilateral involvement usually occurs over the next few days. The parotitis is uncomfortable and children may complain of earache or pain on eating or drinking. Examination of the parotid duct may show redness and swelling. Occasionally, parotid swelling may be absent. The fever usually disappears within 3–4 days. Plasma amylase levels are often elevated and when associated with abdominal pain may be evidence of pancreatic involvement. Infectivity is for up to seven days after the onset of parotid swelling. The illness is generally mild and self-limiting. Although hearing loss can follow mumps, it is usually unilateral and transient.

Central nervous system involvement
Is determined by the presence of lymphocytes in the CSF. It occurs in about 50%, but meningeal signs are seen in 10% and encephalitis in about 1 in 5000. The common clinical features are headache, photophobia, vomiting and neck stiffness.

Orchitis
Is the most feared complication, although it is uncommon in prepubertal males. When it does occur it is usually unilateral. Although there is some evidence of a reduction in sperm count, infertility is actually extremely unusual. Rarely oophoritis, mastitis and arthritis may occur.

RUBELLA (GERMAN MEASLES)
Rubella is generally a mild disease in childhood. It occurs in winter and spring. It is an important infection as it can cause severe damage to the fetus (see Chapter 7). The incubation period is 14–21 days. Spread is by the respiratory route, frequently from a known contact. The prodrome is usually mild, with a low-grade fever or none at all. The maculopapular rash is often the first sign of infection, appearing initially on the face, then spreading centrifugally to cover the whole body. It fades in 3–5 days. Unlike in adults, the rash is not itchy. Lymphadenopathy, particularly the suboccipital and postauricular nodes, is prominent. Complications are rare in childhood but include arthritis, encephalitis, thrombocytopenia and myocarditis. Clinical differentiation from other viral infections is unreliable. Accurate identification during pregnancy requires serological testing. There is no effective antiviral treatment. Prevention lies in immunisation, the aim being to avoid maternal/fetal infection.

THE HUMAN HERPES VIRUSES
There are eight herpes viruses known to infect humans (herpes simplex virus 1 and 2, varicella zoster, cytomegalovirus, Epstein–Barr virus, human herpes viruses 6, 7 and 8). The hallmark of herpes infections is latency with subsequent recurrent disease.

I. HERPES SIMPLEX INFECTIONS
Herpes simplex virus (HSV) usually enters the body through the mucous membranes or skin. The incubation period for primary infection is 2–20 days. After the neonatal period, HSV1 infections predominate. The prevalence of HSV2 increases in early adulthood. HSV1 is transmitted in body fluids such as saliva, while HSV2 is mainly transmitted through the transfer of genital secretions. HSV infections have a wide variety of clinical manifestations.

Asymptomatic
Herpes simplex infections are very common and are mostly asymptomatic.

Gingivostomatitis
This is the most common form of primary HSV illness in children. It usually occurs at 10 months to 3 years of age. There are vesicular lesions on the lips, gums and anterior surfaces of the tongue and hard palate which often progress to extensive, painful ulceration with bleeding (Fig. 12.3). There is a high fever and the child is very miserable. The illness may persist for up to 2 weeks. Eating and drinking are painful, which may lead to dehydration. Management is symptomatic, but severe disease may necessitate intravenous fluids.

Skin manifestations
Mucocutaneous junctions and damaged skin are particularly prone to infection. 'Cold sores' are recurrent HSV1 lesions on the lip margin.

Eczema herpeticum
In this serious condition widespread vesicular lesions develop on eczematous skin (Fig. 12.4). This may be complicated by secondary bacterial infection which may result in septicaemia.

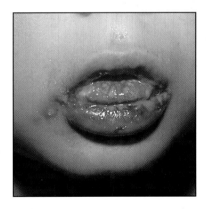

Fig. 12.3 Vesicles with ulceration in gingivostomatitis.

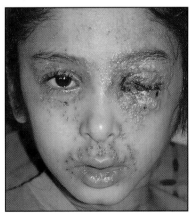

Fig. 12.4 Eczema herpeticum.

Herpetic whitlows

These are painful, erythematous, oedematous white pustules on the site of broken skin on the fingers. Spread is by auto-inoculation from gingivostomatitis and infected adults kissing their children's fingers. In sexually active adolescents HSV2 may be the cause.

Eye disease

Eye disease may cause a blepharitis or conjunctivitis. It may extend to involve the cornea producing dendritic ulceration. This can lead to corneal scarring and ultimately loss of vision.

Central nervous system infection

Aseptic meningitis

Usually a complication of HSV2 infection, occurring within 10 days of a primary infection. It resolves without sequellae.

Encephalitis

By contrast, a very serious condition with a mortality of 70% if untreated. It may follow either primary or recurrent infection. The clinical features and management are described in Chapter 4 and Chapter 24.

Neonatal infection (see Chapter 8)

The infection may be focal, infecting the skin or eyes, may cause encephalitis or may be widely disseminated. Its morbidity and mortality are high.

Infection in the immunocompromised host

Infection is often severe. Cutaneous lesions may spread to involve adjacent sites, e.g. oesophagitis and proctitis. Pneumonia and disseminated infections involving multiple organs are serious complications.

Treatment is with acyclovir, a viral DNA polymerase inhibitor, which is used to treat skin, ophthalmic, cerebral and systemic infections.

2A. VARICELLA ZOSTER (CHICKENPOX)

Varicella zoster shares many features with HSV, as both produce a vesicular rash and latent infections. In contrast to HSV, however, varicella zoster is spread by the respiratory route progressing via the blood and lymphatics to infect the skin.

Clinical features

In normal children, chickenpox is characterised by a pruritic, generalised, vesicular rash which starts on the scalp or trunk, spreading centrifugally over the rest of the body. Lesions may be macular or papular before developing into vesicles which crust soon after their appearance. Depigmentation of black skin is seen at the site of vesicles. Systemic illness is mild or absent. The incubation period is 10 to 21 (usually 14 to 16) days. Children are infectious from 48 hours before and up to 5 days after the onset of the lesions.

Secondary bacterial infection of the skin by staphylococci or streptococci may occur. Other complications are rare. Encephalitis, 3–6 days after the onset of rash, is characterised by cerebellar signs, with marked ataxia. In contrast to the encephalitis caused by HSV, the prognosis is good.

In the immunocompromised, primary varicella infection may result in severe progressive disease. The vesicular eruptions persist and frequently become haemorrhagic (Fig. 12.5). Visceral involvement occurs in the lungs, central nervous system and liver. Secondary bacterial infection may also occur. The mortality may be as high as 20%. The disease in the neonatal period is described in Chapter 8.

Treatment and prevention

Human varicella zoster immunoglobulin (ZIG) is recommended for high-risk individuals following contact with chickenpox. They include:

- bone marrow transplant recipients
- patients on high doses of steroids or other immunosuppressive drugs within the previous three months
- neonates whose mothers develop varicella within five days before or two days after delivery
- neonates born at less than 30 weeks' gestation who have been exposed to varicella.

Acyclovir should be given in severe chickenpox and considered in adolescents, as they are more likely to develop severe disease. Trials in the US have shown some benefit from oral acyclovir in normal children, but the drug is not currently recommended for this purpose in the UK. Although an effective varicella vaccine exists, there are concerns about subsequent zoster infections and that adults may become susceptible to infection when immunity wanes. It is not currently licensed in the UK. Salicylates should be avoided because of the risk of developing Reye syndrome.

2B. HERPES ZOSTER (SHINGLES)

Latent varicella zoster can reactivate, causing a vesicular eruption in the distribution of sensory nerves (shingles). It occurs most commonly in the thoracic region although any dermatome can be affected. (Fig. 12.6). Children, unlike adults, rarely suffer pain, and shingles is not associated with malignancy. In the immunocompromised, reactivated infection can also lead to a severe disseminated form of the disease. This is treated with acyclovir.

3. EPSTEIN–BARR VIRUS

Epstein–Barr virus (EBV) has not only been established as the major cause of the infectious mononucleosis syndrome but is also involved in the pathogenesis of Burkitt lym-

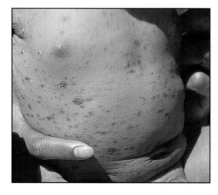

Fig. 12.5 Haemorrhagic chickenpox is seen in malnourished or immunodeficient children. (Courtesy of Dr Sam Walters)

phoma, lymphoproliferative disease in immunocompromised hosts and nasopharyngeal carcinoma. The virus has a particular tropism for B lymphocytes and epithelial cells of the oro- and nasopharynx.

Infectious mononucleosis (glandular fever).

The clinical features of primary EBV disease in young children are non-specific. Older children, and occasionally young children, develop a syndrome of infectious mononucleosis, with the features of:

- fever
- malaise
- tonsillopharyngitis – often severe, limiting the oral ingestion of fluids and food. Rarely, breathing may be compromised
- lymphadenopathy – prominent cervical lymph nodes, often with diffuse adenopathy.

Other features include:

- petechiae on the soft palate
- splenomegaly (50%), hepatomegaly (10%)
- a macular papular rash (5%)
- jaundice.

Diagnosis is supported by:

- atypical lymphocytes (T cells seen on blood film)
- a positive Monospot test
- the presence of heterophile antibodies, i.e. antibodies that agglutinate sheep erythrocytes (Paul–Bunnell reaction). This test is often negative in young children with the disease.

The infection may persist for 1–3 months but ultimately resolves.

Treatment is symptomatic. When respiration is severely compromised corticosteroids may be considered. In 5% of infected individuals Group A streptococcus is grown from the tonsils. This should be treated with penicillin. Ampicillin or amoxycillin may cause a florid macular papular rash in children infected with EBV and should be avoided.

4. CYTOMEGALOVIRUS

Cytomegalovirus (CMV) is a common human pathogen. It is transmitted via the oral and genital routes, by maternal transmission *in utero* and by blood transfusions and organ transplants. It causes mild or asymptomatic infections in normal hosts. In developed countries, about half of the adult population show serological evidence of past infection. However, in immunocompromised individuals and in the fetus, CMV is an important pathogen.

As with EBV and toxoplasmosis, CMV can cause a mononucleosis syndrome. Pharyngitis and lymphadenopathy are not usually as prominent as in EBV infections. Patients may have atypical lymphocytes on blood film but are heterophile antibody negative.

Maternal CMV infection may result in congenital infection (see Chapter 7) which may be present at birth or develop during infancy.

In the immunocompromised host CMV can cause retinitis, pneumonitis, encephalitis, hepatitis, colitis and oesophagitis. It has become a particularly important pathogen following organ transplantation. In order to reduce the risk of transmission, CMV-negative blood is used whenever possible for transfusions in immunodeficient patients and, if possible, CMV-positive organs are not transplanted into CMV-negative recipients.

Treatment with gancyclovir, an analogue of acyclovir, can be effective in the immunocompromised patient. Foscarnet, another antiviral agent may also be used as second-line therapy.

5. HUMAN HERPES VIRUS 6

Nearly all children have acquired antibody to human herpes virus 6 (HHV6) by the age of two. In common with other herpes viruses, reactivation can occur following immunosuppression. After bone marrow transplantation 40% of recipients become viraemic with HHV6 2–3 weeks after transplantation.

In 1988 it was found to be the aetiological agent of exanthem subitum (also known as roseola infantum). The classical description of this condition is of a high fever, lasting a few days, followed by a generalised macular rash which appears as the fever wanes. However, recent studies suggest that HHV6 is a frequent cause of pyrexial illnesses without a rash in young children, and is a common cause of febrile convulsions.

HHV6 has also been associated with aseptic meningitis, encephalitis, hepatitis, infectious mononucleosis-like syndrome and haematological malignancies.

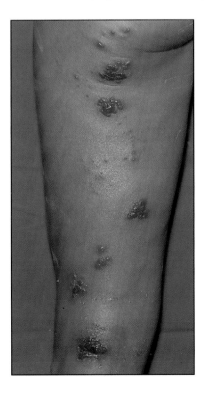

Fig. 12.6 Herpes zoster (shingles) in a child. It is distributed along a dermatome.

 Human herpes virus 6 (HHV 6) infection is a common cause of febrile convulsions.

PARVOVIRUS B19

In 1983 parvovirus B19 was found to be the aetiological agent for erythema infectiosum or fifth disease (so-named because it was the fifth disease to be described with similar rashes), also called slapped cheek syndrome. Infections can occur at any time of the year, although outbreaks are most common during the spring months. Transmission is via respiratory secretions from viraemic patients, by vertical transmission from mother to fetus and by transfusion of contaminated blood products.

It causes a range of clinical syndromes:

- *asymptomatic infection* is common. About 5–10% of preschool children and 65% of adults have antibodies
- *erythema infectiosum* is the most common illness, with a viraemic phase of fever, malaise, headache and myalgia followed by a characteristic rash a week later on the face ('slapped cheek') progressing to a maculopapular, 'lace'-like rash on the trunk and limbs. Complications are rare in children although arthralgia or arthritis is common in adults
- *aplastic crisis* is the most serious consequence of parvovirus infection. It occurs in children with chronic haemolytic anaemias, e.g. sickle cell disease or thalassaemia
- *fetal disease* from maternal parvovirus infection may lead to fetal hydrops and death.

ENTEROVIRUSES

The human enteroviruses coxsackie A, B and echovirus are a common cause of childhood infection. Transmission is primarily by the faecal–oral route. Following replication in the pharynx and gut the virus spreads to infect other organs. Infections occur most commonly in the summer and autumn. Enterovirus infection has a wide range of clinical manifestations.

Asymptomatic or non-specific febrile illness
Over 90% of infections.

Herpangina
Vesicular and ulcerated lesions on the soft palate and uvula causing anorexia, pain on swallowing and fever.

Hand, foot and mouth disease
Painful vesicular lesions on the hands, feet, mouth and tongue. Systemic features are mild. The disease subsides within a few days.

Pleurodynia (Bornholm disease)
An acute illness with fever, pleuritic chest pain and muscle tenderness. There may be a pleural rub but examination is otherwise normal. Recovery is within a few days.

Myocarditis and pericarditis
Heart failure associated with a febrile illness and ECG evidence of myocarditis.

Meningitis/encephalitis
Aseptic meningitis is caused by many of the enteroviruses. There may be an associated skin rash which can be difficult to differentiate from meningococcal infection. A complete recovery can be expected.

Infection in the immunocompromised host
Enteroviruses can cause severe disease in immunocompromised individuals. Echovirus can cause a persistent and sometimes fatal central nervous system infection in agammaglobulinaemic patients.

Polio
Poliovirus infection is uncommon in developed countries with successful immunisation programmes. It falls into four main clinical categories:

- >90% are *asymptomatic*
- 5% have a poliomyelitis *'minor illness'*. The fever, headache, malaise, sore throat and vomiting occur within 4 days of exposure and recovery is uneventful
- 2% of patients progress to *central nervous system involvement*. There is stiffness of the back, neck and hamstrings from meningeal irritation
- in <2% of cases, *paralytic polio* occurs about 4 days after the minor illness has subsided. Involvement of the anterior horn cells and cerebral cortex leads to varying degrees of paralysis which may recover completely or be permanent. Involvement of the muscles of respiration may be fatal.

Effective vaccines are available against the poliovirus. Live attenuated vaccine strains of polio can cause fatal infections in children with severe combined immunodeficiency or agammaglobulinaemia

Staphylococcal and streptococcal infections

Staphylococcal and streptococcal infections are usually caused by direct invasion of the organisms. They may also cause disease by releasing toxins, some of which may act as superantigens. Whereas conventional antigens stimulate only a small subset of T cells which have a specific receptor, superantigens bind to a part of the T cell receptor which is shared by many T cells and therefore stimulates massive T cell proliferation and cytokine release. The wide range of diseases caused by these organisms are shown in Figure 12.7.

IMPETIGO

This is a localised staphylococcal or streptococcal skin infection, most common in infants and young children. It is more common where there is pre-existing skin disease, e.g. atopic eczema. Lesions are usually on the face, neck and hands and begin as erythematous macules which become vesicular (Fig. 12.8). Rupture of the vesicles with exudation of fluid leads to the characteristic confluent honey-coloured crusted lesions. The lesions are sometimes bullous. Infection is readily spread to adjacent areas and other parts of the body by auto-inoculation of the infected exudate. It is also highly contagious. Topical antibiotics (e.g. mupirocin) are effective for mild cases. Systemic antibiotics (e.g. erythromycin or

Organism	Mode	Disease	Mechanism	
Staphylococcal infection	*Direct*	Impetigo Cellulitis Orbital cellulitis Pneumonia Abscess Osteomyelitis Septic arthritis	By release of proteases and attachment to host cells	
	Toxin-mediated	Toxic shock syndrome Food poisoning Toxic epidermal necrolysis (scalded skin syndrome) Kawasaki disease	Toxic shock syndrome toxin (TSST) Staphylococcal enterotoxins Staphylococcal exfoliative toxins It has been postulated that this disease is caused by a bacterial toxin	These toxins cause T cell proliferation and cytokine release
Streptococcal infection	*Direct*	Tonsillitis Otitis media Pneumonia Impetigo Cellulitis Osteomyelitis Septicaemia Meningitis	By release of proteases and attachment to host cells	
	Toxin-mediated	Scarlet fever Erysipelas "Toxic shock-like syndrome"	Streptococcal pyrogenic exotoxins (also called 'erythrogenic toxins')	These toxins cause T cell proliferation and cytokine release
	Post-infectious	Glomerulonephritis Rheumatic fever Arthritis Erythema nodosum	Immunological response to primary infection may cause host damage	

Fig. 12.7 Staphylococcal and streptococcal disease

flucloxacillin) are needed for more severe infections. Affected children should not go to nursery or school until the lesions are dry. Nasal carriage is an important source of infection which can be eradicated with a nasal cream containing mupirocin or chlorhexidine and neomycin.

BOILS

These are infections of hair follicles or sweat glands, usually caused by *Staphylococcus aureus*. Treatment is

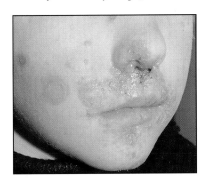

Fig. 12.8 Impetigo showing characteristic confluent honey-coloured crusted lesions. (Courtesy of Dr Paul Hutchins.)

with systemic antibiotics and occasionally surgery. Recurrent boils are usually from persistent nasal carriage in the child or family acting as a reservoir for reinfection. Only rarely are they due to diabetes mellitis or immune deficiency.

PERIORBITAL CELLULITIS

In periorbital cellulitis there is fever with erythema, tenderness and oedema of the eyelid (Fig. 12.9). It is almost always unilateral. In young children, *Haemophilus influenzae* b infection was a common cause before the introduction of the Hib vaccine. It may follow local trauma to the skin.

In older children it may spread from a paranasal sinus infection or dental abscess. Periorbital cellulitis should be treated promptly with intravenous antibiotics to prevent spread of the infection to an orbital cellulitis where there is proptosis, painful or limited ocular movement and reduced visual acuity. This may be complicated by abscess formation, meningitis or cavernous sinus thrombosis.

SCALDED SKIN SYNDROME

This is caused by an exfoliative staphylococcal toxin. It affects infants and young children, who develop fever and malaise and may have a purulent, crusting localised infection around the eyes, nose and mouth with subsequent widespread erythema and tenderness of the skin. Areas of epidermis separate on gentle pressure (Nikolsky sign), leaving denuded areas of skin (Fig. 12.10) which subsequently dry and heal without scarring. Management is with an intravenous anti-staphylococcal antibiotic and monitoring of fluid balance.

TOXIC SHOCK SYNDROME

While this syndrome is best known for its association with staphylococcal-infected tampons in women in the late 1970s, the disease was first described in children. Toxin-producing streptococci can also cause a toxic shock-like illness. The toxin, released from infection at any site including small abrasions, causes a systemic illness characterised by high fever, a diffuse, macular rash, hypotension, shock and multi-organ failure. There may be redness of the mucous membranes (Fig. 12.11), vomiting or diarrhoea, severe myalgia, altered consciousness, thrombocytopenia and abnormal hepatic and renal function. There is desquamation of the palms, soles, fingers and toes 1–2 weeks after the onset of the illness. Without aggressive fluid replacement, removal of infectious foci and intensive care the outcome is poor.

Kawasaki disease

Although uncommon, Kawasaki disease is an important diagnosis to make as aneurysms of the coronary arteries and sudden death are important complications and prompt treatment reduces their incidence.

Kawasaki disease, first described in 1967, mainly affects children of six months to four years old with a peak at the end of the first year. The disease is much more common in children of Asian ethnicity and, to a lesser extent, Afro-Caribbeans as compared with Caucasians. The cause is unknown but the many clinical and immunological similarities with the staphylococcal and streptococcal toxic shock syndromes has led to the recent suggestion that it too is caused by a bacterial toxin acting as a superantigen.

The diagnosis is made on clinical findings (Fig. 12.12). The disease is a vasculitis affecting the small and medium-sized vessels. It affects the coronary arteries in about one-third of affected children within the first six weeks of the illness. This can lead to aneurysms which are visualised on echocardiography. Subsequent narrowing of the vessels from scar formation can result in myocardial ischaemia and sudden death. Mortality is 1–2%.

Treatment with intravenous immunoglobulin (2 g/kg) given within the first ten days has been shown to lower the risk of coronary artery aneurysms. Aspirin is used to reduce the risk of thrombosis. It is given at a high dose until the fever subsides and continued at a low dose where there is an abnormality of the coronary arteries. When the platelet count is very

high, antiplatelet aggregation agents may also be used to reduce the risk of coronary thrombosis. Children suspected of the disease but who do not have all the clinical features should still be considered for treatment. Steroids and antibiotics are of no proven benefit.

 Prolonged fever – is it Kawasaki disease?

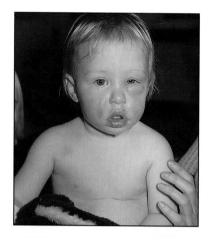

Fig. 12.9 Periorbital cellulitis. It should be treated promptly with intravenous antibiotics to prevent spread into the orbit.

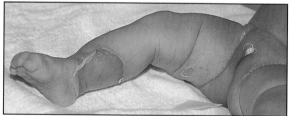

Fig. 12.10 Staphylococcal scalded skin syndrome. Its appearance must not be mistaken for a scald from non-accidental injury.

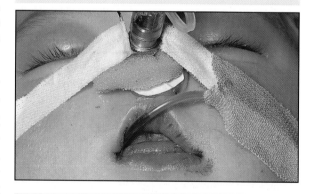

Fig. 12.11 A child with toxic shock syndrome receiving intensive care including artificial ventilation via a nasotracheal tube. The lips are red and the eyelids are oedematous from capillary leak. (Courtesy of Professor Mike Levin.)

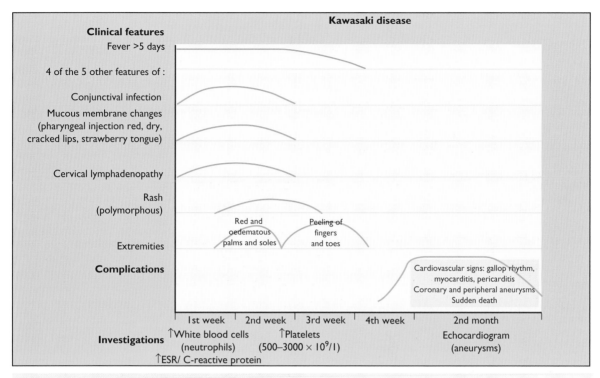

Kawasaki disease

Clinical features

Fever >5 days

4 of the 5 other features of :

Conjunctival infection

Mucous membrane changes
(pharyngeal injection red, dry,
cracked lips, strawberry tongue)

Cervical lymphadenopathy

Rash
(polymorphous)

Extremities

Red and oedematous palms and soles

Peeling of fingers and toes

Complications

Cardiovascular signs: gallop rhythm,
myocarditis, pericarditis
Coronary and peripheral aneurysms
Sudden death

| 1st week | 2nd week | 3rd week | 4th week | 2nd month |

Investigations

↑White blood cells (neutrophils)

↑Platelets (500–3000 × 10^9/l)

Echocardiogram (aneurysms)

↑ESR/ C-reactive protein

Fig. 12.12 Clinical features and investigations in Kawasaki disease.

Case history

KAWASAKI DISEASE

This three-year-old boy had developed a high fever of three days' duration. Examination showed a mild conjunctivitis, a rash and cervical lymphadenopathy. A viral infection was diagnosed and his mother reassured. Four days later she presented to her local hospital. The child's condition was unchanged, but he was noted to have cracked red lips (Fig. 12.12a). He was admitted for observation as he appeared unwell and was not eating. A full septic screen, including a lumbar puncture was performed and antibiotics started. A urine infection was suspected as there were 50–100 WBC/mm³ in the urine sample, though culture proved to be negative. After five days he was still febrile and irritable and the antibiotics were changed after a repeat blood count, blood and urine culture. He remained febrile and irritable. Four days later the neutrophil count was 15×10^9/l, platelet count 800×10^9/l and ESR 125. Sixteen days into the illness, there was peeling of the skin of the fingers and toes (Fig. 12.12b) and Kawasaki disease was suspected. An echocardiogram showed aneurysms of the coronary arteries. He was treated with intravenous immunoglobulins, following which his clinical condition improved and he became afebrile. Delayed diagnosis meant that the maximum benefit from early immunoglobulin therapy in preventing coronary artery aneurysms was missed.

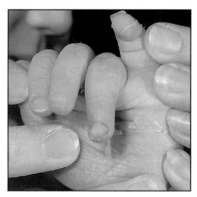

Fig. 12.12a Red, cracked lips and conjunctival inflammation.

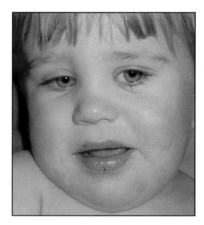

Fig. 12.12b Peeling of the fingers, which developed on the 16th day of the illness.

Tuberculosis

The decline in the incidence and mortality from tuberculosis (TB) in developed countries has been hailed as an example of how public health measures and antimicrobial therapy can dramatically modify a disease. However, tuberculosis is again becoming a public health problem, partly through its increasing incidence in patients with HIV infection and the emergence of multiresistant strains.

With the decline in tuberculosis from infected dairy cattle, the spread of TB is usually by the respiratory route. Close proximity, infectious load and underlying immunodeficiency enhance the risk of transmission. Children, particularly infants and toddlers, are usually infected by adults or adolescents within the same household. Child-to-child spread is rare.

Clinical features
These are outlined in Figure 12.13.

Diagnosis
Diagnosing TB in children is even more difficult than in adults. The clinical features of chronic tuberculous disease, which include prolonged fever, malaise, anorexia, weight loss and focal signs of infection, may be the only clues and empirical treatment may be necessary. Children usually swallow sputum, so gastric washings are required to visualise or culture acid-fast bacilli originating from the lung. Urine, lymph node, CSF and radiological examinations should also be performed where appropriate. Heaf tests are used for screening for TB. In individuals suspected of having TB, a Mantoux test is usually used. Ten units of purified protein derivative of tuberculin (0.1ml of 1:1000) is given intradermally and read after 48–72 hours; 1 unit is only used when there is a likelihood of a hypersensitivity reaction e.g. a child with erythema nodosum. Induration of greater than 10 mm in diameter is positive. When interpreting the result, consideration needs to be given to the child's age, if there are clinical or chest x-ray features of TB, household contact with TB, previous BCG and relative anergy due to immunosuppression or malnutrition.

Treatment
Triple therapy with rifampicin, isoniazid and pyrazinamide remains the most commonly used initial combination. This is usually rationalised to rifampicin and isoniazid after two months. By this time antibiotic sensitivities are often known. Streptomycin is often included for the treatment of tuberculous meningitis in the initial phase. Children who are Mantoux positive but are asymptomatic should be treated; a single agent, usually isoniazid, is often used. Drug resistance is of increasing concern.

Prevention and contact tracing
BCG immunisation has been shown to be helpful in preventing or modifying TB in the UK. However, its usefulness worldwide in preventing the disease is controversial. Currently BCG is recommended at birth for high-risk groups (communities with a relatively high prevalence of TB, i.e. Asian or African origin or TB in a family member in the previous five years) and routinely for all tuberculin negative children between ten and 14 years. BCG should not be given to HIV-positive children due to the risk of dissemination.

As most children are infected from a household contact, it is essential to screen other family members for the disease. Children who are exposed to smear positive individuals (where organisms are visualised on sputum) are given a Mantoux test and treated with a single agent, usually isoniazid. After 3 months, if the child is Mantoux negative on repeat testing, has a normal chest x-ray and is clinically well, drug therapy is stopped and the child given BCG.

Atypical TB
There are numerous mycobacteria found in the environment. Immunocompetent individuals rarely suffer from diseases caused by these organisms. They occasionally cause lymphadenopathy which is usually treated surgically. These organisms, however, may cause disseminated infection in immunocompromised individuals. *Mycobacterium avium complex* (MAC) infections are particularly common in patients with AIDS. These organisms do not respond well to standard mycobacterial treatment and require a cocktail of antituberculous drugs.

Lyme disease

This disease, caused by the spirochaete *Borrelia burgdorferi*, was first recognised in 1975 in a cluster of children with arthritis in Lyme, Connecticut. Some cases have been reported in northern Europe including the UK. The organism is transmitted by the hard tick which has a range of hosts but favours deer and moose. It occurs most commonly in the summer months.

Clinical features
Following an incubation period of 3–32 days, the first stage of the illness consists of a classical skin lesion known as *erythema chronicum migrans*, a painless red expanding lesion with a bright red outer spreading edge. The skin lesion is often accompanied by fever, headache, malaise, myalgia, arthralgia and lymphadenopathy. These features fluctuate over several weeks and then resolve.

The next stage follows weeks to months later and includes neurological, cardiac and joint manifestations. Neurological disease includes meningoencephalitis and cranial (particularly facial nerve) and peripheral neuropathies. Cardiac disease includes myocarditis and heart block. Joint disease occurs in about 50% and varies from brief migratory arthralgia to acute asymmetric mono- and oligoarthritis of the large joints. Recurrent attacks of arthritis are common. In 10%, chronic erosive joint disease occurs months to years after the initial attack.

Diagnosis
This is based on clinical and epidemiological features and on serology (ELISA or western blot analysis), although serological testing is not entirely reliable. Isolation of the organism is difficult.

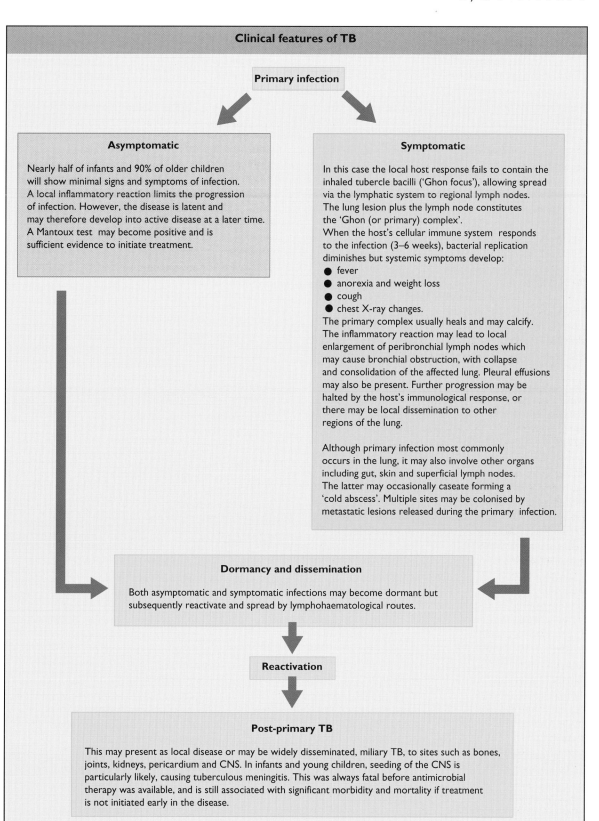

Clinical features of TB

Primary infection

Asymptomatic

Nearly half of infants and 90% of older children will show minimal signs and symptoms of infection. A local inflammatory reaction limits the progression of infection. However, the disease is latent and may therefore develop into active disease at a later time. A Mantoux test may become positive and is sufficient evidence to initiate treatment.

Symptomatic

In this case the local host response fails to contain the inhaled tubercle bacilli ('Ghon focus'), allowing spread via the lymphatic system to regional lymph nodes. The lung lesion plus the lymph node constitutes the 'Ghon (or primary) complex'.
When the host's cellular immune system responds to the infection (3–6 weeks), bacterial replication diminishes but systemic symptoms develop:
● fever
● anorexia and weight loss
● cough
● chest X-ray changes.
The primary complex usually heals and may calcify. The inflammatory reaction may lead to local enlargement of peribronchial lymph nodes which may cause bronchial obstruction, with collapse and consolidation of the affected lung. Pleural effusions may also be present. Further progression may be halted by the host's immunological response, or there may be local dissemination to other regions of the lung.

Although primary infection most commonly occurs in the lung, it may also involve other organs including gut, skin and superficial lymph nodes. The latter may occasionally caseate forming a 'cold abscess'. Multiple sites may be colonised by metastatic lesions released during the primary infection.

Dormancy and dissemination

Both asymptomatic and symptomatic infections may become dormant but subsequently reactivate and spread by lymphohaematological routes.

Reactivation

Post-primary TB

This may present as local disease or may be widely disseminated, miliary TB, to sites such as bones, joints, kidneys, pericardium and CNS. In infants and young children, seeding of the CNS is particularly likely, causing tuberculous meningitis. This was always fatal before antimicrobial therapy was available, and is still associated with significant morbidity and mortality if treatment is not initiated early in the disease.

Fig. 12.13 Clinical features of TB.

Treatment

The drug of choice for all children over eight years old is doxycycline; for younger children it is amoxycillin, with erythromycin for those who are allergic to penicillin. Third-generation cephalosporins are the drug of choice for carditis and neurological disease.

Tropical infections

When assessing an unwell child returning from the tropics, both non-tropical and tropical infections must be considered (Fig. 12.14).

Immunodeficiency disorders

Immunodeficiencies may be *primary*, when there is an intrinsic defect in the immune system or, more commonly, *secondary* to another phenomenon, such as malnutrition, malignant disease, immunosuppresive therapy, splenectomy sickle cell disease, nephrotic syndrome and many bacterial and viral infections, of which infection with HIV is the most severe.

Clinical features

Many of the primary immunodeficiencies (Fig. 12.15) are inherited as X-linked or autosomal recessive disorders. There may be a family history of unexplained death, particularly in boys, and parental consanguinity. Children with an immunodeficiency will usually have a history of infections which are recurrent, persistent or unusual (Fig. 12.16). There may also be evidence of a protein-losing enteropathy and failure to thrive.

Investigation of immunological competence

Is directed towards the most likely cause (fig. 12.17). Investigations can quantify the essential components of the immune system and also provide a functional assessment of immunocompetence.

Treatment

The recent discovery of the genetic basis of many of the primary immunodeficiencies is likely to have a profound impact on future management. Gene therapy, in which a normally functioning gene is transfected into defective progenitor cells, has already been performed for adenosine deaminase deficiency. Until gene therapy becomes available for the other immunodeficiencies, management will continue to comprise:

- antibiotic prophylaxis to prevent infection, e.g. cotrimoxazole to prevent *Pneumocystis carinii* pneumonia
- appropriate antibiotics to treat infection
- immunoglobulin replacement therapy for defects in antibody function or production and replacement of missing factors such as adenosine deaminase or cytokines, e.g. interleukin-2 (IL-2)
- bone marrow transplantation for severe immunodeficiency.

Fig. 12.16 Defects in the components of the immune system that render an individual susceptible to specific types of infection. Only the most common/important are listed.

Immune defect	Infectious susceptibility	
Antibody	Bacteria	Pneumococcus, Staphylococcus, Streptococcus, Haemophilus influenzae
	Viruses	Enteroviruses
Cellular immunity	Bacteria	Mycobacteria, Listeria
	Viruses	CMV, herpes, measles, RSV
	Fungi	Candida, Aspergillus, Pneumocystis carinii
Neutrophils	Bacteria	Gram-positive, Gram-negative
	Fungi	Aspergillus, Candida
Complement	Bacteria	Neisseria, Staphylococcus

Fig. 12.17 Some of the more commonly used tests of immune function in children

Test	Function
Lymphocytes	
Lymphocyte subsets	Determines the number T cells, B cells, monocytes and natural killer (NK) cells
Immunoglobulins	Level of IgG, IgM, IgA and IgE and IgG subclasses
Specific immunoglobulin	Tests the ability to mount an appropriate antibody responses to known antigens, e.g. vaccine response
T cell proliferation in response to mitogens and antigens, e.g. phytohaemaglutinin (PHA) and *Candida*	Functional test of cell-mediated immunity
Neutrophils	
Nitroblue tetrazolium test (NBT)	Defective in chronic granulomatous disease
Adhesion molecules e.g. CD18	Test for leucocyte adhesion deficiency
Complement	
Individual complement components	Reduced in complement deficiency states and other diseases
Total haemolytic complement	Functional test for complement

History

All places visited and duration. Immunisation, malaria prophylaxis. History of food, drink (infected water), accommodation (exposure to vectors), swimming (infected rivers and lakes).

Examination

Particular reference to: fever, jaundice, anaemia, enlarged liver or spleen

Non-tropical causes of fever

Consider non-tropical causes of fever in childhood – urinary tract infection, upper and lower respiratory tract infections, gastroenteritis, septicaemia, meningitis, osteomyelitis, hepatitis, viral infections including the childhood exanthems.

Tropical infections

Malaria

40% of the world's population live in an area where the female *Anopheles* mosquito transmits malaria. Over 1 million children die in Africa each year predominantly from *Plasmodium falciparum* malaria. The clinical features include fever (often not cyclical), diarrhoea, vomiting, flu-like symptoms, jaundice, anaemia and thrombocytopenia. Whilst typically the onset is 7–10 days after inoculation, infections can present many months later. Children are particularly susceptible to severe anaemia and the gravest form of the disease, cerebral malaria. The infection is diagnosed by examination of a thick film. The species (*falciparum, vivax, ovale* or *malariae*) is confirmed on a thin film. Repeated blood films may be necessary.

Typhoid

A child with worsening fever, headaches, cough, abdominal pain, anorexia, malaise and myalgia may be suffering from infection with *Salmonella typhi* or *paratyphi*. Gastro-intestinal symptoms (diarrhoea or constipation) may not appear until the second week. Splenomegaly, bradycardia and rose-coloured spots on the trunk may be present. The serious complications of this disease include gastro-intestinal perforation, myocarditis, hepatitis and nephritis. The recent increase in multi-resistant strains, particularly from the Indian subcontinent, means that treatment with cotrimoxazole, chloramphenicol or ampicillin may be inadequate. A third-generation cephalosporin or ciprofloxacin is usually effective.

Gastroenteritis and dysentery

Gastroenteritis frequently accompanies foreign travel. 'Traveller's diarrhoea' is commonly caused by a change in gut flora, viruses including rotavirus and by *E. coli*. It rarely needs more than attention to rehydration. Fever accompanied by loose stools with blood or mucus suggests dysentery caused by *Shigella, Salmonella, Campylobacter* or *Entamoeba histolytica*. Blood cultures and stool cultures should be taken and appropriate antibiotics started.

Viral haemorrhagic fever

Causes include Dengue fever, and rarely Marburg, Ebola and Lassa fever viruses. These infections are imported, although Hantavirus has recently been isolated from within the UK. Some are highly contagious and strict isolation procedures should be initiated if these infections are suspected.

Quinine is required in nearly all cases seen in the UK because of the emergence of chloroquine-resistant strains worldwide, and primaquine is given (after a G6PD screen) for *Plasmodium vivax* and *ovale* infection to prevent relapse. Travellers to endemic areas should always seek up-to-date information on malaria prevention. Prophylaxis reduces but does not eliminate the risk of infection. Prevention of mosquito bites with repellants and bed nets is also important.

Fig. 12.14 The febrile child returning from the tropics

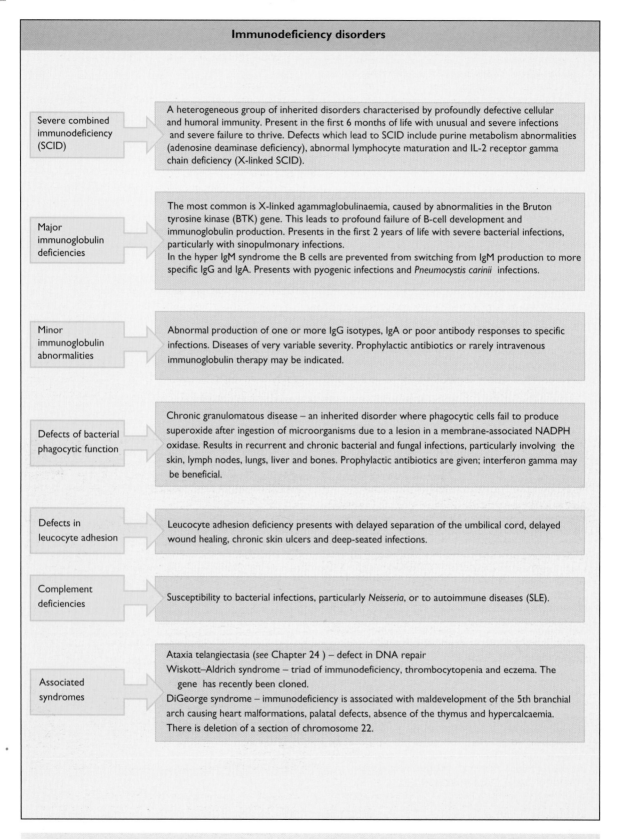

Immunodeficiency disorders

Severe combined immunodeficiency (SCID)

A heterogeneous group of inherited disorders characterised by profoundly defective cellular and humoral immunity. Present in the first 6 months of life with unusual and severe infections and severe failure to thrive. Defects which lead to SCID include purine metabolism abnormalities (adenosine deaminase deficiency), abnormal lymphocyte maturation and IL-2 receptor gamma chain deficiency (X-linked SCID).

Major immunoglobulin deficiencies

The most common is X-linked agammaglobulinaemia, caused by abnormalities in the Bruton tyrosine kinase (BTK) gene. This leads to profound failure of B-cell development and immunoglobulin production. Presents in the first 2 years of life with severe bacterial infections, particularly with sinopulmonary infections.
In the hyper IgM syndrome the B cells are prevented from switching from IgM production to more specific IgG and IgA. Presents with pyogenic infections and *Pneumocystis carinii* infections.

Minor immunoglobulin abnormalities

Abnormal production of one or more IgG isotypes, IgA or poor antibody responses to specific infections. Diseases of very variable severity. Prophylactic antibiotics or rarely intravenous immunoglobulin therapy may be indicated.

Defects of bacterial phagocytic function

Chronic granulomatous disease – an inherited disorder where phagocytic cells fail to produce superoxide after ingestion of microorganisms due to a lesion in a membrane-associated NADPH oxidase. Results in recurrent and chronic bacterial and fungal infections, particularly involving the skin, lymph nodes, lungs, liver and bones. Prophylactic antibiotics are given; interferon gamma may be beneficial.

Defects in leucocyte adhesion

Leucocyte adhesion deficiency presents with delayed separation of the umbilical cord, delayed wound healing, chronic skin ulcers and deep-seated infections.

Complement deficiencies

Susceptibility to bacterial infections, particularly *Neisseria*, or to autoimmune diseases (SLE).

Associated syndromes

Ataxia telangiectasia (*see* Chapter 24) – defect in DNA repair
Wiskott–Aldrich syndrome – triad of immunodeficiency, thrombocytopenia and eczema. The gene has recently been cloned.
DiGeorge syndrome – immunodeficiency is associated with maldevelopment of the 5th branchial arch causing heart malformations, palatal defects, absence of the thymus and hypercalcaemia. There is deletion of a section of chromosome 22.

Fig. 12.15 Immunodeficiency disorders.

HIV INFECTION

The major route of HIV transmission to children is vertically from mother to child, either intrauterine, intrapartum or via breast-feeding. In the UK, Western Europe and the US most mothers become infected from intravenous drug usage, whereas in Africa and other parts of the world, heterosexual spread is the predominant mode of transmission. The virus can also be transmitted to children in infected blood products and contaminated needles. In Europe, approximately 15% of the infants of infected mothers develop HIV infection, but higher rates are reported in other parts of the world.

In children over 18 months old the diagnosis is made by detecting antibodies to HIV. As infants born to infected mothers will have circulating maternal HIV antibodies, the test is unreliable before this age. The HIV-status of these children is commonly referred to as 'indeterminate'. However, HIV infection can be diagnosed in children less than 18 months old by virus culture, detection of viral p24 antigen and detection of viral DNA by polymerase chain reaction (PCR). High immunoglobulin levels, reduced CD4 to CD8 ratio or clinical features may suggest the diagnosis. Even with all these tests persistently negative, an absolute assurance that a child is not infected cannot be given until antibodies to HIV have become undetectable.

Progression to AIDS

Infected children may remain asymptomatic for months or years before progressing to AIDS. Clinical presentation varies with the degree of suppression. Children whose immunosuppression is mild have lymphadenopathy or parotitis; if moderate they have recurrent bacterial infections, candidiasis, chronic diarrhoea and lymphocytic interstitial pneumonitis (LIP) (Fig. 12.18). Severe AIDS-defining disease includes opportunist infections, e.g. *Pneumocystis carinii* pneumonia (PCP), severe failure to thrive, encephalopathy (Fig. 12.19) and malignancy, which is rare in children. More than one clinical feature is often present and an unusual constellation of symptoms, especially if due to an infectious cause, should alert the clinician to consider HIV infection. Even at this stage of the disease, the rate of progression cannot be predicted.

Drug therapy

Prophylaxis against *pneumocystis* pneumonia with cotrimoxazole is widely prescribed for children who are infected or whose infection status is not yet determined. Intravenous immunoglobulin is given in some centres to try to reduce the incidence of bacterial infections, but its efficacy is unproven. Zidovudine (AZT) is the most widely used antiretroviral agent in children. However, combination therapy e.g. AZT with didanosine (ddI) or

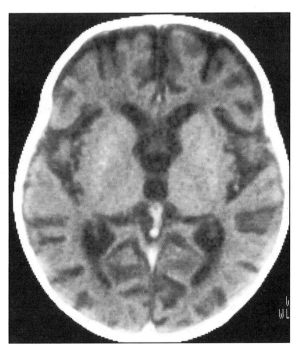

Fig. 12.18 Lymphocytic interstitial pneumonitis (LIP) in a child with HIV infection. There is diffuse reticulonodular shadowing with hilar lymphadenopathy. EBV infection hs been implicated in the pathogenesis of LIP. A similar radiological appearance can be seen with miliary TB, but in contrast to LIP, the child would be acutely unwell.

Fig. 12.19 A CT scan in a child with HIV encephalopathy showing diffuse increase in CSF spaces from cerebral volume loss. The condition may present with developmental delay or as a rapid decline in cerebral function. It responds initially to zidovudine (AZT) therapy.

zalcitabine (ddC) may be superior to zidovudine alone. Antiretroviral agents are usually prescribed at the onset of symptoms as there is some data suggesting that it can modulate disease activity at this stage of the illness. The efficacy of these drugs in asymptomatic children is being assessed.

Recent evidence suggests that AZT given during pregnancy and at the time of delivery may reduce the rate of vertical transmission.

Management of asymptomatic children

Asymptomatic children should be seen regularly to identify disease progression, assess growth and development and monitor immunological function.

Immunisation

All infected children should be immunised according to the normal immunisation schedule. Pneumococcal vaccine should also be given at 18 months–2 years of age. BCG should not be given due to the risk of dissemination. There is also a theoretical risk of infection of immunocompromised care givers if oral polio vaccine is used, and where possible inactivated Salk vaccine should be given.

Social, psychological and family support

Providing coordinated medical, psychological and social support for the whole family is one of the most important aspects of managing HIV-infected children. In nearly all instances at least one parent is also infected. Unless there is a coordinated service for the parents and children, the family will spend a significant proportion of their time travelling to and from hospitals. A multidisciplinary team is required to help the family cope with complicated issues, such as when and what to tell the child, confidentiality, schooling, housing, future pregnancies and planning for the family's future.

It was estimated that in 1993 there were 1 million children and 6 million women with HIV infection throughout the world.

Immunisation

Immunisation is one of the most effective and economic public health measures to improve the health of both children and adults (Fig. 12.20). The most notable success has been the worldwide eradication of smallpox achieved in 1979, but the prevalence of many other diseases has been dramatically reduced by immunisation programmes (Figs 12.21a–e). In many countries the immunisation uptake rate exceeds 90%. If this could be extended worldwide, the deaths of several millions of young children would be prevented.

Although differences exist in the composition and scheduling of immunisation programmes, most are similar to that used in the UK (Fig. 12.22). Following vaccination, there may be swelling and discomfort at the injection site and a mild fever and malaise. Some vaccines, such as measles and rubella, may be followed by a mild form of the disease. More serious reactions, including anaphylaxis, may occur but are very rare.

Local guidelines about vaccination and its contra-indications should be followed. Vaccination should be postponed if the child has an acute illness; however, a minor infection without fever or systemic upset is not a contraindication. Live vaccines should not be given to children with impaired immune responsiveness (except in children with HIV infection in whom MMR vaccine can be given safely).

Following pertussis vaccination, convulsions and encephalopathy are rare complications, but publicity in the UK in the 1970s surrounding this risk resulted in a marked fall in vaccine uptake and was followed by several whooping cough epidemics (see Fig. 12.21b). It is now recognised that in many instances the

Fig. 12.20 Immunisations in children	
Routine immunisations	Diphtheria (T)
	Poliomyelitis – oral (L) parenteral (I)
	Tetanus (T)
	Pertussis (I)
	Measles (L)
	Mumps (L)
	Rubella (L)
	Haemophilus influenzae b (S)
Immunisations available for children at risk	TB (BCG) (L)
	Hepatitis A and B (S)
	Meningococcus (serogroups A, C, Y, W135) (S)
	Pneumococcus (S)
	Influenza (S)
Immunisations available for children travelling abroad	Typhoid – oral (L), parenteral (I)
	Cholera (I)
	Yellow fever (L)
	Rabies (I)
	Japanese encephalitis (I)
	Tick-borne encephalitis (I)
Immunisation under trial or development	Varicella
	Conjugated meningococcal and pneumococcal vaccines
	Diarrhoea pathogens, e.g. rotavirus
	Respiratory viruses, e.g. RSV
	Malaria
	HIV infection
L = live attenuated; I = inactivated ; T = toxoid; S = subunit	

complications were falsely attributed to the vaccine and that the neurological complications from the illness itself are considerably more frequent than after the vaccine.

The main contraindication to pertussis vaccination is if the child has experienced a severe local or general reaction to a preceding dose. If there is an evolving neurological problem, immunisation should be deferred until the condition is stable. A personal or family history of febrile convulsions is not a contraindication, but, advice on fever prevention should be given.

The MMR vaccine is contraindicated in children who are allergic to neomycin or kanamycin, which may be present in small quantities in the vaccine. Children with a history of anaphylaxis to egg (in which the virus for the vaccine is grown) can be immunised, but only under close specialist supervision.

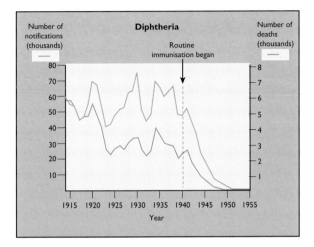

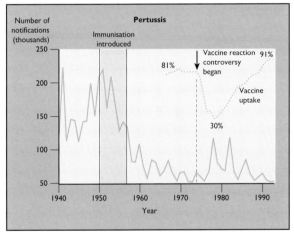

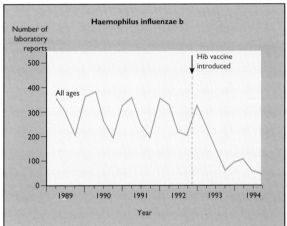

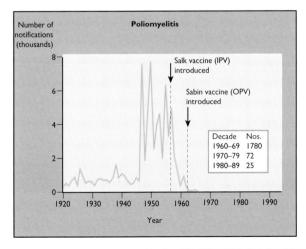

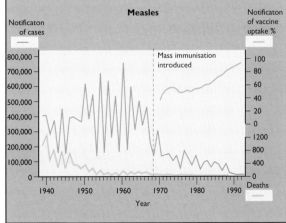

Fig. 12.21 Effect of immunisation on the number of notifications in England and Wales. (a) DIptheria (b) Pertussis (c) Polio (d) Haemophilus influenzae b (e) Measles (courtesy of PHLS Communicable Disease Surveillance Centre).

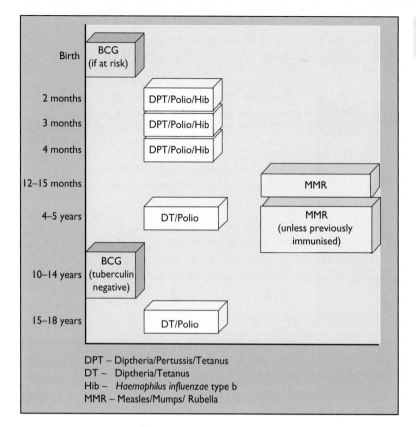

Fig. 12.22 Immunisation schedule in the UK.

DPT – Diptheria/Pertussis/Tetanus
DT – Diptheria/Tetanus
Hib – *Haemophilus influenzae* type b
MMR – Measles/Mumps/ Rubella

FURTHER READING

Davies EG, Elliman DAC, Hart CA, Nicoll A, Rudd PT. *Manual of Childhood Infections.* British Paediatric Association. WB Saunders London 1996.

Department of Health. *Immunisation Against Infectious Disease.* HMSO, London. 1996. Manual on immunisation practice in the UK.

Feigin RD, Cherry JD. *Textbook of Paediatric Infectious Disease.* 3rd edn. WB Saunders, Philadelphia. 1992. Large comprehensive textbook.

Report of the Committee on Infectious Diseases. 'Red Book' 23rd edn. American Academy of Pediatrics. 1994. Manual on paediatric infections and immunisation in the US.

Respiratory Disorders

Respiratory disorders are important as:
- they account for 50% of consultations with general practitioners for acute illness in young children and one-third of consultations in older children
- respiratory illness leads to 20–35% of acute paediatric admissions to hospital
- they are the fifth most common cause of death in children aged between one and 14 years in the UK
- asthma is the most common chronic illness of childhood in the UK and the most frequent single cause for emergency hospital admission
- cystic fibrosis is the most common lethal inherited disorder in Caucasians.

Respiratory infections

These are the most frequent infections of childhood. The pre-school child has on average 6–8 respiratory infections a year. Most are mild, self-limiting illnesses but some, such as bronchiolitis or epiglottitis, are potentially life-threatening.

Pathogens
Viruses cause 80–90% of childhood respiratory infections. The most important are the respiratory syncytial virus (RSV), rhinoviruses, parainfluenza, influenza and adenoviruses. An individual virus can cause several different patterns of illness, e.g. RSV can cause bronchiolitis, croup, pneumonia or a common cold.

The important bacterial respiratory pathogens are *Streptococcus pneumoniae* (pneumococcus) and other streptococci, *Haemophilus influenzae*, *Bordetella pertussis* which causes whooping cough, and *Mycoplasma pneumoniae*. *Mycobacterium tuberculosis* remains an important pathogen. Some pathogens cause predictable epidemics, such as RSV bronchiolitis every winter, whereas others, e.g. pneumococcus, show little seasonal variation.

Host and environmental factors
An increased risk of respiratory infection is associated with:
- poor socio-economic status (such as overcrowded, damp housing and poor nutrition)
- large family size
- maternal smoking
- boys more than girls
- prematurity – especially infants who have required artificial ventilation
- congenital abnormalities of the heart or lungs
- rarely, immune deficiency, either congenital, e.g. agammaglobulinaemia, or acquired, e.g. malignant disease or HIV infection.

The child's age influences the prevalence and severity of infections (Fig. 13.1). It is in infancy that serious respiratory illness requiring hospital admission is most common and the risk of death is greatest. There is an increased frequency of infections when the child or older siblings start nursery or school. Repeated upper respiratory tract infections are rarely an indication of underlying disease.

Classification of respiratory infections
Respiratory infections are classified according to the level of the respiratory tree most involved:
- upper respiratory tract infection
- laryngeal/tracheal infection
- bronchitis
- bronchiolitis
- pneumonia.

UPPER RESPIRATORY TRACT INFECTION (URTI)
80% of respiratory infections involve only the nose, throat, ears or sinuses.

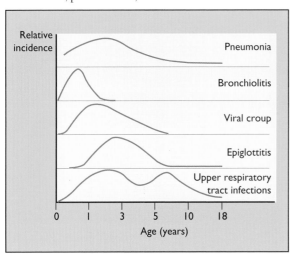

Fig. 13.1 Age distribution of acute respiratory infections in children.

The term URTI embraces a number of different conditions:
- common cold (coryza)
- sore throat (pharyngitis, including tonsillitis)
- acute otitis media
- sinusitis (relatively uncommon).

The most common presentation is a child with a combination of a painful throat, fever, nasal blockage and discharge and earache. Cough is troublesome in many cases. URTIs may cause:
- difficulty in feeding in infants as their noses are blocked and this obstructs breathing
- febrile convulsions
- precipitation of acute asthma.

In infants, hospital admission may be required to exclude a more serious infection.

The common cold (coryza)

The most common infection of childhood. Classical features include a clear or mucopurulent nasal discharge and nasal blockage. The most common pathogens are viruses – rhinoviruses (of which there over a 100 different serotypes), corona viruses and RSV. Health education to advise parents that colds are self-limiting and have no specific curative treatment may reduce anxiety and save unnecessary visits to doctors. Fever and pain are best treated with paracetamol or ibuprofen. Antibiotics are of no benefit as the common cold is not caused by bacteria and secondary bacterial infection is uncommon.

Sore throat (pharyngitis)

Is usually of viral origin. Respiratory viruses, (mostly adenoviruses, enteroviruses and rhinoviruses) are the most common pathogens. In the older child *Group A β-haemolytic streptococcus* is a common pathogen.

Tonsillitis

Is a form of pharyngitis where there is intense inflammation of the tonsils, often with a purulent exudate. *Group A β-haemolytic* streptococci and the Epstein–Barr virus (infectious mononucleosis) are common pathogens.

It is not possible to distinguish clinically between viral and bacterial pharyngitis/tonsillitis. Marked constitutional disturbance such as headache, apathy and abdominal pain, tonsillar exudate and lymphadenopathy are more common with bacterial infection. It is reasonable to give penicillin (or erythromycin if there is penicillin allergy) for severe pharyngitis and tonsillitis even though only one-third are caused by bacteria. Antibiotics may hasten recovery from streptococcal infection, but ten days's treatment is required to eradicate the organism to prevent rheumatic fever. Some doctors restrict the use of antibiotics to those children with positive streptococcal cultures from throat swabs. Amoxycillin and ampicillin are best avoided as they may cause a widespread maculopapular rash if the child has infectious mononucleosis.

 It is not possible to distinguish clinically viral from bacterial tonsillitis

Acute infection of the middle ear (acute otitis media)

Is common; 20% of children under four years old are affected at least once a year. There is pain in the ear and fever. The child is irritable and may pull at the affected ear. Every child with a fever must have their tympanic membranes examined (Fig. 13.2a–d). In acute otitis media the tympanic membrane is seen to be bright red and bulging with loss of the normal light reflection. Occasionally there is acute perforation of the ear drum with pus visible in the external canal. Pathogens include viruses, pneumococcus, *Group A β-haemolytic streptococcus*, *Haemophilus influenzae* and *Moraxella catarrhalis*. Serious complications such as mastoiditis and meningitis are now uncommon.

Pain should be treated with paracetamol. Although many cases of acute otitis media resolve spontaneously within 24 hours, an antibiotic is usually given to shorten the illness and reduce the risk of complications. Amoxycillin is widely used but amoxycillin with clavulanic acid, or cefaclor, are reasonable alternatives in view of the increasing proportion of β-lactamase-producing *H.influenzae* and *M. catarrhalis*. Decongestants are often given to help Eustachian tube drainage, but their efficacy is unproven.

Recurrent ear infections can lead to chronic secretory otitis media (glue ear), the most common cause of conductive hearing loss in children. This can interfere with normal speech development and result in learning difficulties in school. This condition also causes earache due to pressure changes resulting from obstruction to the Eustachian tube.

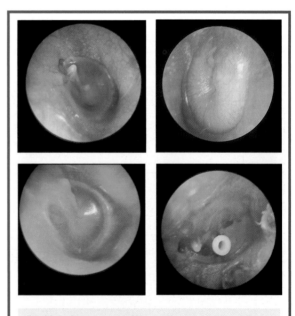

Fig. 13.2 Appearance of the eardrum (a) Normal (b) Acute otitis media (c) Chronic secretory otitis media (d) Grommet. (Courtesy of Mr N. Shah & Mr N. Tolley.)

Sinusitis

Infection of the paranasal sinuses may occur with viral URTIs. Occasionally there is secondary bacterial infection with pain, swelling and tenderness over the cheek from infection of the maxillary sinus. As the frontal sinuses do not develop until late childhood, frontal sinusitis is uncommon in the first decade of life. Antibiotics and analgesia are used for acute sinusitis.

Tonsillectomy and adenoidectomy

Children with recurrent URTIs are often referred for removal of their tonsils and adenoids, one of the most common operations performed in children. Many children have large tonsils, but this in itself is not an indication for tonsillectomy as tonsils shrink spontaneously in late childhood.

The indications for surgery remain controversial, but for tonsillectomy are:
- recurrent tonsillitis (as opposed to recurrent URTIs), particularly if they interfere with the child's development or schooling, despite adequate antibiotic treatment
- a peritonsillar abscess (quinsy)
- obstructive sleep apnoea.

Like the tonsils, adenoids increase in size until about the age of seven years and then gradually regress. They may sufficiently narrow the posterior nasal space to justify adenoidectomy if they cause:
- chronic secretory otitis media and hearing loss from Eustachian tube malfunction. These children may also benefit from the insertion of ventilation tubes (grommets) although there is also debate about the benefit of these procedures

- upper airways obstruction leading to snoring and mouth breathing, hypoxaemia during sleep, and more seriously, obstructive sleep apnoea when the child snores loudly, breathes 'heavily', may struggle for breath and stops breathing for 30–45 seconds when asleep. Sleep disturbance leads to daytime somnolence; in severe cases, pulmonary hypertension, failure to thrive and developmental delay can occur. Adenotonsillectomy is usually curative (Fig. 13.3a,b).

LARYNGEAL AND TRACHEAL INFECTIONS

The mucosal inflammation and swelling produced by these infections can rapidly cause life-threatening obstruction of the airways in young children. Several conditions can cause acute upper airways obstruction (Fig. 13.4). They are characterised by:
- stridor, a rasping sound heard predominantly on inspiration
- hoarseness due to inflammation of the vocal cords
- in most cases a barking cough like a sea lion.

The severity of upper airways obstruction is best assessed clinically by:
- the degree of sternal and subcostal recession (Fig. 13.5)
- respiratory rate
- heart rate
- increasing agitation
- drowsiness, tiredness, exhaustion
- central cyanosis indicating severe hypoxaemia and the need for urgent intervention.

The measurement of oxygen saturation by pulse oximetry is the most reliable objective measure of hypoxaemia.

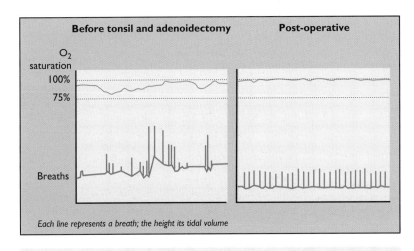

Fig. 13.3 Extract from cardiorespiratory monitoring in a child with obstructive sleep apnoea showing (a) irregular breathing with periodic pauses associated with desaturation. Post adenotonsillectomy (b), the breathing is regular and the desaturation has resolved. (Courtesy of Dr Parviz Habibi)

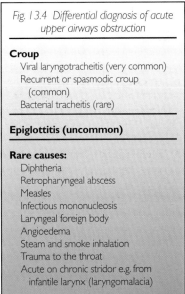

Fig. 13.4 Differential diagnosis of acute upper airways obstruction

Croup
Viral laryngotracheitis (very common)
Recurrent or spasmodic croup (common)
Bacterial tracheitis (rare)

Epiglottitis (uncommon)

Rare causes:
Diphtheria
Retropharyngeal abscess
Measles
Infectious mononucleosis
Laryngeal foreign body
Angioedema
Steam and smoke inhalation
Trauma to the throat
Acute on chronic stridor e.g. from infantile larynx (laryngomalacia)

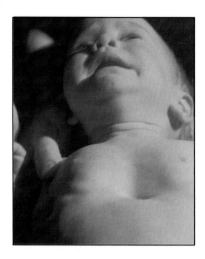

Fig. 13.5 The degree of subcostal, intercostal and sternal recession is a more useful indicator of severity of upper airways obstruction than the respiratory rate. (© Boehringer Ingelheim International GmbH)

Total obstruction may be precipitated by examination of the throat using a spatula – one must avoid looking at the throat of a child with upper airways obstruction unless full resuscitation equipment and personnel are at hand.

 Basic management of upper airways obstruction:
- *don't examine the throat*
- *reduce anxiety by staff being calm, confident and well organised*
- *watch carefully for signs of deterioration*
- *urgent tracheal intubation for respiratory failure from increasing airways obstruction, exhaustion or secretions blocking the airway.*

Viral croup

Viral croup accounts for over 95% of laryngotracheal infections. Parainfluenza viruses are the most common cause but other viruses can produce a similar clinical picture. There is mucosal inflammation and increased secretions affecting the larynx, trachea and bronchi, but it is the narrowing of the subglottic area that is potentially dangerous in young children because of their narrow trachea. The peak incidence of croup is in the second year of life. The typical features are of a barking cough, harsh stridor and hoarseness, usually preceded by fever and coryza. The symptoms often start, and are worse, at night.

The child with mild viral croup can usually be managed at home. When the upper airways obstruction is mild, the stridor and chest recession disappear when the child is at rest. Parents need to observe the child closely for signs of increasing severity. The decision to manage the child at home or in hospital is influenced by the severity of the illness, the time of day, the ease of access to hospital, the age of the child (with a low threshold for those <12 months old) and the parents' understanding and confidence about the disorder.

Inhalation of warm moist air is widely used but is of unproven benefit. Nebulised steroids may be helpful in severe croup; the place of systemic corticosteroids to reduce subglottic inflammation remains uncertain. Nebulised adrenaline can provide transient improvement in severe upper airways obstruction, but cardiorespiratory monitoring should be performed when it is given. About 2–5% of children admitted with croup require tracheal intubation.

Spasmodic or recurrent croup

Some young children suddenly develop a barking cough and stridor at night without preceding respiratory tract symptoms. These children appear to have hyper-reactive upper airways, and some will develop asthma.

Bacterial tracheitis

This rare but dangerous condition is usually caused by infection with *Staph. aureus* or *Haemophilus influenzae*. The clinical picture is similar to severe viral croup except that the child has a high fever, appears toxic and has rapidly progressive airways obstruction. At tracheal intubation copious thick secretions are found.

Acute epiglottitis

Acute epiglottitis is an uncommon life-threatening emergency due to respiratory obstruction. It is caused by *H. influenzae* type b. There is intense swelling of the epiglottis and surrounding tissues. The accompanying septicaemia accelerates the progression of the illness and likelihood of sudden collapse. Epiglottitis is most common in children aged 1–6 years but can affect all age groups. The incidence of the disease has fallen markedly since the introduction of routine immunisation against *H. influenzae* b (Hib). It is imperative to distinguish between epiglottitis and viral croup (Fig. 13.6) as they require quite different treatment.

The onset of epiglottitis is very acute with:
- high fever in an ill, toxic-looking child
- an intensely painful throat that prevents the child from speaking or swallowing. Saliva drools down the chin
- soft inspiratory stridor and rapidly increasing respiratory difficulty over hours
- the child sitting immobile, upright, with an open mouth to maximise the airway.

In contrast to viral croup, cough is minimal or absent.

Fig. 13.6 Clinical features of viral laryngotracheitis (croup) and epiglottitis

	Croup	Epiglottitis
Onset	Over days	Over hours
Preceding coryza	Yes	No
Cough	Severe, barking	Absent or slight
Able to drink	Yes	No
Drooling saliva	No	Yes
Appearance	Unwell	Toxic, very ill
Fever	<38.5°C	>38.5°C
Stridor	Harsh, rasping	Soft, whispering
Voice, cry	Hoarse	Muffled, reluctant to speak

Attempts to lie the child down or examine the throat with a spatula can precipitate total obstruction and death and must be avoided.

Once the diagnosis has been made, urgent hospital admission and treatment are required. A senior anaesthetist, paediatrician and ENT surgeon should be summoned and treatment initiated without delay. The child should be transferred directly to the intensive care unit or an anaesthetic room, and must be accompanied by senior medical staff in case respiratory obstruction occurs. The child should be intubated under a general anaesthetic to maintain a patent airway. Rarely, this is impossible and an urgent tracheostomy is lifesaving. Only after the airway is established should blood be taken for culture and intravenous antibiotics started. A second- or third-generation cephalosporin (e.g. cefuroxime or cefotoxime) is suitable. The tracheal tube can usually be removed after 24 hours and antibiotics given for about five days. With appropriate treatment, most children recover completely within 3–5 days. As with other serious *H. influenzae* infections, prophylaxis with rifampicin is offered to close household contacts.

 Minutes count in acute epiglottitis.

BRONCHITIS

There is some controversy about the term bronchitis in childhood. Whereas a degree of inflammation of the bronchi producing a mixture of wheeze and coarse crackles is a feature of the many respiratory infections, bronchitis in children is very different from the chronic bronchitis of adults. In acute bronchitis in children, cough and fever are the main symptoms. The cough may persist for about two weeks. There is no evidence that antibiotics, cough suppressants or expectorants expedite recovery.

There is also disagreement over the use of the term 'wheezy bronchitis'. Many authorities define this as a presentation of asthma, while others consider that the bronchial inflammation and smooth muscle spasm are related to the effect of the particular infectious organisms affecting infants, rather than to the child's permanent predisposition to bronchial hyper-reactivity. If there is 'recurrent bronchitis' with hyperinflation of the chest or wheeze, the child has asthma and appropriate therapy should be given.

Whooping Cough (pertussis)

Is a specific and highly infectious form of bronchitis, caused by *Bordetella pertussis*. It is endemic, with epidemics every four years. After 2–3 days of coryza, the child develops a

---

Case History

ACUTE EPIGLOTTITIS

This 5-year-old girl developed a severe sore throat, drooling of saliva, a high fever and increasing difficulty breathing over 8 hours (Fig.13.7a). Epiglottitis was diagnosed and treatment started immediately (Fig. 13.7 b, c).

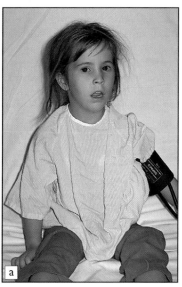 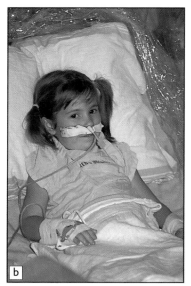 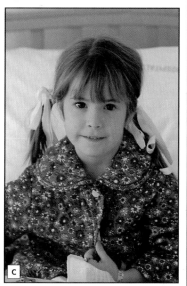

Fig. 13.7 Acute epiglottitis. (a) At presentation. (b) At 14 hours, with nasotracheal and nasogastric tubes and an indwelling cannula for intravenous antibiotics. (c) At 36 hours, following removal of the nasotracheal and nasogastic tubes.

characteristic paroxysmal or spasmodic cough followed by a characteristic inspiratory whoop. The spasms of cough are often worse at night and may culminate in vomiting. During a paroxysm, the child goes red or blue in the face, and mucus flows from the nose and mouth. The whoop at the end of a spasm may be absent in infants. Epistaxes and sub-conjunctival haemorrhages can occur after vigorous coughing. Symptoms may persist for 10–12 weeks.

Complications of pertussis such as pneumonia, convulsions and bronchiectasis are uncommon, but there is still a significant mortality, particularly in infants in whom the infection can cause apnoea and sudden unexpected death. Infants and young children suffering cyanotic attacks should be admitted to hospital.

Characteristically, there is a marked lymphocytosis (>15 000 cells/mm³). The organism can be identified early in the disease from a per-nasal swab.

Although erythromycin eradicates the organism and its early use may reduce family spread, there is no specific treatment that reduces the duration of the illness. Siblings, parents or school contacts may develop a similar cough. Immunisation reduces the risk of an individual developing pertussis by 80–90% but does not guarantee protection.

BRONCHIOLITIS

Bronchiolitis is the most common serious respiratory infection of infancy. Two to three per cent of all infants are admitted to hospital with the disease each year during annual winter epidemics. Ninety per cent are aged 1–9 months – bronchiolitis is rare after one year of age. Respiratory syncitial virus (RSV) is the pathogen in 75–80% cases.

Clinical features

Coryzal symptoms precede a dry cough and increasing breathlessness. Wheezing is often but not always present. Feeding difficulties associated with increasing dyspnoea are often the reason for admission to hospital. Recurrent apnoea is a serious complication in infants in the first few months of life. Infants born prematurely who develop bronchopulmonary dysplasia and infants with congenital heart disease are more severely affected. The findings on examination are characteristic:

- sharp, dry cough
- tachypnoea
- subcostal and intercostal recession
- hyperinflation of the chest
    sternum prominent
    liver displaced downwards
- fine end-inspiratory crackles
- high pitched wheezes
    expiratory > inspiratory
- tachycardia
- cyanosis or pallor.

Investigations

RSV can be identified rapidly using a fluorescent antibody test on nasopharyngeal secretions. The chest X-ray shows hyperinflation of the lungs due to small airways obstruction

and air trapping (Fig. 13.8). Blood gas analysis, which is required in only the most severe cases, shows lowered arterial oxygen and raised CO_2 tension.

Management

Is supportive. Humidified oxygen is delivered into a headbox; the concentration required is ascertained using a pulse oximeter. The child is monitored for apnoea. Mist, antibiotics and steroids are not helpful. Nebulised bronchodilators do not reduce the severity or duration of the illness. The antiviral drug ribavirin only marginally shortens viral excretion and clinical symptoms, and should be considered only for infants with underlying cardiopulmonary disorders or immunodeficiency. Fluids may need to be given by nasogastric tube or intravenously. Mechanical ventilation is required in about 2% of infants admitted to hospital.

Prognosis

Most infants recover from the acute infection within two weeks. However, as many as half will have recurrent episodes of cough and wheeze over the next 3–5 years. Rarely, the illness is very severe and results in permanent damage to the airways (*bronchiolitis obliterans*).

PNEUMONIA

A wide range of pathogens cause pneumonia in childhood and different organisms affect different age groups.

The *newborn* is infected by organisms from the mother's genital tract. The most common is the Group B β-haemolytic streptococcus. Other pathogens are *E. coli* and other Gram-negative bacilli. *Chlamydia trachomatis*, (which is also a cause of neonatal conjunctivitis), is an unusual but important pathogen.

In *infancy*, respiratory viruses, particularly RSV, are the most frequent cause but bacterial infection from *Streptococcus pneumoniae* and *Haemophilus influenzae* are also important. *Staphylococcus aureus* is uncommon but causes severe infection.

As *children* become older, viruses become less frequent pathogens and bacterial infection more prominent. *Mycoplasma pneumoniae* is a common cause of pneumonia in school age children. Tuberculosis should be considered at all ages.

Fever, cough, breathlessness and lethargy following an upper respiratory tract infection are the usual presenting symptoms. Breathing is rapid, shallow and gives the impression that the child is afraid to breathe deeply. Pleuritic chest pain, neck stiffness and abdominal pain may be present if there is pleural inflammation. Classical signs of consolidation with impaired percussion, decreased breath sounds and bronchial breathing are often absent, particularly in infants, and a chest X-ray is needed. The chest X-ray may show lobar consolidation (Fig. 13.9), patchy bronchopneumonia or, less commonly, cavitation of the lung (Fig. 13.10). Pleural effusions are quite common, particularly in bacterial pneumonia. Blood cultures, nasopharyngeal aspirates for viral isolation and a full blood count should also be performed in children needing hospitalisation.

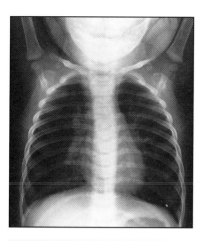

Fig. 13.8 In acute bronchiolitis the chest X-ray shows hyperinflation of the lungs with flattening and depression of the diaphragm, horizontal ribs and increased hilar bronchial markings.

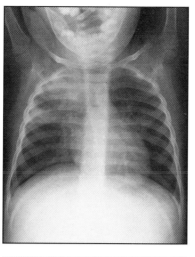

Fig. 13.9 Consolidation of the right upper lobe. Lobar consolidation is a feature of pneumococcal pneumonia.

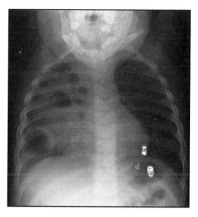

Fig. 13.10 Multiple cavities containing fluid and air in staphylococcal pneumonia.

Management

It is not possible to differentiate reliably between bacterial or viral infection on clinical or radiological grounds, so all children diagnosed as having pneumonia should receive antibiotics. As it is unlikely for the pathogen to be known when treatment is started, the choice of antibiotic is determined by the child's age, severity of illness and appearance of the chest X-ray. If intravenous therapy is required, activity against pneumococci, *H. influenzae* and *Staph. aureus* can be achieved with a second-generation cephalosporin (e.g. cefuroxime). Oral antibiotics (e.g. co-amoxiclav or a second-generation cephalosporin such as cefaclor) are given for less severe infections. If *M. pneumoniae* or *Chlamydia trachomatis* pneumonia is suspected, erythromycin is given. Physiotherapy, an adequate fluid intake and oxygen in severe pneumonia may be required. If a child has recurrent or persistent pneumonia, investigations to exclude an underlying condition such as cystic fibrosis or immunodeficiency is indicated.

 Consider pneumonia in children with neck stiffness or acute abdominal pain.

Asthma

Asthma is the most common chronic respiratory disorder in children, affecting between 11% and 15% of school children. There has been a real increase in the prevalence of asthma in the community. The reasons for this are unclear. In childhood, asthma is twice as common in boys as in girls but by adolescence equal numbers are affected.

Hospital admissions for asthma have increased dramatically in recent years; sevenfold since 1970 for children younger than four years and triple in those 5–14 years old. Asthma is now responsible for 10–20% of all acute medical admissions to paediatric wards in children of 1–14 years. In most children the symptoms of asthma are readily controlled, but asthma is an important cause of school absenteeism, restricted activity and anxiety for the child and family. There are still 20-30 deaths from asthma in children each year in the UK.

Pathophysiology

We now have a better understanding of the pathophysiology of asthma (Fig. 13.11). A combination of a genetic predisposition and environmental influences (e.g. exposure to housedust mite or cigarette smoke) results in chronic inflammation of the bronchial mucosa and airway hyperreactivity. Exposure of the sensitised airway to a number of trigger factors results in bronchoconstriction, mucosal oedema and excessive mucus production which in turn lead to airway narrowing and the clinical features of asthma.

Atopy

The term 'atopy' is not clearly defined but describes a group of disorders that tends to co-exist in individuals and their families (Fig. 13.12).

One-third of children with asthma have or have had eczema. One-half have symptoms of allergic rhinitis – recurrent or persistent obstruction of the nostrils with sniffing, sneezing and nasal discharge. There may be accompanying redness and swelling of the eyes (allergic conjunctivitis). These may occur only in the summer when the grass pollen count is high (hayfever) or throughout the year (perennial rhinitis).

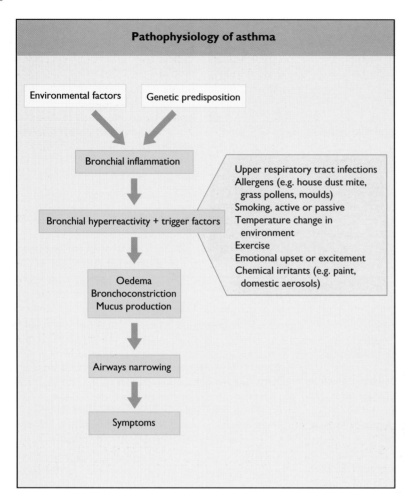

Pathophysiology of asthma

Environmental factors

Genetic predisposition

↓

Bronchial inflammation

↓

Bronchial hyperreactivity + trigger factors

Upper respiratory tract infections
Allergens (e.g. house dust mite,
grass pollens, moulds)
Smoking, active or passive
Temperature change in
environment
Exercise
Emotional upset or excitement
Chemical irritants (e.g. paint,
domestic aerosols)

↓

Oedema
Bronchoconstriction
Mucus production

↓

Airways narrowing

↓

Symptoms

Fig. 13.11 Pathophysiology of asthma.

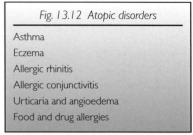

Fig. 13.12 Atopic disorders

Asthma
Eczema
Allergic rhinitis
Allergic conjunctivitis
Urticaria and angioedema
Food and drug allergies

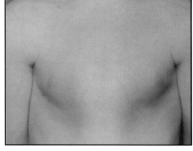

Fig. 13.13 Pectus carinatum ('pigeon chest') deformity is usually associated with chronic airways obstruction, such as asthma. The depressions at the base of the thorax associated with the muscular insertion of the diaphragm are called Harrison sulci.

Many atopic patients have positive skin tests to common allergens (such as housedust mite, pollens and animal danders), eosinophilia and raised serum levels of IgE.

Diagnosis

The diagnosis is primarily clinical and depends on eliciting a history of the typical symptoms of recurrent wheeze, cough and breathlessness. In the pre-school child the main symptom may be a troublesome nocturnal cough. The frequency and severity of symptoms vary enormously, from the child who has infrequent attacks once or twice a year, to the child who is rarely free of debilitating symptoms. The diagnosis is supported by a history of characteristic trigger factors and a personal or family history of atopic disease, although the absence of a family history of atopy does not preclude the diagnosis.

The severity of asthma can be assessed by asking:

• how frequent are the symptoms?
• how is it affecting the child's life?
• how much school has been missed?
• can he play sport normally?
• how often is sleep disturbed?
• what is the longest period he is free from symptoms?

Examination of the chest is usually normal between attacks. In longstanding airways obstruction there may be hyperinflation of the chest and generalised expiratory wheezes. A chest deformity accompanied by Harrison sulci or pectus carinatum (pigeon chest) usually indicates longstanding airways obstruction (Fig. 13.13). Eczema may be present and there may be bogginess of the nasal mucosa from allergic rhinitis. Growth is normal unless the asthma is very severe. The presence of finger clubbing indicates another underlying pathology such as cystic fibrosis or congenital heart disease.

Investigations

Usually the diagnosis is clear from the history and examination, and no investigations are needed. Skin tests are usually positive indicating atopy, but rarely influence management. Similarly a chest X-ray will often show hyperinflation. In infants a chest X-ray is helpful to exclude congenital abnormalities. Most children over the age of five years can use a peak flow meter, and their peak expiratory flow rate (PEFR) should be compared to that predicted for their height (Fig. 13.14 and Appendix). If necessary, the presence of reversible airways obstruction can be demonstrated by measuring the PEFR before and 15 minutes after inhalation of a bronchodilator.

Differential diagnosis

Asthma is still underdiagnosed and undertreated. Many children are labelled as having recurrent chest infections or wheezy bronchitis and receive inappropriate or inadequate treatment. The diagnosis is more difficult in the infant or toddler where other conditions can cause wheeze and breathlessness (Fig. 13.15).

Management

The aim is to allow the child to lead a normal life. This should be achieved with as little medication and disruption to the family's life as possible. The treatment of asthma can be divided into maintenance therapy to control symptoms and the management of acute exacerbations.

Maintenance therapy

The two main groups of drugs used for maintenance therapy are bronchodilators, which give short-term symptomatic relief and prophylactic drugs which reduce bronchial inflammation and hyper-reactivity (Fig. 13.16).

Bronchodilator therapy

The short-acting bronchodilators can be taken orally or by inhalation. The inhaled route is preferable as it gives more rapid onset of action with fewer side-effects. The long-acting β_2-bronchodilators reduce sleep disturbance and exercise-induced symptoms in children with frequent symptoms but they should only be used in conjunction with inhaled steroids. Slow-release oral theophyllines are effective bronchodilators but the high incidence of side-effects (vomiting, insomnia, increased activity, headaches, poor concentration), and the need to monitor drug levels in the blood mean that they are now rarely used in children. Ipratropium bromide, an analogue of atropine, is given to infants when other bronchodilators are found to be ineffective.

Prophylactic therapy

Prophylactic drugs are effective only if taken regularly. Sodium cromoglycate stabilises the mast cell and is exceptionally free of side-effects. Inhaled steroids are the most effective inhaled prophylactic therapy. They have no clinically significant side-effects when given in standard doses. Oral prednisolone, usually given on alternate days to minimise the adverse effect on height, is required only in severe persistent asthma where other treatment has failed. Antibiotics are of no value in the absence of a bacterial infection. Cough medicines and decongestants are unhelpful. Antihistamines, e.g. terfenadine, are useful in the treatment of allergic rhinitis but not in asthma.

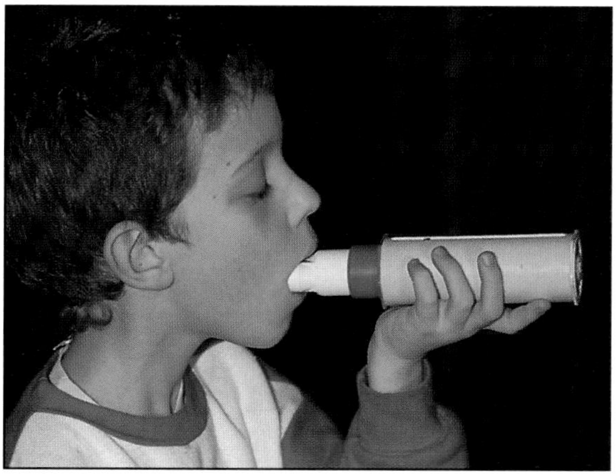

Fig. 13.14 Measurement of the peak expiratory flow rate (PEFR) provides an objective measurement of the severity of airflow obstruction in asthma. Normal values of PEFR are related to height.

Fig. 13.15 Causes of recurrent wheeze in infancy

Asthma
Following bronchiolitis
Recurrent aspiration of feeds
Ex-preterm infant
Cystic fibrosis
Maternal smoking
Cow's milk protein intolerance
Inhaled foreign body
Congenital abnormality of lung, airway or heart
Idiopathic

Fig. 13.16 Drugs in asthma

Type of drug	Drug
β_2 bronchodilators	
Short-acting	Salbutamol
	Terbutaline
Long-acting	Salmeterol
Anticholinergic bronchodilator	
Short-acting	Ipratropium bromide
Preventative/prophylactic treatment	
Inhaled steroids	Budesonide
	Beclomethasone
	Fluticasone
Sodium cromoglycate	
Methyl xanthines	Theophylline
Oral steroids	Prednisolone

All are given by inhalation, except prednisolone and theophylline preparations.

Types of chronic asthma

There is a logical step wise progression to treatment (Fig. 13.17). This is determined by the frequency and severity of symptoms.

1. Infrequent episodic asthma

Three-quarters of asthmatic children have fewer than four episodes a year. Between attacks they are free from symptoms. They need no regular treatment and episodes should be treated with β_2-bronchodilators, given by the inhaled route. If attacks are severe they may need nebulised bronchodilators and a short course of prednisolone.

2. Frequent episodic asthma

One-fifth of children have symptoms every 2–4 weeks. They need regular inhaled prophylactic therapy. Initially this can be with sodium cromoglycate. In addition, an inhaled bronchodilator is used intermittently as required. If this does not control the child's symptoms prophylaxis should be changed to an inhaled steroid.

3. Persistent asthma

Less than 5% of asthmatic children have persistent symptoms. All require inhaled prophylaxis. Sodium cromoglycate is less effective in this group and prophylaxis with inhaled steroids is required. Regular bronchodilators may be needed. A long-acting β_2-bronchodilator may be useful. If symptoms persist, oral prednisolone will be required in a dose titrated against the clinical response so that the minimum is used. Such children need regular monitoring of their asthma and growth and for any side-effects of medication in a specialist clinic. Regular recording of symptoms and of peak expiratory flow rate on a diary card is helpful in assessing progress.

4. Exercise-induced asthma

Some children with asthma have symptoms only on exertion. Mild exercise induced symptoms can be controlled by giving a bronchodilator before exercise. For more severe exercise problems, if symptoms are not controlled, regular sodium cromoglycate with an extra inhalation before exercise is usually effective. Warm up exercises lessen exercise-induced bronchoconstriction.

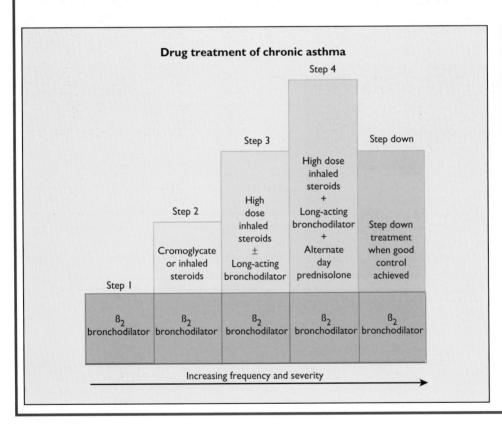

Drug treatment of chronic asthma

Fig. 13.17 A stepwise approach to the treatment of chronic asthma.

Non-pharmacological treatment

The value of many commonly used allergen-avoidance measures such as regular dusting, removal of feather or woollen bedding and wrapping of mattresses in plastic is unproven. Pets present a difficult problem. Some children react immediately and obviously to exposure to a pet, in others exposure results in chronic bronchial hyper-reactivity which may not be attributed to the pet.

Choosing the correct inhaler

Many children fail to gain the benefit of their treatment because they cannot use the inhaler they have been given. The child's age is often the best guide as to whether they will be able to use a particular device. Of all the inhalers available, the pressurised metered-dose inhaler (MDI) requires the greatest coordination and is the least efficient and effective. MDIs should not be used by themselves in children. Dry powder inhalers – e.g. terbutaline sulphate (Bricanyl Turbohaler), sodium chromoglycate (Intal Spincaps), salbutamol (Ventolin Disc-haler) – require less coordination than the MDIs (Fig. 13.18). Using an MDI through a spacer device (such as the Nebuhaler or Volumatic) increases the proportion of the drug reaching the airways and requires less coordination. In children below the age of four years, a soft face mask can be attached to the spacer (Fig. 13.19). Spacers are effective at delivering bronchodilators, cromoglycate and inhaled steroids to the preschool child. Children who need inhaled therapy, but who are unable to use any of these devices, should use a nebuliser for drug delivery at home (Fig. 13.20).

 The correct way to use an inhaler must be demonstrated and the child's ability to use it checked.

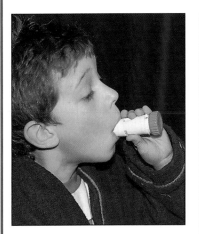

Fig. 13.18 4–10 years old: dry-powder inhaler as shown or metered dose inhaler with spacer.

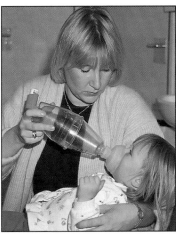

Fig. 13.19 <4 years old: metered dose inhaler with spacer and mask.

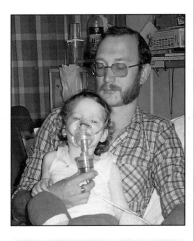

Fig. 13.20 >4years old: nebulised therapy if unable to use any of the other devices.

A trial period of several months without the pet can be considered but may cause great upset and blame. It is reasonable to suggest a thorough cleaning of carpets and furniture to remove danders. Parents should be advised about the effects of smoking in the house. Parental cigarette smoking markedly increases the frequency and severity of childhood asthma. Although exercise improves general fitness, there is no evidence that physical training improves asthma. Hyposensitisation injections, although popular in some countries for hayfever and of benefit after severe allergic reactions to bee stings, are of no value in asthma and can produce fatal anaphylactic reactions.

ACUTE ASTHMA

With each acute attack, the duration of symptoms, the treatment already given and the course of previous attacks should be noted. It can be difficult to assess the severity of an acute asthma attack:

- wheeze and respiratory rate are poor indicators of severity
- contraction of the sternomastoids, chest recession and pulse rate are better guides
- the presence of pulsus paradoxus, the difference between systolic pressure on inspiration and expiration, indicates significant airways obstruction
- cyanosis is a late sign indicating life-threatening asthma.

Investigation of severity:
- oxygen saturation (SaO_2) should be measured with a pulse oximeter in all children presenting to hospital with acute asthma
- measurement of peak expiratory flow rate should be a routine part of assessment in school age children.

The features of a severe and life-threatening acute attack are shown in Figure 13.21.

Criteria for hospital admission

Children require hospital admission if, after nebulised bronchodilator therapy, they:

- have not responded adequately clinically
- are exhausted
- still have a marked reduction in their predicted (or usual) peak flow rate
- have a reduced SaO_2.

A chest X-ray is indicated only if there is severe dyspnoea or unusual features (e.g. asymmetry of chest signs suggesting pneumothorax, lobar collapse) or signs of a chest infection. In children arterial blood gases are only indicated in life-threatening or refractory cases.

Treatment

Acute breathlessness is frightening for both the child and the parents. Calm and skilful management is the key to their reassurance (Fig. 13.22). Nebulised bronchodilators, steroids and oxygen form the foundation of therapy of severe acute asthma.

As soon as the diagnosis has been made the child should be given a nebulised β_2 bronchodilator. This can be repeated every one to two hours until there is improvement. If nebulised treatment is unavailable, 5–10 puffs of bronchodilator from a pressurised aerosol can be given through a spacer. A spacer can be improvised simply by using a polystyrene cup. Oxygen is given when there is any evidence of oxygen desaturation. A short course (2–5 days) of oral prednisolone expedites recovery from severe acute asthma.

Intravenous aminophylline has a role in the minority of children who fail to respond adequately to nebulised therapy. A loading dose is given over 20 minutes followed by continuous infusion. Seizures, severe vomiting and fatal cardiac arrhythmias may follow a rapid infusion. If the child is already on oral theophylline the aminophylline level in the blood should be checked or the loading dose should be omitted. Alternatively, an intravenous salbutamol infusion can be used. Adequate fluids should be given either orally or intravenously, especially if vomiting is a feature.

Antibiotics should only be given if there are signs of bacterial infection. Occasionally these measures are insufficient and artificial ventilation is required.

After each acute exacerbation, a child's maintenance treatment and inhaler technique should be reviewed and altered if inadequate. Follow-up arrangements should be made to monitor progress by the general practitioner or, for more problematic patients, by a paediatrician.

Patient education

In order for families to make rational decisions, they need to know:

- when drugs should be used (regularly or 'as required')
- how to use the drug (inhaler technique)
- what each drug does (relief vs prevention)
- how often and how much can be used (frequency and dosage)
- what to do if asthma worsens (management of acute attacks).

Patients and parents need to know that increasing cough, wheeze and breathlessness and difficulty in walking, talking and sleeping all indicate worsening asthma. Decreasing relief from their bronchodilator indicates worsening asthma. Some asthmatics find it difficult to be aware of gradual deterioration – measurement of peak expiry flow rate at home allows earlier recognition. Parents need to know when to start steroids at home and what dose to give. A personal written self-management plan from the doctor reduces confusion, improves compliance and reduces hospital admissions. Information booklets about asthma for children and parents are useful, but are not a replacement for individual explanation.

Fig. 13.22 Summary of the treatment of acute severe or life-threatening asthma

Immediate treatment	Oxygen via a face mask
	Salbutamol (5 mg) or terbutaline
	(10 mg) via oxygen-driven
	nebuliser (half dose if
	<5 years old)
	Oral prednisolone (1–2 mg/kg;
	maximum dose 40 mg)
Life-threatening features	Intravenous aminophylline
	(5 mg/kg over 20 mins, then
	continuously 1mg/kg/h)
	Intravenous hydrocortisone
	(100 mg qid)
	Consider ipratropium bromide
	(nebulised 0.25 mg)
Subsequent management	Oxygen
	Repeat β_2 agonist 1–4 hourly
	Monitor peak flow and
	oxygen saturation

Fig. 13.21 Features of severe and life-threatening acute asthma

Severe	Too breathless to talk or feed
	Respirations >50/min
	Pulse >140/min
	Peak flow <50% predicted or best value
Life-threatening	Peak flow < 33% predicted or best value
	Fatigue, agitation, drowsiness
	Cyanosis, silent chest or poor respiratory effort

Recurrent cough

Cough is the most common symptom of respiratory disease and indicates irritation of nerve receptors in the pharynx, larynx, trachea or large bronchi. While recurrent cough may simply indicate that the child is having recurrent respiratory infections, other causes need to be considered (Fig. 13.23).

Asthma is the most common cause of recurrent cough in childhood. Although there is often associated wheeze and breathlessness triggered by characteristic factors, in the pre-school child a troublesome night-time cough may be the only symptom. Many children with asthma have a persistent nasal discharge due to allergic rhinitis – their nocturnal cough may be attributed to a post-nasal drip, when in fact it is due to the associated asthma.

Certain infections (e.g. pertussis, RSV and *Mycoplasma* infection) can cause a cough that persists for weeks or months, long after the infective organism has disappeared. Persistent cough after an acute infection may indicate cystic fibrosis or unresolved lobar collapse which will be seen on a chest X-ray. In any child with a severe, persistent cough, TB should be excluded and a chest X-ray and tuberculin test performed.

Aspiration of feeds may cause coughing and wheeze. This may be caused by gastro-oesophageal reflux in infants or as a result of swallowing disorders, e.g. in children with cerebral palsy.

Some older children and adolescents develop a barking, unproductive, habit cough after an infection or an asthma attack which can result in them being sent home from school. The cough characteristically disappears during sleep. Reassurance and explanation after a thorough examination are usually effective.

The importance of parental smoking on children is generally underestimated. If both parents smoke, young children are twice as likely to have recurrent cough and wheeze than if the parents do not smoke. In the older child, active smoking is common – 10% of 13 year olds and 21% of 15 year olds smoke regularly.

Chronic lung infection

In all children with recurrent pneumonia or chronic suppurative lung disease (bronchiectasis) in which purulent sputum is produced, cystic fibrosis must be excluded. Bronchiectasis following severe pneumonia, particularly tuberculosis, pertussis or measles, has now become uncommon. Nevertheless, it can follow pneumonia and it is prudent to do a repeat chest X-ray 4–6 weeks after an acute pneumonia to ensure that any collapse or consolidation has resolved, particularly if cough persists.

Tuberculosis remains an important cause of chronic lung infection and all children with a persistent productive cough should have a chest X-ray and tuberculin skin test.

Fig. 13.23 Causes of recurrent or persistent cough
Recurrent respiratory infections
Asthma
Prolonged infection (e.g. pertussis)
Recurrent aspiration
Habit cough
Cigarette smoking (active or passive)
Inhaled foreign body
Suppurative lung disease
Tuberculosis

Failure of pneumonia to resolve may indicate an inhaled foreign body (e.g. peanut), in which case a bronchoscopy should be carried out to remove the object.

Persistent infection also occurs where there are congenital abnormalities of the lungs, such as congenital cysts or a sequestrated lobe.

The microcilia of the respiratory epithelium are an important defence against infection. Children with primary ciliary dyskinesia, in which there are abnormalities of ciliary structure or function, have recurrent infection of the upper and lower respiratory tract – 50% also have dextrocardia and situs inversus (Kartagener syndrome). Ciliary structure can be assessed by electron microscopy of nasal or tracheal mucosa.

Children who have an immunodeficiency may develop severe, unusual or recurrent chest infections. Their immune deficiency may be from their illness, e.g. malignant disease or its treatment with chemotherapy or radiotherapy or from HIV infection. Less commonly it is due to primary immunodeficiency.

Case history

FOREIGN BODY INHALATION

A previously well three-year-old boy presented with a five-day history of severe cough and wheeze. His symptoms developed after choking on some peanuts. A chest X-ray revealed a hyperlucent right lung (Fig. 13.24). Bronchoscopy was performed and revealed a peanut wedged in the right main bronchus.

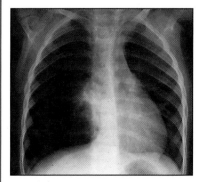

Fig. 13.24 Hyperlucency of the right lung and mediastinal shift to the left. (Courtesy of Dr Abbas Khakoo)

Cystic fibrosis

Cystic fibrosis (CF) is the most common cause of chronic suppurative lung disease in Caucasians. In the past, CF led to death in early childhood from progressive bronchiectasis and respiratory failure, but with improved antibiotic and nutritional therapy survival into early adult life can now be expected for most patients.

CF is an autosomal recessive disease. In Caucasians it affects 1 in 2500 births and the carrier rate is 1 in 25. The disease is much less common in other ethnic groups. A gene located on chromosome 7 (at ΔF508 in 78% of UK CF patients) codes for the protein called cystic fibrosis transmembrane regulator (CFTR) which is defective in CF. CFTR acts as a cyclic AMP-activated chloride channel blocker. Over 200 different gene mutations have been discovered in CF. Identification of the gene mutation involved within a family allows antenatal diagnosis and carrier detection in the majority of families with a child with CF.

In CF the abnormal ion transport across the epithelial cells of the exocrine glands of the respiratory tract and pancreas results in increased viscosity of secretions. Abnormal function of the sweat glands results in excessive concentrations of sodium and chloride in the sweat (80–125 mmol/l in CF, 10–14 mmol/l in normal children). This forms the basis of the essential diagnostic procedure, the sweat test, in which sweating is stimulated by iontophoresing pilocarpine onto the skin. The sweat is collected into a special capillary tube or absorbed onto a weighed piece of filter paper. To minimise diagnostic errors there should be two reliable sweat tests performed by experienced staff.

Fig. 13.25 Clinical features of cystic fibrosis	
Respiratory	Recurrent chest infections
	Bronchiectasis
	Pneumothorax
	Sinusitis
	Nasal polyps
	Haemoptysis
	Aspergillosis
Gastrointestinal	Steatorrhoea, malabsorption
	Failure to thrive/poor growth
	Meconium ileus (neonate)
	Distal intestinal obstruction syndrome (DOS, meconium ileus equivalent)
	Rectal prolapse
	Cirrhosis and portal hypertension (late)
Other	Diabetes mellitus (late)
	Sterility in males (obstructed vas deferens)
	Psychological (child and family)

Clinical features

Most children with CF present with malabsorption and failure to thrive accompanied by recurrent or persistent chest infections (Fig. 13.25). In the lungs viscid mucus in the smaller airways predisposes to chronic infection, particularly with *Staphylococcus aureus* and *Haemophilus influenzae*, and subsequently with *Pseudomonas* species. This leads to damage of the bronchial wall, bronchiectasis and abscess formation (Fig. 13.26). The child has a persistent, loose cough productive of purulent sputum. On examination there is hyperinflation of the chest due to air trapping, coarse crepitations or expiratory rhonchi. With established disease there is finger clubbing.

About 10–20% of CF infants present in the neonatal period with meconium ileus in which inspissated meconium causes intestinal obstruction with vomiting, abdominal distension and failure to pass meconium in the first few days of life.

Over 90% of children with CF have malabsorption and steatorrhoea due to insufficiency of the pancreatic exocrine enzymes (lipase, amylase and proteases). This leads to failure to thrive (Fig. 13.27). Affected children usually have a voracious appetite and frequently pass large, pale, very offensive and greasy stools.

Management

The effective management of CF requires a multidisciplinary team approach including paediatricians, physiotherapists, dieticians, nursing staff, the primary care team, teachers and most importantly the child and parents. All patients with CF should be periodically reviewed in a specialist centre. The condition cannot be cured. The principle aims of therapy are to prevent progression of lung disease and to maintain adequate nutrition and growth.

Respiratory management

Children should have physiotherapy 2–4 times a day depending on the amount of sputum they produce. Parents are taught to perform chest percussion and postural drainage

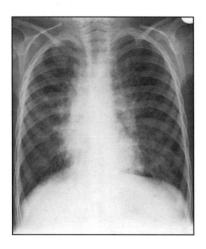

Fig. 13.26 A chest X-ray in cystic fibrosis showing hyperexpansion, marked peribronchial shadowing, bronchial wall thickening and ring shadows.

at home to reduce the accumulation of secretions. Older patients can carry out their own physiotherapy using self-percussion, postural drainage and deep breathing exercises. Physical exercise should be encouraged as it helps strengthen chest muscles and avoids reaccumulation of secretions.

Persistent bacterial chest infection is the major problem. Most centres recommend continuous oral antibiotics with prompt and vigorous intravenous therapy for acute exacerbations to limit lung damage. The role of nebulised antibiotics and mucolytics remains controversial. Up to one-third of children have reversible airways obstruction and may benefit from bronchodilators.

Nutritional management

Dietary status should be assessed regularly. Pancreatic insufficiency is treated with oral enteric-coated pancreatic supplements taken with all meals and snacks. Dosage is adjusted according to clinical response. A high-calorie diet is essential not only to compensate for malabsorption but because the energy requirement of children with CF is 30–40% above normal. Vitamin supplements are routinely given.

Teenagers and adults

Improved survival into adult life has been accompanied by a change in the range of problems seen. In addition to recurrent chest infections other late complications include pneumothorax, haemoptysis, diabetes and liver disease. In distal intestinal obstruction syndrome (meconium ileus equivalent), viscid mucofaeculent material obstructs the bowel. Most adolescents have persistent *Pseudomonas* infection and require intermittent intravenous antibiotic therapy. With appropriate support in the community this can often be given at home through an indwelling intravenous cannula. Males are infertile due to abnormalities of the vas deferens. Women have reduced fertility but many have had successful pregnancies. They should be cautioned that their breast milk has a high sodium concentration The psychological repercussions on the child and family of a chronic and ultimately fatal illness which requires regular physiotherapy and drugs, frequent hospital admissions and missing school should not be lost sight of. The team should provide psychological and emotional support. Heart-lung transplantation has been successful in patients with CF in terminal respiratory failure, but is available to only a minority. Gene therapy (see Chapter 6) is currently being assessed.

Screening

Screening of all newborn infants for CF is possible, but its benefits remain controversial and it is not routinely performed throughout the UK. Immunoreactive trypsin (IRT) is raised in CF patients and can be measured in the routine blood taken for biochemical screening of all babies. Any positive tests require counselling and further investigation with a sweat test. In selected cases, screening may be performed using gene analysis. As with all screening tests the false positive and false negative rates are important. Identification in the neonatal period allows the early introduction of prophylactic antibiotics and prompt recognition and treatment of any respiratory infections. It also enables genetic counselling for the parents about the 1 in 4 risk of recurrence and the possibility of antenatal diagnosis.

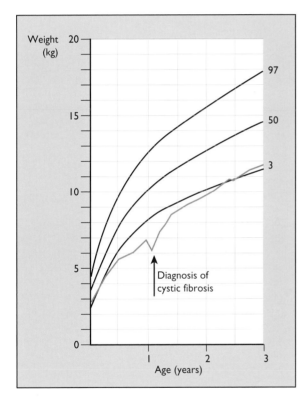

Fig. 13.27 Growth chart of a child with cough and recurrent wheeze. Only when the diagnosis of cystic fibrosis was made and appropriate treatment started did he gain weight.

 Cystic fibrosis should be considered in any child with recurrent chest infections, loose stools and failure to thrive.

FURTHER READING

British Thoracic Society. Guidelines on the management of asthma. *Thorax* 1993; 1–24(Suppl).

Couriel JM. Respiratory infections in children. In Ellis M, Friend JA (eds). *Infections of the Respiratory Tract.* Cambridge University Press. Cambridge, 1996. Review chapter.

Phelan PD, Olinsky A, Robertson C. *Respiratory Illness in Children*, 4th ed. Blackwell, Oxford, 1994. Comprehensive textbook.

Rakshi K, Couriel JM. The management of bronchiolitis. *Arch Dis Child* 1994; **71**:463–469. Review article.

CHAPTER 14

Cardiac Disorders

• *Aetiology* • *Circulatory changes at birth* • *Presentation* • *Diagnosis* • *Non-cyanotic congenital heart disease*
• *Cyanotic congenital heart disease* • *Cardiac arrhythmias* • *Rheumatic fever* • *Sub-acute bacterial endocarditis*
• *Myocarditis/cardiomyopathy* • *Postoperative care*

Whereas heart disease in adults is mostly ischaemic in origin, in children it is mostly congenital. The exception is rheumatic heart disease, which is rare in developed countries but remains a major cause of heart disease in some developing countries.

Congenital heart disease is the most common single group of structural malformations in infants:
- 6–8 per 1000 liveborn infants have significant malformations
- some abnormality of the cardiovascular system, e.g. a bicuspid aortic valve, is present in 10–20 per 1000 live births
- about 1 in 10 stillborn infants have a cardiac anomaly.

Infants with the eight most common anomalies account for over 80% of all lesions (Fig. 14.1) but:
- about 10–15% have complex lesions with more than one cardiac abnormality
- about 10–15% also have a non-cardiac abnormality.

Until relatively recently, the investigation of congenital heart lesions involved invasive catheter studies and the outcome for most serious lesions was poor. This situation has been transformed and now:
- antenatal ultrasound increasingly offers early diagnosis
- most structural defects are diagnosed non-invasively by echocardiography
- even complex defects can often be corrected completely at the initial operation, e.g. transposition of the great arteries
- an increasing number of defects are treated without surgery, by transvenous catheter techniques e.g. closure of a patent ductus arteriosus
- the overall infant surgical mortality has been reduced from approximately 20% in 1970 to 5% in 1993.

Aetiology

Little is known about the aetiology of congenital heart disease. A small proportion are related to external teratogens (Fig. 14.2). About 8% are associated with major chromosomal abnormalities (Fig. 14.3), but recently more subtle chromosomal abnormalities have been identified, e.g. abnormalities of chromosome 22 have been detected in many patients with aortic arch abnormalities. These less obvious and polymorphic abnormalities probably explain why family members of affected individuals have a slightly higher incidence of congenital heart disease.

 Congenital heart disease is the most common group of structural malformations in children.

Fig. 14.1	*The eight most common congenital heart lesions.*
Acyanotic	Ventricular septal defect (VSD) 32%
	Patent ductus arteriosus (PDA) 12%
	Pulmonary stenosis 8%
	Atrial septal defect (ASD) 6%
	Coarctation of the aorta 6%
	Aortic stenosis 5%
Cyanotic	Tetralogy of Fallot 6%
	Transposition of the great arteries 5%

Fig. 14.2 Some important exogenous cardiovascular teratogens.

Teratogen	Cardiac abnormalities	Frequency
Maternal disorders		
Rubella	Peripheral pulmonary stenosis, PDA	30–35%
SLE	Complete heart block (anti-Rho antibody)	35%
Alcoholism (Fetal alcohol syndrome)	ASD, VSD, Tetralogy of Fallot	25%
Diabetes	Incidence increased overall	2%
Drugs		
Warfarin	Pulmonary valve stenosis, PDA	5%

SLE = systemic lupus erythematosus PDA = patent ductus arteriosus ASD = atrial septal defect VSD = ventricular septal defect

Chromosomal abnormality	Incidence	Type
Down syndrome (Trisomy 21)	40%	Atrioventricular septal defect (40%), VSD (30%), ASD (10%), Tetralogy of Fallot (6%)
Edward syndrome (Trisomy 18)	60–80%	Complex
Patau syndrome (Trisomy 13)	60–80%	Complex
Turner syndrome (45XO)	15%	Aortic valve stenosis, coarctation of the aorta
Chromosome 22 microdeletion	–	Aortic arch anomalies, truncus arteriosus

Fig. 14.3 Chromosomal abnormalities and congenital heart disease

Circulatory changes at birth

In the fetus, as relatively little blood returns from the lungs, left atrial pressure is lower than that of the right atrium which receives all the systemic venous return, including blood from the placenta. The flap valve of the foramen ovale is pushed open and blood flows across the atrial septum and into the left ventricle which, in turn, pumps it to the upper body (Fig. 14.4).

With the first breaths, resistance to pulmonary blood flow falls and the volume of blood flowing through the lungs increases sixfold. The left atrial pressure rises because of this, while the volume of blood returning to the right atrium falls as the placenta is excluded from the circulation. The flap valve of the foramen ovale is pushed across to close it. The ductus arteriosus will normally close within the first few hours or days. Children with congenital heart lesions who rely on blood flow through the duct will deteriorate dramatically when this occurs. These infants with a duct-dependent circulation require emergency treatment.

Presentation

Congenital heart disease may present with:
- antenatal cardiac ultrasound diagnosis
- detection of a heart murmur
- cyanosis
- heart failure
- shock.

Antenatal diagnosis

The four-chamber view of the heart has become a routine part of the fetal anomaly scan widely performed in the UK between 18 and 20 weeks' gestation. It allows the detection of hypoplasia of the right or left side of the heart. Interpretation is highly operator dependent and requires high-quality equipment. At tertiary referral centres, more detailed fetal echocardiography is performed for high risk pregnancies, e.g. a previous child with heart disease or if a cardiac abnormality has been identified on routine scanning. Most, but not all, complex abnormalities can be diagnosed. This

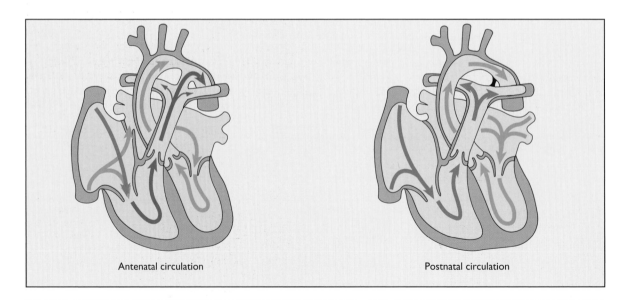

Antenatal circulation

Postnatal circulation

Fig. 14.4 Changes in the circulation from the fetus to the newborn. When congenital heart lesions rely on blood flow through the duct – a duct-dependent circulation – there will be a dramatic deterioration in their clinical condition when the duct closes.

detailed echocardiography allows the parents to be be reassured or counselled appropriately and, if the pregnancy is continued, postnatal management can be planned.

Heart murmurs

The most common presentation of congenital heart disease is with a heart murmur. However, the vast majority of children with murmurs have a normal heart. They have an 'innocent murmur', which can be heard at some time in almost 30% of children. It is obviously important to be able to distinguish an innocent murmur from a pathological one. There are two types of innocent murmurs:

- ejection murmurs – generated in the outflow tracts and great vessels on either side of the heart by turbulent blood flow. They are not associated with any structural abnormality
- venous hums – from turbulent blood flow in the head and neck veins. It is a continuous low pitched rumble heard beneath either clavicle. It may increase on inspiration and will be louder after exercise. It may be mistaken for a patent ductus arteriosus, but can be distinguished by its disappearance on lying flat or with compression of the jugular veins on the ipsilateral side.

Hallmarks of an innocent ejection murmur are:

- soft blowing murmur (usually from the right side pulmonary outflow in the second left interspace) or short 'buzzing' murmur (usually from the left side of the heart – aortic blood flow – in the fourth left interspace)
- localised to left sternal edge
- no diastolic component
- no radiation
- normal heart sounds with no added sounds
- no parasternal thrill
- asymptomatic patient.

Many newborn infants with potential shunts have no symptoms or murmur at birth as the pulmonary vascular resistance is still high. Therefore, conditions such as a ventricular septal defect or patent ductus arteriosus may only become apparent at several weeks of age when the pulmonary vascular resistance falls. During a febrile illness innocent murmurs are often heard because of increased cardiac output.

Differentiating between innocent and significant murmurs can be extremely difficult. If a murmur is thought to be significant, or there is uncertainty if it is innocent, a chest X-ray and ECG should be performed and the child seen by an experienced paediatrician or paediatric cardiologist.

Cyanosis

Peripheral cyanosis (blueness of the hands and feet) may occur when a child is cold or crying or unwell from any cause. This should be distinguished from central cyanosis, seen on the tongue, which is associated with a fall in arterial oxygen tension. It can be recognised clinically if the concentration of reduced haemoglobin in the blood exceeds 5 g/dl, so it is less pronounced if the child is anaemic.

Persistent arterial desaturation in an otherwise well infant is nearly always a sign of structural heart disease. An exception to this is pulmonary hypertension of the newborn (persistent fetal circulation) when there may be profound cyanosis due to failure of the pulmonary vascular resistance to fall after birth. In infants with respiratory distress, cyanosis may also be due to respiratory disease or polycythaemia.

In the neonatal period, cyanosis may be caused by (Fig. 14.5):

- reduced pulmonary blood flow – infants have a duct-dependent pulmonary circulation and rely on blood flowing from left to right across the ductus arteriosus (e.g. see Fig. 14.6). They become severely cyanosed when the duct closes shortly after birth. The lower the pulmonary blood flow the greater the cyanosis. Maintenance of ductal patency is the key to the early survival of these children. This is achieved with intravenous prostaglandin (E_1 or E_2) (dose range 5–20 ng/kg/min), while monitoring its side-effects – apnoea, jitteriness and seizures, flushing/vasodilatation/hypotension and abdominal colic and diarrhoea
- abnormal mixing of systemic venous and pulmonary venous blood – most infants present with cyanosis in the first day or two of life. Cyanosis may not be readily apparent if the pulmonary blood flow is increased from a large left to right shunt and so may present with co-existent heart failure.

The diagnosis of cyanotic congenital heart disease is confirmed by the nitrogen washout test. The infant is placed in 100% oxygen for ten minutes. If the right radial arterial PO_2 is less than 15 kPa (113 mmHg) after this time, a

Fig. 14.5 Causes of neonatal cyanosis
1. Duct-dependent pulmonary circulation
Tetralogy of Fallot (severe)
Pulmonary atresia
Tricuspid atresia
2. Abnormal mixing
Transposition of the great arteries
Total anomalous pulmonary venous drainage
'Univentricular' heart (e.g. double inlet left ventricle)

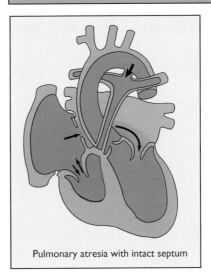

Fig. 14.6 The pulmonary circulation is maintained by blood flowing left to right across the duct – a duct-dependent pulmonary circulation.

Pulmonary atresia with intact septum

diagnosis of 'cyanotic' congenital heart disease can be confidently made, assuming lung disease and pulmonary hypertension of the newborn (persistent fetal circulation) have been excluded. Alternatively, if the oxygen saturation on a pulse oximeter is less than 85%, cyanotic congenital heart disease is likely, but this is a less sensitive indicator.

Heart failure

Heart failure is difficult to define, but in children is best summarised as a clinical syndrome with the following symptoms and signs.

Symptoms:
- breathlessness (particularly on feeding or exertion)
- sweating
- poor feeding
- recurrent chest infections.

Signs:
- slow weight gain or 'failure to thrive'
- cool peripheries
- tachypnoea
- tachycardia
- enlarged heart
- heart murmur, gallop rhythm
- hepatomegaly.

Heart failure in the neonatal period (Fig. 14.7) usually results from left heart obstruction. If the obstructive lesion is very severe, then arterial perfusion may be predominantly by right to left flow of blood via the arterial duct, so-called duct-dependent systemic circulation (e.g. see Fig. 14.8). Closure of the duct under these circumstances rapidly leads to severe acidosis, collapse and death unless ductal patency is restored.

Fig. 14.7 Causes of heart failure
1. Neonates – obstructed duct-dependent systemic circulation
Hypoplastic left heart syndrome
Critical aortic valve stenosis
Severe coarctation of the aorta
Interruption of the aortic arch
2. Infants
Ventricular septal defect
Atrioventricular septal defect
Large patent ductus arteriosus

After the neonatal period, progressive heart failure is most likely due to a left to right shunt. During the first few weeks of life, as the pulmonary vascular resistance falls, there is a progressive increase in pulmonary blood flow. Symptoms of heart failure will increase up to the age of about six months, but may subsequently improve as the pulmonary vascular resistance rises in response to the left to right shunt. If left untreated, some of these children may develop Eisenmenger syndrome, with an irreversibly raised pulmonary vascular resistance resulting from chronically raised pulmonary arterial pressure and flow.

Diagnosis

If congenital heart disease is suspected, a chest X-ray and ECG (Fig. 14.10) should be performed. Although they rarely diagnose the lesion, they may be helpful in establishing that

---

Case history

SHOCK (Fig. 14.8)

A three-day-old baby had been discharged home the day after delivery, following a normal routine examination. He suddenly collapsed and was rushed to hospital. He was pale, with grey lips. The right brachial pulse could just be felt, the femoral pulses were impalpable. Blood gases showed a severe metabolic acidosis. He was given artificial ventilation, plasma, inotropes and sodium bicarbonate. Blood cultures were taken, a suprapubic aspiration of urine performed and antibiotics started for possible sepsis. Blood and urine samples were taken for an amino acid screen and urine for organic acids. As the femoral pulses remained impalpable, a prostaglandin infusion was started. Within two hours he was pink and well perfused and the acidosis had almost resolved. Severe coarctation of the aorta was diagnosed on echocardiography. He had developed shock from left heart obstruction with closure of the arterial duct.

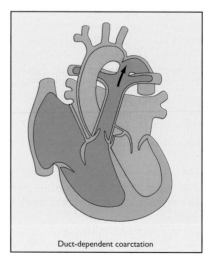

Fig. 14.8 The systemic circulation is maintained by blood flowing right to left across the ductus arteriosus – a duct dependent systemic circulation.

Duct-dependent coarctation

 Maintaining ductal patency is the key to early survival in neonates with a duct-dependent circulation.

Case history

HEART FAILURE

A five-week-old female infant was referred to hospital because of wheezing, poor feeding and poor weight gain during the previous two weeks. Before this, she had been well. Her routine neonatal examination had seen normal. She was tachypnoeic (50–60 breaths/min) and there was some sternal and intercostal recession. The pulses were normal. There was a thrill, a loud pansystolic murmur at the lower left sternal edge and a slightly accentuated pulmonary component to the second heart sound. There were scattered wheezes. The liver was enlarged, palpable at 4 cm below the costal margin. The ECG was unremarkable. The chest X-ray showed cardiomegaly and increased pulmonary vascular markings. An echocardiogram showed a moderate-sized VSD (Fig. 14.9). Treatment was with diuretics. The VSD closed spontaneously at 11 months.

This infant developed heart failure from a ventricular septal defect (VSD) presenting at several weeks of age when the peripheral resistance fell.

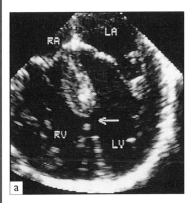
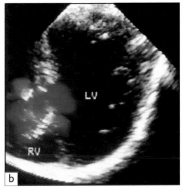
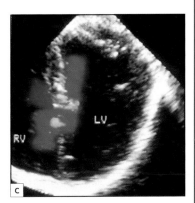

Fig. 14.9 (a) Echocardiogram showing a medium-sized muscular ventricular septal defect, shown with an arrow. (b) The colour Doppler shows a left to right shunt (blue) during systole. (c) There is also a small right to left shunt (red) during diastole. (RA = right atrium, LA = left atrium, RV = right ventricle, LV = left ventricle)

Fig. 14.10 ECGs in children	
Important features	Arrythmias
	Superior QRS axis (negative deflection in AVF)
	Right ventricular hypertrophy (upright T wave in V_1, over 1 month of age)
	Left ventricular strain (inverted T wave in V_6)
Pitfalls	P wave morphology is rarely helpful in children
	Partial right bundle branch block is more often seen in normal children than in those with an ASD
	Left ventricular hypertrophy is difficult to define
ASD = atrial septal defect	

there is an abnormality of the cardiovascular system and as a baseline for assessing future changes. Echocardiography, combined with Doppler ultrasound, enables almost all causes of congenital heart disease to be evaluated. Cardiac catheterisation is almost never required to make the diagnosis and is now reserved for haemodynamic measurements and therapy.

 A normal chest X-ray and ECG do not exclude congenital heart disease.

Non-cyanotic congenital heart disease

ATRIAL SEPTAL DEFECT

There are two main types of atrial septal defect (ASD):
- ostium secundum (Fig. 14.11a)
- ostium primum (Fig. 14.11b).

Both present with similar symptoms and signs, but their anatomy is quite different. The ostium secundum defect

is a deficiency of the foramen ovale and the surrounding atrial septum. The ostium primum defect is a deficiency of the atrioventricular septum and is characterised by:
- an abnormal atrioventricular junction
- abnormal atrioventricular valves (a trileaflet left atrio-ventricular valve being its hallmark)
- an interatrial communication between the bottom end of the atrial septum and the atrioventricular valves.

Clinical features
Symptoms:
- none (commonly)
- recurrent chest infections/wheeze
- heart failure
- arrhythmias (fourth decade onwards).

Physical signs (Fig. 14.11c):
- a fixed and widely split second heart sound – due to the

right and left atrial pressure and volume being equal both in inspiration and expiration
- an ejection systolic murmur best heard in the third left intercostal space – due to increased flow across the right ventricular outflow tract because of the left to right shunt
- a rumbling mid-diastolic murmur best heard at the lower left sternal edge – due to increased flow across the tricuspid valve, because of the left to right shunt at atrial level.

Investigations
Chest X-ray (Fig. 14.11d)
May show cardiomegaly and/or an enlarged pulmonary artery with increased pulmonary vascular markings; all non-specific features.
ECG (Fig. 14.11e)
May provide a strong diagnostic clue. With an ostium secundum ASD there will be sinus rhythm with right axis

Atrial septal defect

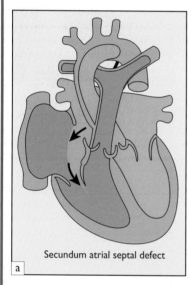

Secundum atrial septal defect

a

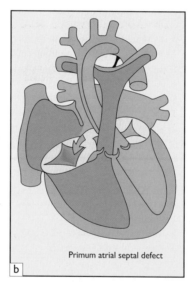

Primum atrial septal defect

b

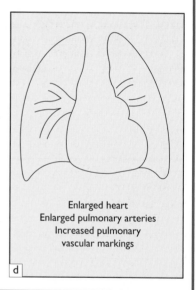

Enlarged heart
Enlarged pulmonary arteries
Increased pulmonary vascular markings

d

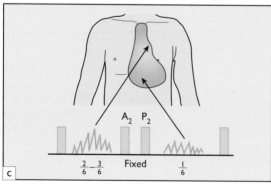

A₂ P₂

$\frac{2}{6}$–$\frac{3}{6}$ Fixed $\frac{1}{6}$

c

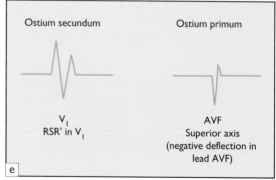

Ostium secundum

V₁
RSR' in V₁

Ostium primum

AVF
Superior axis
(negative deflection in lead AVF)

e

Fig. 14.11 (a) The ostium secundum atrial septal defect (ASD) is a deficiency of the foramen ovale and surrounding atrial septum. (b) The ostium primum ASD is a deficiency of the atrioventricular septum. (c) Murmur. (d) Chest X-ray. (e) ECG.

deviation due to right ventricular enlargement. Right ventricular hypertrophy is uncommon. Partial or complete right bundle branch block is common but may occur in normal children. When there is a primum atrial septal defect the most characteristic feature is the presence of left axis deviation, or a so-called 'superior' QRS axis.

Cross-sectional echocardiography

Will delineate the anatomy, although in some older teenagers and adults transoesophageal echocardiography may be required to demonstrate the atrial septum with precision.

Management

All children with symptoms and most with evidence of right atrial and right ventricular volume overload will be offered surgery. In general this is a low-risk procedure, when the lesion is closed by suturing or by insertion of a patch of pericardium. It is usually electively performed in the fourth or fifth year of life, with the intention of preventing right heart failure and arrhythmias in later life. This is a controversial issue – it has become routine to close nearly all atrial septal defects but there are little data supporting the effectiveness of this procedure.

VENTRICULAR SEPTAL DEFECTS

Ventricular septal defects (VSD) are common, accounting for 32% of all cases of congenital heart disease. There are two main types:

- perimembranous (close to the tricuspid valve)
- muscular (completely surrounded by muscle) (Fig. 14.12a).

Presentation is usually early with a loud murmur heard during routine clinical examination, but may be with symptoms of heart failure. Most will close spontaneously during the first few years of life, with less than 10% requiring surgical closure.

Clinical features

Symptoms:
- asymptomatic
- heart failure/failure to thrive
- recurrent chest infections
- cyanosis (due to pulmonary vascular disease – now rare)
- endocarditis (late).

Physical signs (Fig. 14.12b):
- parasternal thrill
- heart murmur at lower left sternal edge
  – loud pansystolic murmur when small defect

Ventricular septal defect

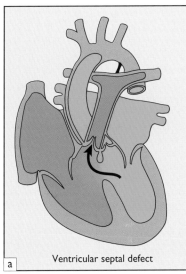

Ventricular septal defect

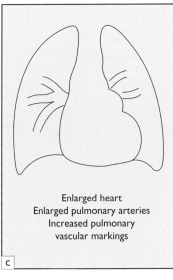

Enlarged heart
Enlarged pulmonary arteries
Increased pulmonary
vascular markings

Fig. 14.12 (a) Ventricular septal defect showing a left to right shunt. (b) Murmur. (c) Chest X-ray. (d) ECG.

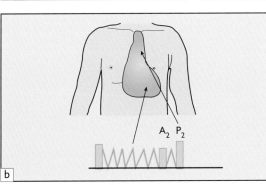

A₂ P₂

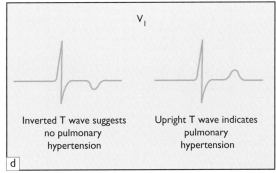

V₁

Inverted T wave suggests
no pulmonary
hypertension

Upright T wave indicates
pulmonary
hypertension

– unimpressive ejection murmur when large defect
* variable pulmonary component of second sound:
  – normal when small defect
  – loud when large with pulmonary hypertension
* tachypnoea, tachycardia, enlarged liver from heart failure.

Investigations

Chest X-ray (Fig. 14.12c)
Will vary from normal (small defects) to grossly abnormal with cardiomegaly, enlarged pulmonary arteries and increased pulmonary vascular markings from pulmonary oedema.

ECG (Fig. 14.12d)
Will vary from normal to grossly abnormal. The most important abnormality is the presence of right ventricular hypertrophy, which always requires further investigation.

Echocardiography
Will almost invariably demonstrate the precise anatomy of the defect. It should also be possible to assess its haemodynamic effects using Doppler ultrasound.

Management

Drug therapy for heart failure is only required for children with symptoms. Commonly used diuretics are frusemide or a thiazide and spironolactone. More recently, angiotensin converting enzyme (ACE) inhibitors have been used in conjunction with diuretics. There is little evidence to suggest that digoxin is useful, but it is still widely prescribed. There are two main reasons for performing surgery within the first year of life:

* severe symptoms with failure to thrive
* pulmonary hypertension with possible progression to pulmonary vascular disease.

In children with a a large left to right shunt, increased pulmonary blood flow and pulmonary hypertension will ultimately lead to irreversible damage of the pulmonary capillary vascular bed. This pulmonary vascular disease usually becomes established in the second year of life but Eisenmenger syndrome, with cyanosis due to intracardiac shunting from right to left, rarely evolves until the second decade (Fig. 14.13). It is, therefore, of critical importance to be able to diagnose the presence of pulmonary hypertension during infancy. The clinical hallmarks of pulmonary hypertension are:

* right ventricular hypertrophy on ECG
* a loud pulmonary component to the second heart sound.

In general, a child with a long, loud pansystolic murmur and a normal pulmonary component to the second heart sound will not require surgery, even if symptomatic early in life. Even if asymptomatic, surgery will be required for any child with an unimpressive murmur but a loud pulmonary component to the second heart sound, implying a raised pulmonary arterial diastolic pressure.

 Symptoms of heart failure from a VSD may resolve because of the development of pulmonary hypertension rather than the success of drug therapy.

ATRIOVENTRICULAR SEPTAL DEFECTS

This is a special form of ventricular septal defect (Fig. 14.14) most commonly seen in children with Down syndrome. There are many different forms, ranging from a simple primum atrial septal defect to a complete atrio-ventricular septal defect (AVD) with a coexisting large VSD and a single common atrioventricular valve. In these children, assessment and management are the same as for simple VSD, although early surgical correction is more hazardous because of the complexity of the intracardiac repair.

 All children with a VSD must be given antibiotic prophylaxis to prevent bacterial endocarditis.

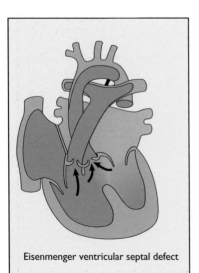

Fig. 14.13 Eisenmenger syndrome with right to left shunting from pulmonary vascular disease following increased pulmonary blood flow and pulmonary hypertension.

Eisenmenger ventricular septal defect

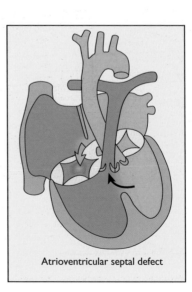

Fig. 14.14 Atrioventricular septal defect.

Atrioventricular septal defect

PATENT DUCTUS ARTERIOSUS

The ductus arteriosus connects the pulmonary artery to the descending aorta. Failure to close shortly after birth frequently occurs in preterm or sick neonates. In other children it is due to a defect in the muscle of the duct. The flow of blood across a patent ductus arteriosus (PDA) is left to right, from the aorta to the pulmonary artery, following the fall in pulmonary vascular resistance after birth.

Clinical features

In preterm infants a PDA may be suspected by detecting a collapsing pulse and a systolic murmur at the left sternal edge. When severe, the resulting heart failure may make it difficult to wean the infant from artificial ventilation.

Most other children with a PDA present in the first few years of life with a continuous murmur beneath the left clavicle (Fig. 14.15a). The murmur continues into diastole because the pressure in the pulmonary artery is lower than in the aorta throughout the cardiac cycle. The pulse pressure is increased, causing a collapsing pulse. Symptoms are rare, but when the duct is large there will be increased pulmonary blood flow with heart failure and even pulmonary hypertension.

Investigations

The findings on chest X-ray (Fig. 14.15b) and ECG (Fig. 14.15c) with a large symptomatic PDA will be indistinguishable from those seen in a patient with a large ventricular septal defect, but the duct should be readily identified with cross-sectional echocardiography assisted by Doppler ultrasound.

Management

In the preterm infant the duct will ultimately close, but if symptomatic, treatment is with fluid restriction, indomethacin (a prostaglandin synthetase inhibitor) or surgical ligation. In the young child with an asymptomatic PDA, closure is recommended to abolish the lifelong risk of bacterial endocarditis. Surgical ligation was previously the method of choice but it is now possible to close most ducts by transvenous umbrella occlusion (Fig. 14.15d–f).

Patent ductus arteriosus

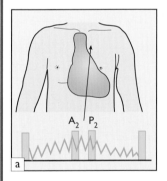

A_2 P_2

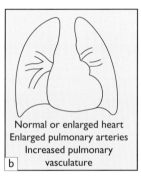

Normal or enlarged heart
Enlarged pulmonary arteries
Increased pulmonary vasculature

ECG

- Usually normal

- Left ventricular hypertrophy with large left to right shunt

- Right ventricular hypertrophy with pulmonary hypertension

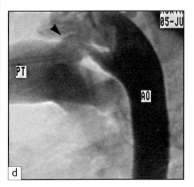

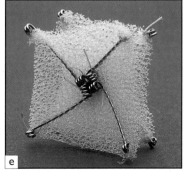

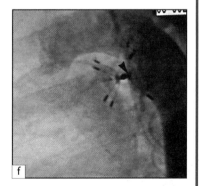

Fig. 14.15 Patent ductus arteriosus. (a) Murmur. (b) Chest X-ray. (c) ECG. (d) A patent ductus arteriosus visualised on echocardiography. (e) A small (12 or 17 mm diameter) double umbrella device which is passed through a catheter via the femoral vein. (f) The distal and proximal umbrellas are deployed in the aortic and pulmonary arterial end of the duct respectively. PT = Pulmonary trunk, AO = Aorta.

PULMONARY VALVE STENOSIS

A small number of neonates will present with critical pulmonary stenosis and a duct-dependent pulmonary circulation.

Clinical features

Most children with pulmonary valve stenosis (Fig. 14.16a) are asymptomatic. It is diagnosed clinically.

Physical signs (Fig. 14.16b):
- an ejection systolic murmur best heard in the second and third left intercostal space, radiating to the back
- an ejection click best heard in the second and third left intercostal space
- when severe, a prolonged right ventricular impulse, with delayed pulmonary valve closure on auscultation.

Investigations

Chest X-ray (Fig. 14.16c)
Shows post-stenotic dilatation of the pulmonary artery.
ECG (Fig. 14.16d)
Shows evidence of right ventricular hypertrophy.

Management

Although most children are asymptomatic, progressive right ventricular hypertrophy and reduced exercise tolerance eventually occur. When the pressure gradient across the pulmonary valve becomes markedly increased (greater than about 50 mmHg), intervention will be required. Transvenous balloon dilatation is the treatment of choice for older children. In the sick neonate with critical pulmonary valve stenosis, as the results of surgery are very poor, transvenous balloon dilatation is considered to be the treatment of choice by most cardiologists although it is technically more difficult.

AORTIC VALVE STENOSIS

Aortic valve stenosis (Fig. 14.17a) may not be an isolated lesion. It is often associated with mitral valve stenosis and coarctation of the aorta, and their presence should always be actively excluded.

Clinical features

Symptoms are more common than in pulmonary valve stenosis. In the neonatal period there may be a duct-dependent systemic circulation or severe heart failure. In later life most children with mild or moderate stenosis present with an asymptomatic murmur. Those with severe stenosis may present with reduced exercise tolerance, chest pain on exertion or syncope.

Physical signs (Fig. 14.17b):
- small volume, slow rising, plateau-type pulses
- apical ejection click
- delayed and soft aortic second sound
- ejection systolic murmur maximal in the aortic area and radiating to the neck
- carotid thrill.

Investigations

There is a prominent left ventricle with post-stenotic dilatation of the ascending aorta on chest X-ray (Fig. 14.17c) and left ventricular hypertrophy on ECG (Fig. 14.17d).

Management

In neonates, balloon valvotomy, avoiding the need for surgery, is frequently performed, but it is less widely accepted than in pulmonary stenosis. This is because of concerns about arterial damage and occlusion following

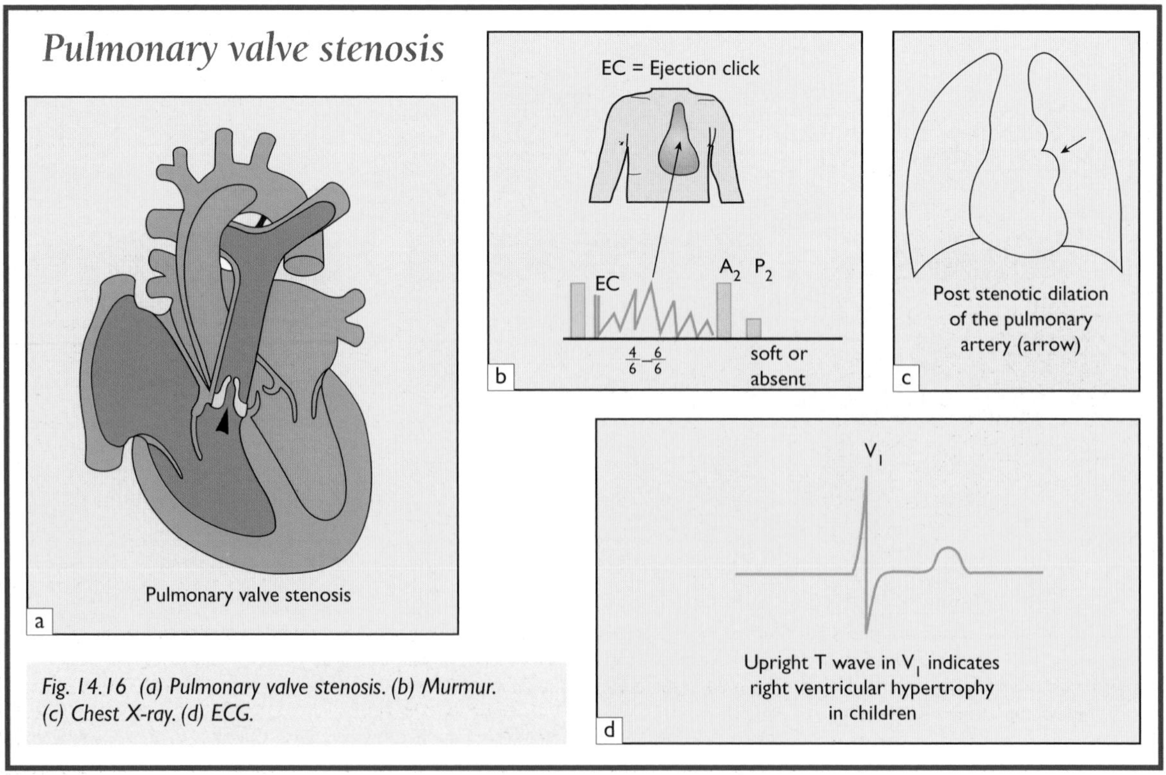

Pulmonary valve stenosis

Pulmonary valve stenosis

EC = Ejection click

EC

A_2 P_2

$\frac{4}{6} - \frac{6}{6}$

soft or absent

Post stenotic dilation of the pulmonary artery (arrow)

V_1

Upright T wave in V_1 indicates right ventricular hypertrophy in children

Fig. 14.16 (a) Pulmonary valve stenosis. (b) Murmur. (c) Chest X-ray. (d) ECG.

percutaneous insertion of a large balloon through the femoral artery and the risk of severe aortic incompetence due to disruption of the aortic valve.

In older children, regular clinical and echocardiographic assessment is required in order to assess when to intervene. Children with symptoms on exercise or who have a high resting pressure gradient (more than 50–60 mmHg) across the aortic valve will either undergo balloon or surgical valvotomy. Balloon dilatation in this age group is generally safe and uncomplicated.

Most neonates and children with significant aortic valve stenosis requiring treatment in the first few years of life will eventually require aortic valve replacement. Early treatment is therefore palliative and directed towards delaying this for as long as possible.

COARCTATION OF THE AORTA

Coarctation of the aorta (Fig. 14.18a) is often associated with other lesions, the most common being a bicuspid aortic valve and ventricular septal defect.

Clinical features

In the neonatal period, severe coarctation presents with duct-dependent systemic circulation and circulatory collapse. If less severe, it may present with symptoms of heart failure or with a heart murmur between the shoulder blades. In older children or adults it may present with hypertension. The key to the clinical diagnosis is the recognition of weak or absent femoral pulses. The blood pressure in the arms will be markedly higher than in the legs.

Palpation of the femoral pulses must be performed routinely during the cardiovascular examination of any child. There may be an ejection systolic murmur between the shoulder blades (Fig. 14.18b).

Investigations

Chest X-ray (Fig. 14.18c)

Is usually normal but may show cardiomegaly and increased vascular markings in children with heart failure. In older children there may also be 'rib-notching' due to the effect of large collateral arteries running under the ribs posteriorly to by-pass the obstruction.

ECG

In the neonatal period, shows right ventricular hypertrophy because the right ventricle is supplying the descending aorta in fetal life. In older children there will be left ventricular hypertrophy (Fig. 14.18d).

Management

The majority will undergo surgery. There are several different operations, but the most common is the subclavian flap procedure, when the left subclavian artery is transected and used as a flap to relieve the coarctation just distal to it. This is performed via a left thoracotomy and although the left arm pulses are lost, the arm develops normally. There is a small incidence (approximately 5–10%) of recoarctation after surgery, but the mortality is now low (less than 2%). Balloon dilatation, avoiding the need for surgery, is performed at some centres but its exact role remains uncertain. If restenosis occurs after operation, balloon dilatation is the treatment of choice.

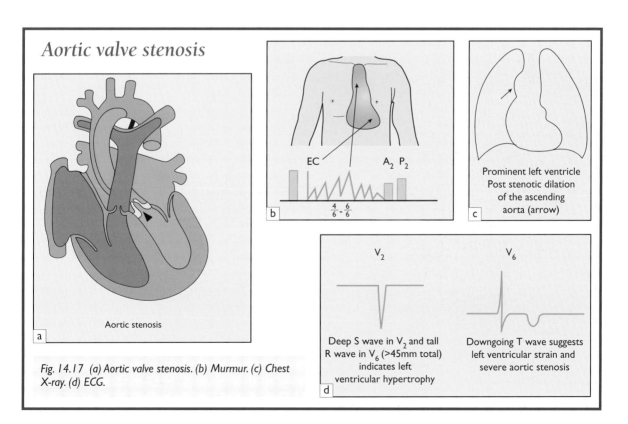

Aortic valve stenosis

Aortic stenosis

EC   A₂ P₂

4/6 - 6/6

Prominent left ventricle
Post stenotic dilation
of the ascending
aorta (arrow)

V₂   V₆

Deep S wave in V₂ and tall R wave in V₆ (>45mm total) indicates left ventricular hypertrophy

Downgoing T wave suggests left ventricular strain and severe aortic stenosis

Fig. 14.17 (a) Aortic valve stenosis. (b) Murmur. (c) Chest X-ray. (d) ECG.

Coarctation of the aorta

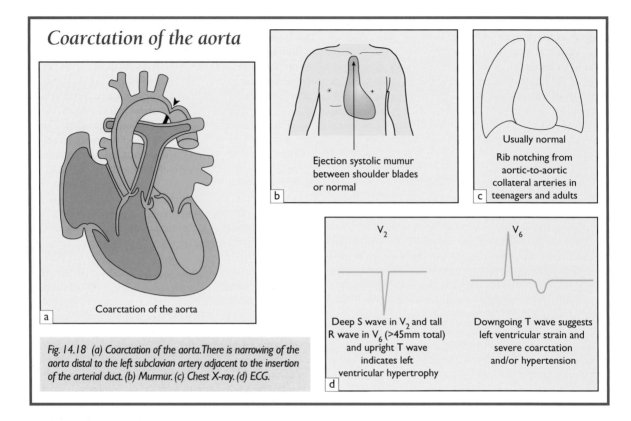

Ejection systolic mumur between shoulder blades or normal

Usually normal
Rib notching from aortic-to-aortic collateral arteries in teenagers and adults

V_2

V_6

Deep S wave in V_2 and tall R wave in V_6 (>45mm total) and upright T wave indicates left ventricular hypertrophy

Downgoing T wave suggests left ventricular strain and severe coarctation and/or hypertension

Coarctation of the aorta

Fig. 14.18 (a) Coarctation of the aorta. There is narrowing of the aorta distal to the left subclavian artery adjacent to the insertion of the arterial duct. (b) Murmur. (c) Chest X-ray. (d) ECG.

INTERRUPTION OF THE AORTIC ARCH

This is a severe form of coarctation with no connection between the aorta proximal and distal to the arterial duct. A ventricular septal defect (VSD) is usually present. Presentation is almost invariably in the neonatal period with features of a duct-dependent circulation (Fig. 14.19). Complete correction, with closure of the VSD and repair of the aortic arch, is usually performed within the first few days of life. The risk of death is higher than that for simple coarctation of the aorta, being in the order of 20%.

HYPOPLASTIC LEFT HEART SYNDROME

In this condition there is under-development of the entire left side of the heart (Fig. 14.20). The mitral valve is small or atretic, the left ventricle is diminutive and there is usually aortic valve atresia. The ascending aorta is small, there

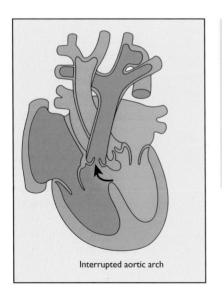

Interrupted aortic arch

Fig. 14.19 Interruption of the aortic arch. The lower body circulation is maintained by right to left flow of blood across the duct.

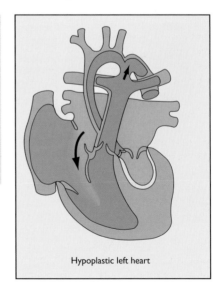

Hypoplastic left heart

Fig. 14.20 Hypoplastic left heart syndrome. The entire left side of the heart is under-developed.

is almost invariably associated coarctation of the aorta or interruption of the aortic arch and so there is a duct-dependent systemic circulation.

Clinical features

These are the sickest of all neonates presenting with a duct-dependent systemic circulation. There is no flow through the left side of the heart so ductal constriction leads to profound acidosis and rapid cardiovascular collapse. The weakness or absence of all peripheral pulses, rather than simply loss of the femoral pulses, will differentiate the condition from coarctation of the aorta. The infant will fail the nitrogen washout test as there is common mixing of pulmonary venous and systemic venous blood at atrial level. The diagnosis must be established urgently by echocardiography, when it will need to be differentiated from other causes of a duct-dependent systemic circulation (e.g. coarcation of the aorta and interruption of the aortic arch).

Management

This condition has been inoperable, but recently two surgical approaches have been adopted in North America. Neonatal heart transplantation is one option and a palliative approach with a series of difficult and demanding operations is another. The long-term outcome of both approaches is uncertain.

Cyanotic congenital heart disease

In congenital heart disease there are two causes of cyanosis:
- decreased pulmonary blood flow with a right to left shunt, e.g. Tetralogy of Fallot
- normal or increased pulmonary blood flow with abnormal mixing or streaming of systemic and pulmonary venous return, e.g. transposition of the great arteries, tricuspid atresia and double inlet ventricle.

TETRALOGY OF FALLOT

This is the most common cause of cyanotic congenital heart disease (Fig. 14.21a).

Clinical features

In Tetralogy of Fallot there are four cardinal anatomical features:
- a large outlet ventricular septal defect
- overriding of the aorta with respect to the ventricular septum
- right ventricular outflow tract obstruction (infundibular and valvar pulmonary stenosis)
- right ventricular hypertrophy.

Symptoms

A few children present with severe cyanosis in the first few days of life with a duct-dependent pulmonary circulation, but most are diagnosed in the first month or two of life following the identification of a murmur. Cyanosis at this stage may not be obvious. The classical description of severe cyanosis, hypercyanotic spells and squatting on exercise developing in late infancy is now rare. However, it is important to recognise hypercyanotic spells as they may lead to myocardial infarction, cerebrovascular accidents and even death if left untreated. They are characterised by a rapid increase in cyanosis, usually associated with irritability or inconsolable crying because of severe hypoxia and breathlessness and pallor because of tissue acidosis.

Signs

A long, loud ejection systolic murmur is best heard in the third left intercostal space, usually with a single second heart sound (Fig. 14.21b). With increasing right ventricular outflow tract obstruction, which is predominantly muscular and below the pulmonary valve, the murmur will shorten and cyanosis will increase. During a hypercyanotic spell the murmur will be very short or inaudible as the pressure in the two ventricles becomes similar. Clubbing of the fingers and toes may develop.

Investigations

Chest X-ray (Fig. 14.21c)
Will show a relatively small heart, possibly with an uptilted apex due to right ventricular hypertrophy. There may be a right sided aortic arch, but characteristically there is a pulmonary artery 'bay', a concavity on the left heart border where the normally convex main pulmonary artery and right ventricular outflow tract is profiled. There may also be decreased pulmonary vascular markings reflecting reduced pulmonary blood flow.

ECG (Fig. 14.21d)
Will show right axis deviation and right ventricular hypertrophy.

Echocardiography
Will demonstrate the cardinal features, but cardiac catheterisation is usually required to show the detailed anatomy of the pulmonary arteries, which may be small or stenosed.

Management

Hypercyanotic spells are usually self-limiting and followed by a period of sleep. If prolonged, they require prompt treatment with:
- sedation and pain relief (morphine is excellent)
- intravenous propranolol, which probably works both as a peripheral vasoconstrictor and by relieving the sub-pulmonary muscular spasm which is the cause of reduced pulmonary blood flow
- bicarbonate to correct acidosis
- muscle paralysis and artificial ventilation in order to reduce metabolic oxygen demand. If the above measures are unsuccessful, more potent peripheral vasoconstrictor agents (such as noradrenaline) may be used to increase systemic vascular resistance, thereby increasing flow into the pulmonary artery rather than the aorta. At this stage emergency surgery is usually required.

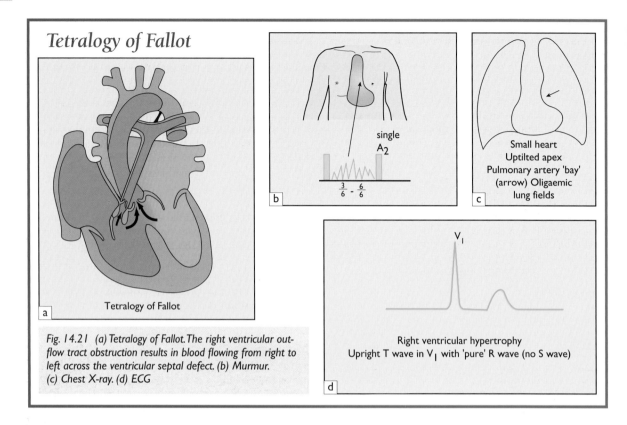

Tetralogy of Fallot

single
A₂

$$\frac{3}{6} - \frac{6}{6}$$

Small heart
Uptilted apex
Pulmonary artery 'bay'
(arrow) Oligaemic
lung fields

V₁

Right ventricular hypertrophy
Upright T wave in V₁ with 'pure' R wave (no S wave)

Tetralogy of Fallot

Fig. 14.21 (a) Tetralogy of Fallot. The right ventricular outflow tract obstruction results in blood flowing from right to
left across the ventricular septal defect. (b) Murmur.
(c) Chest X-ray. (d) ECG

Corrective surgery can now be performed after 4–6 months
of age. It involves closing the ventricular septal defect and
relieving right ventricular outflow tract obstruction with
an artificial patch which sometimes extends across the pulmonary valve. The operative risk is approximately 2–5%.
Most children are free from significant symptoms for up to
20 or 30 years after surgery. Infants who become symptomatic in the first few months of age require palliative
surgery to increase pulmonary blood flow. This is usually
done by surgical placement of an artificial tube between
the subclavian artery and the pulmonary artery (a modified Blalock–Taussig shunt) or sometimes by balloon dilatation of the right ventricular outflow tract. Complete
correction is performed when the infant is older.

TRANSPOSITION OF THE GREAT ARTERIES

In transposition of the great arteries there are two parallel
circulations: the systemic venous return passes from the
right atrium into the right ventricle then into the aorta, and
there is a separate circulation of pulmonary venous blood
returning to the left atrium via the left ventricle and back
into the pulmonary arteries (Fig. 14.22a). If there is no
mixing of blood between the two circulations then this condition is incompatible with life. Fortunately, there are a
number of naturally occurring associated anomalies, e.g.
ventricular septal defects, atrial septal defect, patent ductus,
as well as therapeutic interventions which can achieve this.

Clinical features

Symptoms

Cyanosis is the predominant symptom. It may be profound
and life-threatening; a PaO_2 of 1–3 kPa is not unusual.
These children usually present within the first day or two
of life when spontaneous closure of the ductus arteriosus
leads to a marked reduction in mixing of the desaturated
and saturated blood flowing around the aorta and pulmonary artery respectively. Cyanosis will be less severe and
presentation delayed if there is more mixing of blood from
associated anomalies.

Physical signs (Fig. 14.22b)

There will always be some cyanosis, and in the occasional
child presenting after the first year of life, there may be
finger clubbing. The remainder of the cardiovascular examination will vary depending on the associated abnormalities. The second heart sound is often closely split or single.
There may be a systolic murmur, due to increased flow or
stenosis within the left ventricular (pulmonary) outflow
tract, but there may be no murmur.

Investigations

Chest X-ray (Fig. 14.22c)

May be the classic findings of a narrow upper mediastinum with an 'egg on side' appearance of the cardiac
shadow (due to the anteroposterior relationship of the
great vessels and right ventricular hypertrophy respectively). Increased pulmonary vascular markings are
common.

Transposition of the great arteries

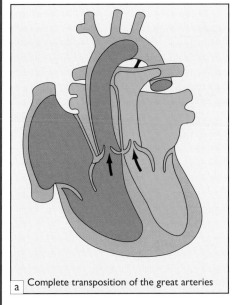

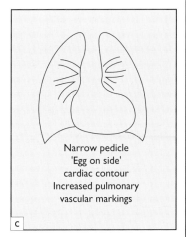

a Complete transposition of the great arteries

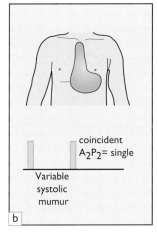

coincident
A₂P₂= single

Variable
systolic
mumur

b

Narrow pedicle
'Egg on side'
cardiac contour
Increased pulmonary
vascular markings

c

ECG

Usually normal neonatal pattern

d

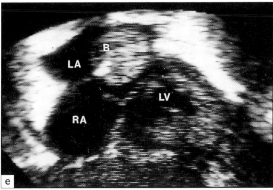

e

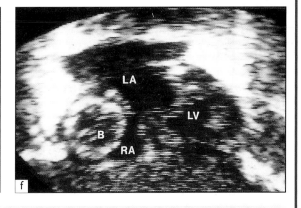

f

Fig. 14.22 (a) Transposition of the great arteries. There must be mixing of blood between the two circulations for this to be compatible with life. (b) Murmur. (c) Chest X-ray. (d) ECG. (e,f) Echocardiogram showing balloon atrial septostomy in transposition of the great arteries. A balloon (about 2 ml) is pulled through the atrial septum from the left atrium (e) across the atrial septum to the right atrium (f) in order to increase the size of the atrial septum. (B = balloon, LA = left atrium, RA = right atrium, LV = left ventricle)

ECG (Fig. 14.22d)

Is rarely helpful in establishing the diagnosis.

Echocardiography

Is essential and demonstrates the abnormal arterial connections and associated abnormalities, and helps assess the degree of mixing of systemic and pulmonary venous blood.

Management

In the sick cyanosed neonate, the key is to improve mixing of saturated and desaturated blood. Maintaining the patency of the ductus arteriosus with a prostaglandin infusion is mandatory. A balloon atrial septostomy is a life-saving procedure which is now virtually routine in children with all forms of transposition of the great arteries (Fig. 14.22e,f). It was first performed by Rashkind in the US, and was one of the most important advances in treating congenital heart disease. A catheter, with an expandable balloon at its tip, is passed through the umbilical or femoral vein and then on through the right atrium and foramen ovale. The balloon is inflated within the left atrium and then pulled through the atrial septum. This tears the atrial septum, renders the flap valve of the foramen ovale incompetent, and so allows mixing of the systemic and pulmonary venous blood within the atrium.

All patients with transposition of the great arteries will ultimately require some form of surgery. Until the 1980s a 'corrective' operation was performed by placing a baffle within the atrium to divert the systemic venous blood towards the left ventricle and then on to the pulmonary artery, thus allowing the pulmonary venous blood to pass into the right ventricle and then on to the aorta (the Mustard or Senning procedure). This 'physiological' correction was usually performed at about nine months of age and had a low early risk. Long-term concerns regarding the ability of the right ventricle to perform as a systemic pump, as well as late problems with stenosis of the intra-atrial baffle and frequent atrial dysrhythmias, have led to the widespread introduction of the arterial switch procedure, so-called anatomical correction. In this operation, performed in the first few weeks of life, the pulmonary artery and aorta are transected above the arterial valves and switched over. In addition, the coronary arteries have to be transferred across to the new aorta. Thus the left ventricle acts as the systemic ventricle, pumping fully oxygenated blood into the aorta, and the right ventricle assumes its more normal role of pumping blood to the lungs. This is a technically demanding operation, and the early surgical risk was initially high. However, with increasing experience, the risk has fallen and the long-term prospects are probably better than that of the atrial redirection procedure.

TRICUSPID ATRESIA AND DOUBLE INLET VENTRICLE

In tricuspid atresia (Fig. 14.23) and double inlet ventricle there is only one effective ventricle (usually the left), the other being small and non-functional.

Clinical features

In all cases there is 'common mixing' of systemic and pulmonary venous return, either in the atrium in tricuspid atresia, or in the ventricle when there is a double inlet ventricle. The degree of cyanosis will therefore depend on the amount of pulmonary blood flow, and hence pulmonary venous return. If there is reduced pulmonary blood flow, as in tricuspid atresia, the child will be cyanosed. If there is a large pulmonary blood flow, as often in double inlet ventricle, the desaturated systemic venous blood is 'diluted' by a large amount of saturated pulmonary venous blood and the child will be relatively pink.

Management

Early palliation is required:
- a Blalock–Taussig shunt in most children with tricuspid atresia
- pulmonary artery banding, to reduce pulmonary blood flow, in most children with double inlet left ventricle.

Completely corrective surgery is not possible as there is only one effective functioning ventricle. They therefore undergo 'physiologically corrective' surgery. The Fontan operation connects the right atrium directly to the pulmonary arteries and closes the atrial septal defect. It produces a more normal circulation with the left ventricle pumping exclusively fully oxygenated blood returning from the lungs. There have been many modifications of this operation, but the basic principle of a venopulmonary connection is the same in all. The Fontan operation results in a less than ideal functional outcome, but has the advantages of relieving cyanosis and removing the long-term volume load on the single functional ventricle. Many of the children lead normal, or near normal, lives. These operations were first performed in the early 1970s so the late outcome is unknown.

Cardiac arrhythmias

Sinus arrhythmia is very common in normal children and is detectable as a cyclical change in heart rate with respiration. There is slowing on inspiration and acceleration during expiration (the heart rate changing by up to 30 beats/min).

SUPRAVENTRICULAR RE-ENTRY TACHYCARDIA

This is the most common childhood arrhythmia. The heart rate is rapid, between 250 and 300 beats per minute. It can cause poor cardiac output, left atrial hypertension and pulmonary oedema. It typically presents with symptoms of heart failure in the neonate or young infant. It is a cause of hydrops fetalis and intrauterine death. This arrhythmia is known as a re-entry tachycardia because a circuit of conduction is set up, with premature activation of the atrium via an accessory pathway. There is rarely a structural heart problem but these children should have an echocardiogram.

Investigation

The ECG will generally show a narrow complex tachycardia of 250–300 beats per minute (Fig. 14.24). It may be possible to discern a P wave after the QRS complex due

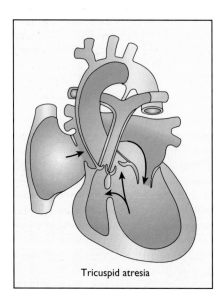

Fig. 14.23 In tricuspid atresia and double inlet ventricle there is only one effective ventricle. In tricuspid atresia there is usually complete absence of the tricuspid valve.

Tricuspid atresia

to retrograde activation of the atrium via the accessory pathway. If heart failure is severe there may be changes suggestive of myocardial ischaemia, with T wave inversion in the lateral precordial leads. When in sinus rhythm, there may be a delta wave due to early antegrade activation of the ventricle via the pathway and, consequently, a shortened P–R interval (Wolff–Parkinson–White, WPW syndrome).

Management

In the severely ill child, prompt restoration of sinus rhythm is the key to improvement. This is achieved by:

- circulatory support – tissue acidosis is corrected, positive pressure ventilation if required
- vagal stimulating manoeuvres – carotid sinus massage, eyeball pressure, submersion. Although the very sick neonate rarely responds, they should always be tried. The most effective of these manoeuvres in the less ill child is immersion head first into ice cold water: it will terminate 80% of supraventricular tachycardias but is difficult to perform in the older child to whom it may be unacceptable
- intravenous adenosine – the treatment of choice. This is safe and effective, inducing atrioventricular block after rapid intravenous injection. It terminates the tachycardia by breaking the re-entry circuit that is set up between the atrioventricular node and accessory pathway. It is given in incrementally increasing doses (up to a total dose of 0.5 mg/kg)
- electrical cardioversion with a DC shock (1–2 joules/kg bodyweight) is the next step.

Once sinus rhythm is restored, maintenance therapy will be required. Digoxin can be used and is probably safe when there is no overt pre-excitation wave (delta wave) on the resting ECG. Alternatively, flecainide is highly effective but blood levels need to be closely monitored. Even though the resting ECG may remain abnormal, 90% of children will have no further attacks after infancy. Treatment is therefore stopped at one year of age and chronic treatment reserved for those who relapse thereafter.

CONGENITAL COMPLETE HEART BLOCK

This is a rare condition (Fig. 14.25) which may remain asymptomatic for many years. However, it is increasingly recognised during fetal scanning and may cause fetal hydrops and death *in utero*. There may be associated complex congenital heart disease, but in most there is no discernible structural abnormality. Complete heart block is usually related to the presence of anti-Rho antibodies in maternal serum. These mothers will either have a manifest or latent connective tissue disorder. Subsequent pregnancies are nearly always affected. This antibody appears to prevent normal development of the electrical conduction system in the developing heart, with atrophy and fibrosis of the atrioventricular node. A few neonates develop heart failure. Most, however, remain symptom free for many years but a few become symptomatic with pre-syncope or syncope. All children with symptoms require insertion of an endocardial or epicardial pacemaker.

OTHER ARRHYTHMIAS

Prolonged Q-T syndrome may be associated with sudden loss of consciousness during exercise, stress or emotion, usually in late childhood. It may be mistakenly diagnosed as epilepsy. If unrecognised sudden death from ventricular tachycardia may occur. It may be autosomal dominant or autosomal recessive accompanied by deafness

Atrial fibrillation, atrial flutter, ectopic atrial tachycardia, ventricular tachycardia and ventricular fibrillation occur in children but all are rare. They are most often seen in children who have undergone surgery for complex congenital heart disease, and in general their treatment is similar to that of adults.

Rheumatic fever

Worldwide, this remains the most important cause of heart disease in children. Improvements in sanitation, social factors, the more liberal use of antibiotics and diminished streptococcal virulence have led to its virtual disappearance in developed countries. In susceptible individuals there is an abnormal immune response to a preceding infection with Group A β-haemolytic streptococcus. It mainly affects children 5–15 years old. The diagnosis is clinical (Fig. 14.26).

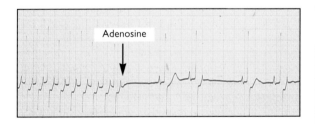

Fig. 14.24 Rhythm strip showing supraventricular re-entry tachycardia, in which there is a narrow complex tachycardia (<120 msec or 3 small squares) of 250–300 beats/min., and response to treatment with adenosine.

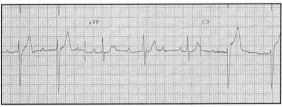

Fig. 14.25 ECG of congenital complete heart block. The P waves and QRS complexes are dissociated.

Fig. 14.26 Jones criteria for diagnosis of rheumatic fever

Major manifestations

Pancarditis (50%)

Polyarthritis (80%)

Erythema marginatum (<5%)

Sydenham chorea (10%)

Subcutaneous nodules (rare)

Minor manifestations

Fever

Polyarthralgia

History of rheumatic fever

Raised acute phase reactants: ESR, C-reactive protein,
leucocytosis

Prolonged P–R interval on ECG

Required to make the diagnosis

Two major, or one major and two minor, criteria

plus supportive evidence of preceding Group A streptococcal
infection (markedly raised ASO titre or other streptococcal
antibodies, or Group A streptococcus on throat culture)

Clinical features

After a latent interval of 2–6 weeks following a pharyngeal infection, polyarthritis, mild fever and malaise develop.

Polyarthritis

The ankles, knees and wrists rapidly become exquisitely tender but with only moderate redness and swelling. The arthritis is 'flitting', lasting less than a week in an individual joint, but migrating to other joints over 1–2 months. It does not cause long-term damage.

Pancarditis

Endocarditis

May be detected by the presence of a significant murmur and may lead to marked valvular dysfunction within the heart, e.g. severe mitral incompetence.

Myocarditis

May accompany the endocarditis and lead to severe heart failure and death.

Pericarditis

May be associated with a pericardial friction rub, pericardial effusions and tamponade.

Chorea

Chorea occurs 2–6 months after the streptococcal infection. There are typical involuntary movements and emotional lability lasting 3–6 months.

Erythema marginatum

This rash over the trunk and limbs is an uncommon, early manifestation. Pink macules spread outwards, giving rise to a pink border with a fading centre. The borders may unite to give a map-like outline to the rash.

Subcutaneous nodules

These are painless, pea-sized and hard and are mainly found over the extensor surfaces.

Chronic rheumatic heart disease

The most common form of long-term damage from scarring and fibrosis of the valve tissue of the heart is mitral stenosis. If there have been repeated attacks of rheumatic fever with carditis this may occur as early as the second decade of life, but usually symptoms do not develop until later adult life. Although the mitral valve is the most frequently affected, aortic, tricuspid and, rarely, pulmonary valve disease may occur.

Management

The acute episode is usually treated by bed rest and anti-inflammatory agents. While there is evidence of active myocarditis (echocardiographic changes with a raised ESR), bed rest and limitation of exercise are essential. Aspirin is very effective at suppressing the inflammatory response of the joints and heart. It needs to be given in high dosage and serum levels monitored. If the fever and inflammation do not resolve rapidly, corticosteroids will be required. Symptomatic heart failure is treated with diuretics and ACE inhibitors, and significant pericardial effusions will require pericardiocentesis. Antistreptococcal antibiotics may be given if there is any evidence of persisting infection.

Following resolution of the acute episode, recurrence should be prevented. Monthly injections of benzathine penicillin is the most effective prophylaxis. Alternatively, the penicillin can be given orally every day, but compliance may be a problem. Oral erythromycin can be substituted in those sensitive to penicillin. The length of treatment is controversial. Most recommend treatment to the age of 18 or 21 years, but more recently lifelong prophylaxis has been advocated. The severity of eventual rheumatic valvular disease relates to the number of childhood episodes of rheumatic fever.

Subacute bacterial endocarditis

All children with congenital heart disease of any age, including neonates, are at risk of bacterial endocarditis. The risk is highest when there is a turbulent jet of blood, as with a ventricular septal defect, coarctation of the aorta and patent ductus arteriosus or if prosthetic material has been inserted at surgery. It may be difficult to diagnose, but should be suspected in any child or adult with a sustained fever, malaise, raised ESR, unexplained anaemia or haematuria. The presence of the classical peripheral stigmata of bacterial endocarditis should not be relied upon.

Clinical signs

These are:

- fever
- anaemia and pallor
- splinter haemorrhages

- clubbing (late)
- necrotic skin lesions (Fig. 14.27)
- changing cardiac signs
- splenomegaly
- neurological signs from cerebral infarction
- retinal infarcts
- arthritis/arthralgia
- haematuria (microscopic).

Diagnosis

Detailed cross-sectional echocardiography may confirm the diagnosis by identification of vegetations but can never exclude it. The vegetations consist of fibrin and platelets and contain infecting organisms. If in doubt, children should be admitted to hospital for frequently repeated blood cultures. Acute phase reactants are raised and can be useful to monitor response to treatment.

The most common causative organism is α-haemolytic *Streptococcus (viridans)*. Bacterial endocarditis is usually treated with high-dose penicillin in combination with an aminoglycoside, giving six weeks of intravenous therapy and checking that the serum level of the antibiotic will inhibit growth of the organism. If there is infected prosthetic material, e.g. prosthetic valves, VSD patches or shunts, there is less chance of complete eradication and surgical removal may be required.

Prophylaxis

The most important factor in prophylaxis against endocarditis is good dental hygiene, and this should be encouraged in all children with congenital heart disease. Antibiotic prophylaxis will be required for:

- dental treatment, however trivial
- surgery which is likely to be associated with bacteraemia (e.g. appendicectomy, ENT surgery). A standard protocol is shown in Figure 14.28.

 Antibiotic prophylaxis is essential for dental and surgical treatment in almost all children with congenital heart disease.

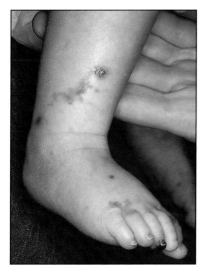

Fig. 14.27 Widespread infected emboli and infarcts in a child with subacute bacterial endocarditis. The tip of the third toe is gangrenous.

Myocarditis/cardiomyopathy

Dilated cardiomyopathy (a large, poorly contracting heart) may result from a viral infection of the myocardium. It is rare but should be suspected in any child with an enlarged heart and heart failure who has previously been well. The diagnosis is readily made on echocardiography. Treatment is symptomatic with diuretics. The role of steroids and immunoglobulin infusion is controversial. The condition usually improves spontaneously, but some children ultimately require heart transplantation. Other cardiomyopathies (hypertrophic/ restrictive) are rare in childhood and are usually related to a systemic disorder (Hurler, Pompe or Noonan syndromes).

Fig. 14.28 Prophylaxis against bacterial endocarditis			
Dental/oropharyngeal procedures			
Local/no anaesthetic, not had penicillin more than once in previous month	*Dose & time*	*< 5 years old*	*< 10 years old*
Amoxycillin po	3g, 1 hour before	1/4 adult	1/2 adult
Clindamycin (if allergic to penicillin) po	600mg, 1 hour before	1/4 adult	1/2 adult
General anaesthetic			
Amoxycillin iv	1g iv before and	1/4 adult	1/2 adult
or	0.5g po 6 hours later		
Amoxycillin po	3g po before and	1/4 adult	1/2 adult
	3g po 6 hours later		
Dental (ga) procedures in patients with prosthetic valves or had endocarditis or gastro-intestinal procedures or genitourinary surgery			
Amoxycillin iv and	1g at op	1/4 adult	1/2 adult
Gentamicin	120mg iv	2mg/kg	2mg/kg
If allergic to penicillin or penicillin more than once in previous month – vancomycin and gentamicin or teicoplanin and gentamicin.			
British Society for Antimicrobial Chemotherapy, Recommendations for endocarditis prophylaxis. Lancet 1992; 339: 1292–3.			

Postoperative care

Most children recover rapidly from cardiac surgery and are back at nursery or school within a month. Almost all will require antibiotic prophylaxis against subacute bacterial endocarditis. Exercise tolerance will be variable and most children can be allowed to find their own limits. RestICted exercise is advised only for children with severe residual aortic stenosis and hypertrophic cardiomyopathy.

Most of the children are followed up in specialist cardiac clinics. The majority lead normal, unrestricted lives, but any change in symptoms, e.g. decreasing exercise tolerance or an arrythmia, requires further investigation. An increasing number of adolescents and young adults require revision of surgery performed in early life. The most common reason for this is replacement of artificial valves and relief of post-surgical suture line stenosis, e.g. re-coarctation or pulmonary artery stenosis.

FURTHER READING AND ACKNOWLEDGEMENT

Anderson LRH et al. Paediatric Cardiology. Churchill Livingstone, Edinburgh, 1987.
Jordan SC, Scott O. Heart Disease in Paediatrics. Butterworth/Heinemann, Oxford, 1989.

The anatomical illustrations used in this chapter are based on artwork provided by Dr Yen Ho, Royal Brompton National Heart & Lung Hospital, London, UK.

CHAPTER 15

Kidney and Urinary Tract

• Antenatal diagnosis • Urinary tract infection • Enuresis • Proteinuria • Haematuria • Renal masses • Renal calculi • Renal tubular disorders • Acute renal failure • Hypertension • Chronic renal failure

The spectrum of renal disease in children differs from adults:

- many structural abnormalities of the kidneys and urinary tract are identified on antenatal ultrasound screening
- urinary tract infection, vesicoureteric reflux and urinary obstruction have the potential to damage the growing kidney
- post-streptococcal nephritis, Henoch–Schönlein nephritis and haemolytic uraemic syndrome (HUS) are more common in childhood and have a better prognosis
- nephrotic syndrome is usually steroid-sensitive and only rarely leads to renal failure
- chronic renal disorders may adversely affect physical growth and emotional development
- dialysis and transplantation are more difficult, but recent advances enable even neonates to be treated.

Renal blood flow in the fetus is very low. The glomerular filtration rate (GFR) at 28 weeks' gestation is only 25% of that at term. Over the first two weeks of life, the GFR doubles, increasing sixfold from birth to one year of age when the adult rate (120 ml/min/1.73m^2) is achieved. Assessment of renal function in children is listed in Figure 15.1 and radiological investigation of the renal and urinary tract in Figure 15.2.

Fig. 15.1 Assessment of renal function in children

Plasma creatinine concentration

Rises progressively throughout childhood according to height and muscle bulk

Plasma creatinine does not rise until renal function has fallen to less than half of normal

Glomerular filtration rate (GFR)

In suspected renal failure, a rough estimate of GFR can be obtained using the formula:

$$\frac{\text{height (cm)} \times 40}{\text{plasma creatinine (micromol/l)}}$$

More accurate measurement of GFR is by measuring the clearance from the plasma of a substance that is freely filtered at the glomerulus and is not secreted or reabsorbed by the tubules (e.g. inulin, chromium EDTA)

Creatinine clearance

Rarely measured in children because of the difficulties in collecting a complete, timed urine sample

---

Fig. 15.2 Radiological investigation of the renal and urinary tract

Ultrasound

Provides a non-invasive anatomical assessment of the whole urinary tract. It is now the standard imaging procedure of the kidneys and urinary tract, but it does not give information about function and its accuracy is operator-dependent

Functional scanning

Radioisotopes give a lower radiation dose than conventional X-rays and allow comparison of individual kidney function. Good images cannot be obtained until several weeks of age

Static nuclear medicine scanning uses an isotope-labelled substance (e.g. DMSA) that is incorporated into the functioning renal tissue. It is particularly good for the detection of renal scars

Dynamic nuclear medicine scanning uses an isotope-labelled substance (e.g. MAG 3, DTPA) that is excreted by glomerular filtration, and gives information on blood flow, renal function and drainage. It is particularly useful for detecting urinary obstruction. It can also be used to detect vesicoureteric reflux in the older child who can cooperate by stopping and starting micturition on command (indirect cystography)

Intravenous urography (IVU)

Is rarely indicated in children unless detailed anatomy of the calyces or ureter is required

Micturating cystourethrography (MCUG)

Filling the bladder with contrast via a urethral catheter outlines the bladder and is used to identify vesicoureteric reflux

Urethral obstruction is demonstrated on views during voiding without the catheter. Its disadvantages are that infection may be introduced, that urethral catheterisation is unpleasant and the radiation dose is high, particularly to the gonads. Using radioisotope scanning lowers the radiation dose but will not identify urethral obstruction

---

Antenatal diagnosis of urinary tract anomalies

Antenatal ultrasound scanning has markedly altered the presentation of congenital abnormalities of the kidneys and urinary tract, which in the past were identified only when symptoms developed during childhood or adult life. Abnormalities can be identified in approximately 1 in 400 fetuses. These abnormalities are important as:

- they may be associated with abnormal renal development or function
- they may predispose to postnatal infection
- urinary obstruction may require surgical treatment.

The early detection and treatment of urinary tract anomalies provides an exciting opportunity to minimise or prevent damage to the kidneys. A disadvantage is that mild abnormalities are also detected, which do not require treatment or resolve spontaneously but engender unnecessary investigations, treatment and parental anxiety.

Anomalies detectable on antenatal ultrasound screening

Absence of both kidneys (renal agenesis) results in Potter syndrome (Fig. 15.3). Failure of union of the ureteric bud (which forms the ureter, pelvis, calyces and collecting ducts) with the nephrogenic mesenchyme produces a nonfunctioning structure with large fluid-filled cysts, no renal tissue and no connection with the bladder, a multicystic kidney (Fig. 15.4a). Bilateral involvement results in Potter syndrome. Other causes of large cystic kidneys are autosomal recessive infantile polycystic kidney disease; autosomal dominant adult-type polycystic disease and tuberous sclerosis. These disorders can be distinguished from multicystic kidneys as some or normal renal function is maintained, and there are different appearances on imaging.

Abnormal caudal migration of the kidneys may result in a pelvic kidney or a horseshoe kidney (Fig. 15.4b). The abnormal position may predispose to infection or obstruction to urinary drainage. Premature division of the ureteric bud gives rise to a duplex system, which can vary from a bifid renal pelvis to complete division with two ureters. These ureters frequently have abnormal drainage so that the ureter from the lower pole moiety often refluxes, whereas the upper pole ureter may drain ectopically into the urethra or vagina or may prolapse into the bladder (ureterocoele) and obstruct urine flow (Fig. 15.4c).

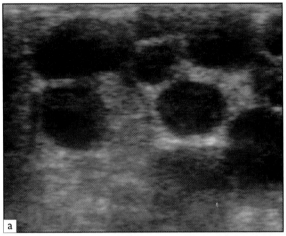

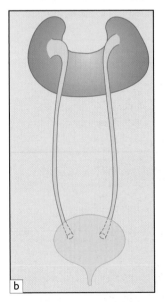

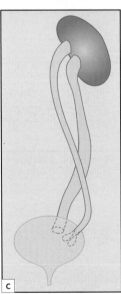

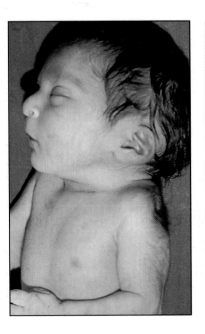

Fig. 15.3 Potter syndrome. Intrauterine compression of the fetus from oligohydramnios caused by lack of fetal urine causes characteristic facies, large and low-set ears, lung hypoplasia and postural deformities including severe talipes. The infant may be stillborn or dies soon after birth from respiratory failure.

Fig. 15.4 Some anomalies of the urinary tract detectable on antenatal ultrasound: (a) multicystic kidney on ultrasound; (b) horseshoe kidney; (c) duplex kidney showing ureterocele of upper moiety ureter and reflux into lower pole moiety.

Failure of fusion of the infraumbilical mid-line structures results in exposed bladder mucosa (bladder extrophy). Absent abdominal musculature is associated with a large bladder and dilated ureters (megacystis-megaureters) and cryporchidism, the prune belly syndrome (Fig. 15.5).

Obstruction to urine flow may occur at the pelviureteric or vesicoureteric junction, at the bladder neck, e.g. due to disruption of the nerve supply (neuropathic bladder), or at the posterior urethra in a boy due to mucosal folds or a membrane, called a posterior urethral valve. The consequences of obstruction to urine flow are shown in Figure 15.6. Intrauterine obstruction may be associated with a dysplastic kidney which is small, poorly functioning and may contain cysts and aberrant embryonic

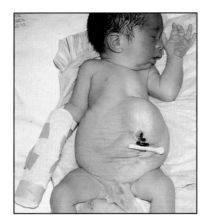

Fig. 15.5 Prune belly syndrome. The name arises from the wrinkled appearance of the abdomen. It is associated with a large bladder, dilated ureters and cryptorchidism. (Courtesy of Dr Jane Deal.)

Urinary tract obstruction

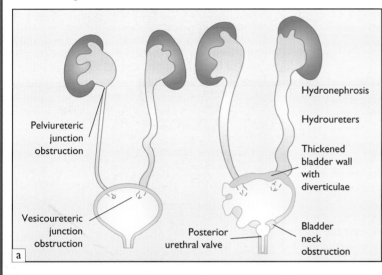

Pelviureteric junction obstruction

Vesicoureteric junction obstruction

Posterior urethral valve

Hydronephrosis

Hydroureters

Thickened bladder wall with diverticulae

Bladder neck obstruction

a

Fig. 15.6a Obstruction to urine flow results in dilatation of the urinary tract proximal to the site of obstruction. Obstruction may be at the pelviureteric or vesicoureteric junction or bladder neck or urethra.

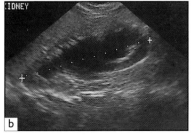

b

Fig. 15.6b An ultrasound showing a dilated renal pelvis from pelviureteric junction obstruction.

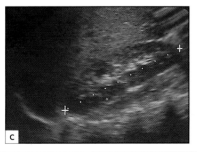

c

Fig. 15.6c A normal ultrasound of the kidney is shown for comparison.

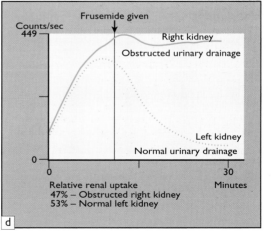

Frusemide given

Counts/sec
449

Right kidney

Obstructed urinary drainage

Left kidney

Normal urinary drainage

0

0   30

Relative renal uptake   Minutes
47% – Obstructed right kidney
53% – Normal left kidney

d

Fig. 15.6d Graph from dynamic nuclear medicine scan (MAG 3) showing delayed excretion from right pelviureteric junction obstruction.

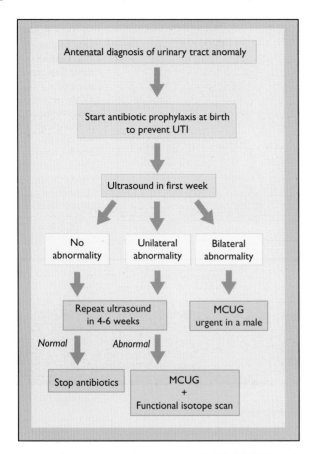

Fig. 15.7 An example of a protocol for the management of infants with antenatally diagnosed urinary tract anomalies.

tissue such as cartilage and hair. Renal dysplasia can also occur in association with severe intrauterine vesicoureteric reflux or may occur in isolation.

Antenatal treatment

The male fetus with a posterior urethral valve may develop severe urinary outflow obstruction, resulting in progressive bilateral hydronephrosis, poor renal growth and declining liquor volume. Intrauterine bladder drainage procedures have been attempted but have not improved the prognosis, possibly because severe renal damage has already occurred. Early delivery is rarely indicated; it is only performed if there is evidence of progressive renal damage.

Postnatal management

An example of a protocol for infants with antenatally diagnosed anomalies is shown in Figure 15.7. Prophylactic antibiotics should be started at birth to prevent urinary tract infection and an ultrasound performed within the first week of life. As the newborn kidney has a low glomerular filtration rate, urine flow is low and mild outflow obstruction may not be evident. The scan should therefore be repeated several weeks later. Bilateral hydronephrosis in a male infant

warrants urgent further investigation to exclude a posterior urethral valve (Fig. 15.8) which always requires surgery. The decision to operate on urinary tract obstruction from other causes is difficult as the natural history of these conditions is not yet known. Indications currently are recurrent urinary tract infection in spite of prophylactic antibiotics, deterioration of renal function, or progressive increase in the size of the hydronephrosis.

Case history

POSTERIOR URETHRAL VALVE

Bilateral hydronephrosis was noted on antenatal ultrasound at 20 weeks' gestation in a male fetus. Because of poor renal growth, progressive dilatation and decreasing volume of amniotic fluid (Fig. 15.8a), labour was induced at 35 weeks' gestation. After birth prophylactic antibiotics were started. An urgent ultrasound showed bilateral hydronephrosis with small dysplastic kidneys. The bladder and ureters were grossly distended. Plasma creatinine was raised. A micturating cystourethrogram (MCUG) (see Fig.15.8b) showed vesicoureteric reflux and a posterior urethral valve which was fulgurated. Renal function initially improved but then progressed to chronic renal failure. He had a renal transplant at ten years of age.

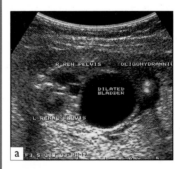

Fig. 15.8a Antenatal ultrasound scan in an infant with urinary outflow obstruction from a posterior urethral valve. (Courtesy of Mr Karl Murphy.)

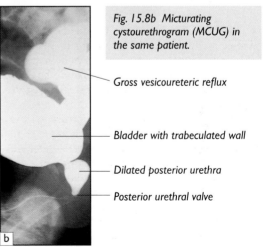

Fig. 15.8b Micturating cystourethrogram (MCUG) in the same patient.

Gross vesicoureteric reflux

Bladder with trabeculated wall

Dilated posterior urethra

Posterior urethral valve

Bilateral hydronephrosis in a male requires urgent investigation to exclude a posterior urethral valve.

Urinary tract infection

Three per cent of girls and 1% of boys have a symptomatic urinary tract infection (UTI) before the age of 11 years and 50% of them have a recurrence within a year. All children should be thoroughly assessed and investigated following their first UTI as:

- up to half have a structural abnormality of the urinary tract
- a UTI may damage the growing kidney by forming a scar, predisposing to hypertension and chronic renal failure if scarring is bilateral.

Clinical features

Presentation of UTI varies with age (Fig. 15.9). In the newborn, symptoms are non-specific and septicaemia may develop rapidly. The classical symptoms of dysuria, frequency and loin pain are rarely seen in young children. Dysuria without fever is often due to vulvitis in girls or balanitis in boys rather than a UTI. Symptoms suggestive of a UTI may also occur following sexual abuse.

Collection of urine samples

It is essential that the diagnosis of UTI is made correctly. Contamination of a urine specimen may lead to a false positive diagnosis which will commit the child to unnecessary investigations. For the child in nappies, urine can be collected by:

- a 'clean-catch' sample into a waiting sterile pot when the nappy is removed
- an adhesive plastic bag applied to the perineum after careful washing
- by suprapubic aspiration (SPA), the method of choice in the severely ill infant under one year old requiring urgent diagnosis and treatment and in those where previous samples have suggested contamination (Fig. 15.10). Catheter samples are used as an alternative in some centres.

In the older child, urine can be obtained by collecting a mid-stream sample. Careful cleaning and collection are necessary, as contamination with both white cells and bacteria can occur from under the foreskin in boys and by reflux of urine into the vagina during voiding in girls.

Diagnosis

Ideally the urine sample should be microscoped and cultured straight away. If not, it should be refrigerated to prevent overgrowth of contaminating bacteria. Alternatively, delay in culture can be circumvented by the use of boric acid or dipslides. Microscopy can demonstrate pyuria and organisms. Pyuria is virtually always present with a UTI. However, as cell lysis may occur if the sample is not microscoped immediately, and as white cells may be present in febrile children without a UTI and in children with balanitis or vulvovaginitis, the urinary white cell count alone is not a reliable feature in the diagnosis of UTI. Positive testing with sticks for nitrite and white cell

esterase is also suggestive of infection, but there may be false negative results.

A bacterial culture of $>10^5$ colony-forming units of a single species/ml in a properly collected specimen gives a 90% probability of infection. If the same result is found in a second sample, the probability rises to 95%. A growth of mixed organisms in the absence of white blood cells usually represents contamination, but if there is doubt, another sample should be collected.

Fig. 15.9 *Presentation of UTI in infancy and childhood*

Infancy	Childhood
Fever	Fever with/without rigors
Lethargy or irritability	Dysuria and frequency
Vomiting and/or diarrhoea	Lethargy and anorexia
Poor feeding/failure to thrive	Vomiting and/or diarrhoea
Prolonged neonatal jaundice	Abdominal or loin pain
Septicaemia	Febrile convulsion (not to be
Febrile convulsion (>6 months)	confused with rigors)
	Recurrence of enuresis

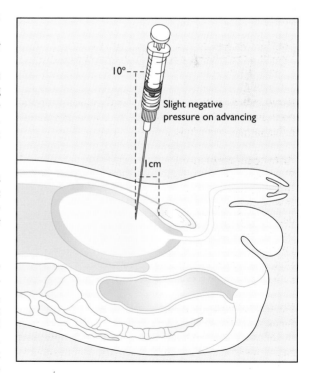

$10°$

Slight negative pressure on advancing

1 cm

Fig. 15.10 *Suprapubic aspiration. In an infant, the bladder extends into the abdomen. Negative pressure is applied to the syringe while advancing the needle until urine appears. This should avoid puncture of the rectum.*

Bacterial and host factors that predispose to infection

1. Infecting organism

UTI is usually the result of bowel flora entering the urinary tract via the urethra. The most common organism to do this is *E. coli*, followed by *Proteus* and *Pseudomonas*. The virulence of *E. coli* varies with its cell wall antigens and possession of endotoxin. *Proteus* infection is more common in boys, possibly because of its presence under the prepuce. *Proteus* infection predisposes to the formation of triple phosphate stones. *Pseudomonas* infection usually indicates that there is a structural abnormality in the urinary tract.

2. Incomplete bladder emptying

Contributing factors in some children are:

- infrequent voiding, resulting in bladder enlargement
- hurried micturition
- obstruction by a loaded rectum from constipation
- neuropathic bladder.

3. Vesicoureteric reflux

Vesicoureteric reflux is a developmental anomaly of the vesicoureteric junctions. The ureters are displaced laterally and enter directly into the bladder rather than at an angle, with a shortened intramural course. Severe reflux may be associated with renal dysplasia. It is familial, with a 10% chance of occurring in first-degree relatives. It may also occur with bladder pathology, e.g. a neuropathic bladder or urethral obstruction. Its severity varies from that occurring into the lower end of the ureter during micturition to the severest form with reflux during bladder filling and voiding, with a distended ureter, renal pelvis and clubbed calyces (Fig. 15.11). With growth, reflux resolves in 10% each year. Reflux is important as:

- urine returning to the bladder from the ureters after voiding results in incomplete bladder emptying which encourages infection

- the kidneys may become infected (pyelonephritis)
- bladder voiding pressure is transmitted to the renal papillae. This may contribute to renal damage if the bladder pressure is abnormally high.

Infection may destroy renal tissue, leaving a scar, resulting in a shrunken, poorly functioning segment of kidney. If scarring is bilateral and severe, chronic renal failure may develop. A renal scar may produce increased quantities of renin leading to hypertension. The risk for this is around 10% in childhood.

Management

Prompt treatment reduces the risk of renal scarring. Most children can be treated with oral antibiotics (e.g. amoxicillin for five days or for ten days if the child was systemically unwell), adjusting the choice of antibiotic according to sensitivity on urine culture. All infants, and any child who is severely ill, require intravenous antibiotic therapy (e.g. cefotaxime or ampicillin and an aminoglycoside such as gentamicin, monitoring serum levels) until the temperature has settled, when oral treatment is substituted. The urine should be recultured to ensure that infection has been eradicated.

All children should be investigated following their first confirmed UTI. The aim is to identify:

- serious structural abnormalities and urinary obstruction
- renal scars
- vesicoureteric reflux.

The investigations performed include:

- prelimary ultrasound to identify serious structural abnormalities
- abdominal X-ray to identify renal stones, or occult spinal abnormalities
- static radioisotope scanning to identify renal scars
- cystourethrography to identify reflux or urethral obstruction.

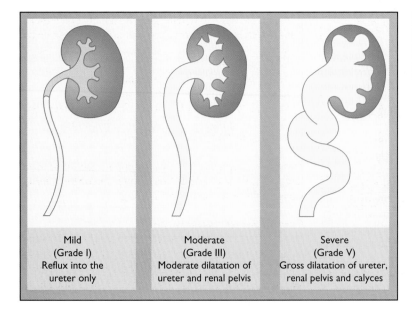

| Mild (Grade I) Reflux into the ureter only | Moderate (Grade III) Moderate dilatation of ureter and renal pelvis | Severe (Grade V) Gross dilatation of ureter, renal pelvis and calyces |

Fig. 15.11 Grades of vesicoureteric reflux during a micturating cystourethrogram (MCUG) (International Classification).

The number of investigations should be kept to a minimum, particularly direct cystography which is unpleasant for the child and the radiation dosage is relatively high. Ultrasound is performed on all children. An abdominal X-ray is indicated if there is a history suggestive of renal stones or if bladder emptying is abnormal suggesting a spinal abnormality. The choice of further investigations is adjusted to the child's age:

- all infants less than one year old are fully investigated as the incidence of abnormalities is highest at this age and the rapidly growing kidney is most susceptible to damage
- young children beyond infancy have a static radioisotope scan but cystography is used selectively
- older children, in whom new scar formation is uncommon, have a radioisotope scan and cystography only if there is a specific indication. A suggested scheme of investigations is outlined in Figure 15.12, although protocols differ between centres.

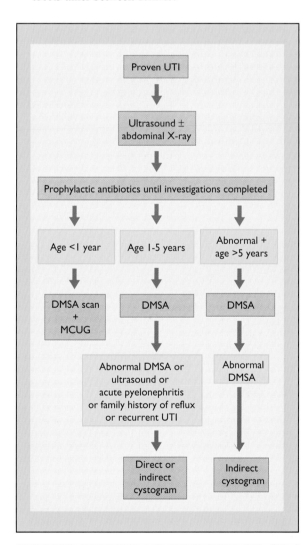

Fig. 15.12 An example of a protocol for the investigation of a first UTI.

The initial ultrasound of the kidneys and urinary tract should be performed promptly. Cystography and functional scans should be deferred for about three months after a UTI to avoid missing a newly developed renal scar and false positive results due to reflux or inflammation that may resolve. Recurrence of infection can be prevented by prophylactic antibiotic therapy while awaiting the results of the investigations.

Several simple measures can be taken to try to prevent recurrence of UTI. These are:

- high fluid intake to produce a high urine output
- regular voiding
- complete bladder emptying using double micturition to empty any residual or refluxed urine returning to the bladder
- avoidance of constipation
- good perineal hygiene.

> All children need investigation after a first urinary tract infection

Follow-up of children with recurrent UTIs, renal scarring or reflux

These children require:

- urine culture to be checked with any non-specific illness
- routine urine culture every 3–4 months
- long term low dose antibiotic prophylaxis. Trimethoprim (2 mg/kg at night) is used most often; but nitrofurantoin or nalidixic acid may be given
- circumcision in boys to be considered as there is some evidence that it reduces the incidence of UTI
- surgical reimplantation of refluxing ureters if medical management fails
- blood pressure to be checked twice a year if renal scarring is present
- regular assessment of renal growth and function if there is bilateral scarring because of the risk of chronic renal failure.

Investigations are usually repeated after two years:

- to check renal growth (by ultrasound)
- to check for new scar formation if there have been further UTIs
- to determine if reflux has resolved.

Antibiotic prophylaxis can be stopped once reflux has resolved or if the child has been asymptomatic for at least a year in the absence of renal scarring.

Asymptomatic bacteriuria

Asymptomatic bacteriuria may be detected during routine screening. Although treatment with antibiotics will eradicate the bacteriuria, recurrence is common. Asymptomatic bacteriuria does not need treatment as it does not cause renal damage.

Case history

URINARY TRACT INFECTION

A two-month-old infant stopped feeding and had a high intermittent fever. She was referred to hospital, where she had an infection screen. Urine examination showed >100 white blood cells, >10^5 *E. coli*/ml. She was treated with intravenous antibiotics. An ultrasound showed a small right kidney with a dilated renal pelvis and a dilated ureter. She was started on prophylactic antibiotics. A DMSA scan (Fig. 15.13) confirmed bilateral renal scarring, with the right kidney contributing only 17% of renal function. The MCUG (Fig. 15.14) showed bilateral vesicoureteric reflux (Grade IV on the right, III on the left). At five years of age the reflux had resolved and antibiotic prophylaxis was stopped. Her blood pressure and renal function continue to be monitored.

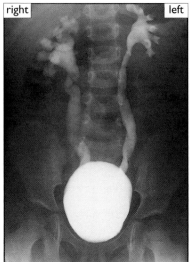

Fig. 15.14 Micturating cystourethrogram showing bilateral vesico-ureteric reflux with ureteric dilatation and dilated, clubbed calyces on the right.

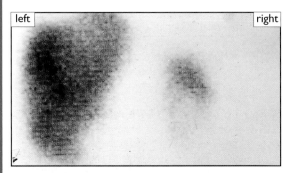

Fig. 15.13 DMSA scan showing a small scarred right kidney and scars at the upper and lower poles of the left kidney.

Enuresis

Primary nocturnal enuresis

This is considered in Chapter 20.

Diurnal enuresis

Diurnal (day and night) enuresis may be due to lack of attention to bladder sensation in the younger child, detrusor instability or bladder neck weakness. These children may benefit from bladder training, pelvic floor exercises and star charts. A small portable alarm with a pad in the pants which is activated by urine is also available. Anticholinergic or adrenergic drugs (e.g. oxybutynin to damp down bladder contractions or ephedrine to increase tone at the bladder neck) may be helpful if other measures fail. A constant dribble of urine is suggestive of an ectopic ureter. Girls who are dry at night but wet on getting up suggests overnight pooling of urine from an ectopic ureter opening in the vagina.

Secondary enuresis

The loss of previously achieved urinary continence may be due to:

- emotional upset, the most common cause
- UTI
- polyuria from an osmotic diuresis in diabetes mellitus or a concentrating disorder e.g. sickle cell disease or chronic renal failure.

Investigation should include:

- checking a urine sample for glycosuria and proteinuria and culture
- assessment of urinary concentrating ability by measuring the osmolality of an early morning urine
- ultrasound of the renal tract.

Proteinuria

Proteinuria may be detected by urine 'dipstick' testing incidentally in an asymptomatic child or when checked during a systemic disease. Transient proteinuria may occur during febrile illnesses or after exercise and does not require investigation. Persistent proteinuria can be quantified either by a 24-hour urine or a timed collection (protein excretion should not exceed 4 mg/h/m²) or, more usefully in younger children, by measuring the urine protein to creatinine ratio in an early morning sample (protein should not exceed 20 mg/mmol of creatinine).

A common cause is orthostatic proteinuria, when proteinuria is only found when the child is upright, i.e. during the day. It can be diagnosed by measuring the urine protein to creatinine ratio on the first morning urine and daytime urine specimens. Renal function is normal and the prognosis is good. Other causes of proteinuria are listed in Figure 15.15.

NEPHROTIC SYNDROME

Heavy proteinuria results in a low plasma albumin and oedema – the nephrotic syndrome. In over 90% of children the proteinuria resolves with corticosteroid therapy (steroid-sensitive nephrotic syndrome) and these children do not progress to renal failure, unlike some of the remaining 10% who have steroid-resistant nephrotic syndrome. The cause of the condition is unknown, but a few cases are secondary to systemic diseases such as Henoch-Schönlein purpura (HSP), vasculitis, e.g. systemic lupus erythematosus, infections, e.g. malaria, or allergens, e.g. bee sting.

Clinical signs of the nephrotic syndrome are:
- periorbital oedema (particularly on waking), the earliest sign
- scrotal, leg and ankle oedema (Fig. 15.16)
- ascites
- breathlessness due to pleural effusions and abdominal distension.

The initial investigations are listed in Figure 15.17.

Steroid-sensitive nephrotic syndrome

Steroid-sensitive nephrotic syndrome is more common in boys and in atopic families. It is often precipitated by respiratory infections. Features suggesting steroid-sensitive nephrotic syndrome are:
- age between one and ten years
- no macroscopic haematuria
- normal blood pressure
- normal complement levels
- normal renal function.

Management

At clinical presentation, treatment is begun with oral corticosteroids (60 mg/m²/day) unless there are atypical features. The average time for the urine to become free of protein is ten days. Once in remission, when the urine has been protein free for three days, the corticosteroid dose is reduced and then stopped after 4–6 weeks. Children who do not respond to four weeks of corticosteroid therapy or have atypical features may have a more sinister diagnosis and require a renal biopsy. Renal histology in steroid-sensitive nephrotic syndrome is usually normal on light microscopy but podocyte fusion is seen on electron microscopy. For this reason it is called minimal change disease. In most of these children the protein leak is mainly of low molecular weight proteins and is referred to as selective proteinuria, although this is no longer measured

routinely as it does not reliably predict steroid responsiveness.

The child with nephrotic syndrome is susceptible to several serious complications at presentation or relapse.

1. Hypovolaemia

During the initial phase of oedema formation the intravascular compartment may become volume-depleted. The child who becomes hypovolaemic characteristically complains of abdominal pain and may feel faint. There is peripheral vasoconstriction and urinary sodium retention. A low urinary sodium (<20 mmol/l), a high packed cell volume and a peripheral temperature more than 2°C cooler than

---

Fig. 15.15 Causes of proteinuria

Orthostatic proteinuria
Glomerular abnormalities
    Minimal change disease
    Glomerulonephritis
    Abnormal glomerular basement membrane
      (familial nephritides)
Increased glomerular perfusion pressure
    Reduced renal mass
    Hypertension
Tubular proteinuria

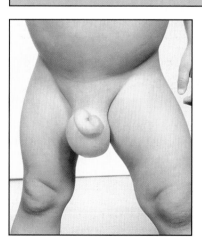

*Fig. 15.16
Gross oedema of the scrotum and legs as well as abdominal distension from ascites.*

Fig. 15.17 Investigations performed at presentation of nephrotic syndrome

Urine protein – on test strips ('Dipstick')
Full blood count and ESR
Urea, electrolytes, creatinine, albumin
Complement levels – C3, C4
Antistreptolysin O titre and throat swab
Urine microscopy and culture
Urinary sodium concentration
Hepatitis B antigen

the central temperature are indications of hypovolaemia which requires urgent treatment with intravenous albumin, as the child is at risk of vascular thrombosis.

Increasing peripheral oedema, assessed clinically and by daily weight, may cause striae, discomfort and respiratory compromise, which if severe needs treatment with albumin and diuretics. Care must be taken in the use of colloid, as it may precipitate pulmonary oedema and hypertension from fluid overload, and with giving diuretics which may cause or worsen hypovolaemia.

2. Thrombosis
A hypercoagulable state due to urinary losses of antithrombin III, increased synthesis of clotting factors and increased blood viscosity from the raised haematocrit, predisposes to renal vein and cerebral thrombosis.

3. Infection
Urinary loss of immunoglobulins renders the child susceptible to infection, particularly pneumococcal. Peritonitis may occur. Penicillin prophylaxis should be given to all children while they have hypoalbuminaemia.

4. Hypercholesterolaemia
Hypercholesterolaemia correlates inversely with the serum albumin, but the cause of the hyperlipidaemia is not fully understood.

Prognosis

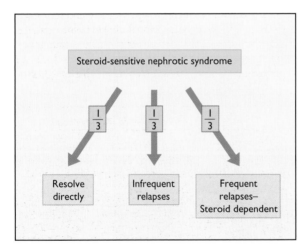

Fig. 15.18 Clinical course in steroid-sensitive nephrotic syndrome.

This is summarised in Figure 15.18. Relapses are identified by parents on urine tesing. Corticosteroid therapy may cause serious side-effects if relapses are frequent or if a high maintenance dose is required, though the side-effects are reduced by an alternate day regimen. Involvement of a paediatric nephrologist in the care of these children is advisable, and other drug therapy may be considered. Levamisole, an immunomodulator, may maintain remission. Cyclophosphamide maintains remission in 75% of cases for one year and 50% at five years, but its its toxicity restricts its use to the most severely affected children. Cyclosporin maintains remission while it is being taken but relapse often occurs when it is stopped. Renal biopsy is necessary before starting cyclosporin because of its nephrotoxicity.

Steroid-resistant nephrotic syndrome (Fig. 15.19)
These children should be managed by a paediatric nephrologist. Management of the oedema is by diuretic therapy, salt restriction and captopril which may reduce proteinuria.

Congenital nephrotic syndrome
Congenital nephrotic syndrome presents in the first three months of life. It is rare. It is associated with early end stage renal failure and a high mortality. When renal failure develops, nephrectomy and dialysis are instituted until the child is large enough for transplantation.

 An oedematous child – test for proteinuria to diagnose nephrotic syndrome.

Haematuria

Urine which is red in colour or tests positive for haemoglobin on test strips (dipstick) should be examined under the microscope to confirm haematuria (>10 red blood cells per high power field). Glomerular haematuria is suggested by brown urine, the presence of deformed red cells (occurs when red cells pass through the basement membrane) and casts, and is often accompanied by proteinuria. Lower urinary tract haematuria is usually red, occurs at the end of the urinary stream, is not accompanied by proteinuria and is unusual in children.

Urinary tract infection is the most common cause of

Fig. 15.19 Steroid-resistant nephrotic syndrome		
Cause	**Specific features**	**Prognosis**
Focal segmental glomerulosclerosis	Most common	30% progress to end-stage renal failure in 5 years; 20%
	Familial or idiopathic	respond to cyclophosphamide, vincristine or cyclosporin
Mesangiocapillary glomerulonephritis (membranoproliferative glomerulonephritis)	More common in older children	Decline in renal function over many years
	Haematuria and low complement level present	
Membranous nephropathy	Associated with hepatitis B	Most remit spontaneously within 5 years. May precede SLE

haematuria (Fig. 15.20). The history and examination may suggest the diagnosis, e.g. a family history of urinary stone formation or nephritis or a history of trauma. A plan of investigation is outlined in Figure 15.21.

A renal biopsy is indicated if:
- microscopic haematuria persists for over a year
- there is recurrent macroscopic haematuria
- a familial nephritis is suspected
- renal function is abnormal
- complement levels are persistently abnormal
- there is heavy proteinuria.

ACUTE NEPHRITIS

Acute nephritis in childhood usually follows a streptococcal sore throat or skin infection. Streptococcal nephritis remains a common condition in the developing world, but has become uncommon and mild in the UK. Other less common causes of acute nephritis are listed in Figure 15.22. In acute nephritis, increased glomerular cellularity restricts glomerular blood flow and therefore filtration is decreased. This leads to:
- decreased urine output and volume overload
- hypertension, which may cause seizures
- oedema, characteristically around the eyes

- haematuria and proteinuria.

Management is by attention to water and electrolyte balance and the use of diuretics when necessary. Rarely, there may be a rapid deterioration in renal function (rapidly progressive glomerulonephritis). This may occur with any cause of acute nephritis, but is uncommon with post-streptococcal, and characteristic of anti-glomerular basement membrane disease. If left untreated, irreversible renal failure will occur over weeks or months, so renal biopsy and treatment with immunosuppression must be undertaken promptly.

Post-streptococcal nephritis

This is diagnosed by a raised ASO titre and low complement C3 levels that return to normal after 3–4 weeks. Long-term prognosis is good.

Henoch-Schönlein purpura

Henoch-Schönlein purpura (HSP) is the combination of:
- characteristic skin rash
- arthralgia
- periarticular oedema
- abdominal pain
- glomerulonephritis.

It usually occurs between the ages of three and ten years, is twice as common in boys, peaks during the winter months and is often preceded by an upper respiratory tract infection. It is postulated that genetic predisposition and antigen exposure increase circulating IgA levels and disrupt IgG syn-

Fig. 15.20 Causes of haematuria	
Non-glomerular	Infection (bacterial, viral, TB, schistosomiasis)
	Trauma to genitalia, urinary tract or kidneys
	Stones
	Tumours
	Sickle cell disease
	Bleeding disorders
	Renal vein thrombosis
	Hypercalcuria
Glomerular	Acute glomerulonephritis
	Chronic glomerulonephritis
	IgA nephropathy
	Familial nephritis
	Thin basement membrane disease

Fig. 15.22 Causes of acute nephritis
Post infectious (including streptococcus)
Vasculitis (Henoch-Schönlein purpura or rarely SLE, Wegener granulomatosis, microscopic polyarteritis, polyarteritis nodosa)
IgA nephropathy and mesangiocapillary glomerulonephritis
Anti-glomerular basement membrane disease (Good pasture syndrome), very rare

Fig. 15.21 Investigation of haematuria	
All patients	Urine microscopy (with phase contrast) and culture
	Protein and calcium excretion
	Kidney and urinary tract U/S and abdominal X-ray
	Plasma urea, electrolytes, creatinine, calcium, phosphate, albumin
	Full blood count, platelets, clotting screen, sickle cell screen
If suggestive of glomerular haematuria	ESR complement levels and anti-DNA binding
	Throat swab and anti-streptolysin O titre
	Hepatitis B antigen
	Renal biopsy if indicated
	Test mother's urine for blood } If Alport
	Hearing test and eye check } syndrome suspected

thesis. The IgA and IgG interact to produce complexes that activate complement and are deposited in affected organs, precipitating an inflammatory response with vasculitis.

Clinical findings

At presentation, affected children often have a fever. The most obvious feature is the *rash* which is symmetrically distributed over the buttocks (Fig. 15.23), extensor surfaces of the arms and legs and the ankles. The trunk is spared unless lesions are induced by trauma. The rash may initially be urticarial, rapidly becoming maculopapular and purpuric, and may recur over several weeks. The rash is the first clinical feature in about 50% and is the cornerstone of the diagnosis, which is clinical.

Joint pain occurs in two-thirds of patients, particularly in the knees and ankles. There is *periarticular oedema.* Long-term damage to the joints does not occur, and symptoms usually resolve before the rash goes.

Colicky abdominal pain occurs in many children, and if severe can be treated with corticosteroids. Gastrointestinal petechiae can cause haematemesis and melaena. Intussusception can occur and can be particularly difficult to diagnose under these circumstances. Ileus, protein losing enteropathy, orchitis and occasionally central nervous system involvement are other rare complications.

Renal involvement is rarely the first symptom, but is common. Over 80% have microscopic or macroscopic haematuria or mild proteinuria. These children usually make a complete recovery. If proteinuria is more severe nephrotic syndrome may result. Risk factors for progressive renal disease are heavy proteinuria, oedema, hypertension and deteriorating renal function, when a renal biopsy will determine if immunosuppressive treatment is necessary. All these children are followed for a year to detect those with persisting urinary abnormalities (5–10%). Long-term follow-up is necessary in those with persistent urinary abnormalities as hypertension and declining renal function

may develop after an interval of several years.

IgA nephropathy

This may present with episodes of macroscopic haematuria, commonly in association with upper respiratory tract infections. Histological findings and treatment are as for HSP, which may be a variant of the same pathological process but is not restricted to the kidney.

Familial nephritis

The most common familial nephritis is Alport syndrome, which is a sex-linked recessive disorder. It progresses to end-stage renal failure by early adult life in males and is associated with nerve deafness and ocular defects. The mother may have haematuria.

Renal masses

An abdominal mass identified on palpating the abdomen should be investigated promptly by ultrasound scan (Fig. 15.24). Bilaterally enlarged kidneys in early life are most frequently due to autosomal recessive polycystic kidney disease, which is associated with hypertension, hepatic fibrosis and progression to chronic renal failure. This form of polycystic kidney disease must be distinguished from the autosomal dominant adult-type polycystic kidney disease which has a more benign prognosis and from tuberous sclerosis.

Renal calculi

Renal stones are uncommon in childhood. When they occur, predisposing causes must be sought:
- UTI
- structural anomalies of the urinary tract
- metabolic abnormalities.

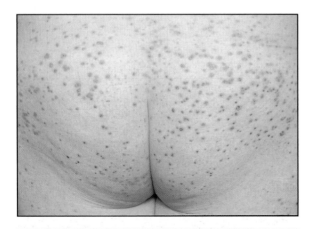

Fig. 15.23 Rash in Henoch-Schönlein purpura on the buttocks. It also occurs on the legs and extensor surface of the arms. (Courtesy of Dr Michael Markiewicz.)

Fig. 15.24 Causes of palpable kidneys	
Unilateral	Multicystic kidney
	Compensatory hypertrophy
	Obstructed hydronephrosis
	Renal tumour (Wilms tumour)
	Renal vein thrombosis
Bilateral	Autosomal recessive (infantile) polycystic kidneys
	Autosomal dominant (adult) polycystic kidneys
	Tuberous sclerosis
	Renal vein thrombosis

Infective stones, composed of magnesium ammonium phosphate and calcium phosphate, are the most common and are associated with *Proteus* urinary tract infections. Calcium-containing stones occur in idiopathic hypercalciuria, the most common metabolic abnormality, and with increased urinary urate and oxalate excretion. Deposition of calcium in the parenchyma (nephrocalcinosis) may occur with hypercalcuria, hyperoxaluria and distal renal tubular acidosis. Nephrocalcinosis may be a complication of frusemide therapy in the neonate. Cystine and xanthine stones are rare.

Presentation may be with haematuria, loin or abdominal pain, UTI or passage of a stone.

Stones that are not passed spontaneously should be removed, either by lithotripsy or surgically and any predisposing structural anomaly repaired. A high fluid intake is recommended in all affected children. If the cause is a metabolic abnormality, specific therapy may be possible.

Renal tubular disorders

Abnormalities of renal tubular function may occur at any point along the length of the nephron and affect any of the substances handled by it.

Generalised proximal tubular dysfunction (Fanconi syndrome)
The cardinal features are excessive urinary loss of amino acids, glucose, phosphate, bicarbonate, sodium, calcium, potassium and urate. The causes are listed in Figure 15.25.

Fanconi syndrome should be considered in a child presenting with:
* polydipsia and polyuria
* salt depletion and dehydration
* hyperchloraemic metabolic acidosis
* rickets and osteoporosis
* failure to thrive/poor growth.

Fig. 15.25 Causes of Fanconi syndrome

Idiopathic
Secondary to inborn errors of metabolism:
  Cystinosis (an autosomal recessive disorder causing
    intracellular accumulation of cystine)
  Glycogen storage disorders
  Lowe syndrome (oculocerebrorenal dystrophy)
  Galactosaemia
  Fructose intolerance
  Tyrosinaemia
  Wilson disease
Acquired
  Heavy metals
  Drugs and toxins
  Vitamin D deficiency

Specific transport defects
See Figure 15.26 overleaf.

Acute renal failure

Acute renal failure is a sudden reduction in renal function (Fig. 15.27). Oliguria (<0.5 ml/kg/h) is usually present. It can be classified as:
* prerenal – the most common cause in children
* renal – there is salt and water retention; blood, protein and casts are often present in the urine, and there may be symptoms specific to an accompanying disease (e.g. HSP)
* postrenal – from urinary obstruction.

Acute on chronic renal failure is suggested by the child having growth failure, anaemia and a bone mineralisation disorder (osteodystrophy).

Management
Children with acute renal failure should have their circulation and fluid balance meticulously monitored. Investigation by ultrasound scan will identify obstruction of the

---

Fig. 15.27 Causes of acute renal failure

Prerenal
Hypovolaemia
  Gastroenteritis
  Burns
  Sepsis
  Haemorrhage
  Nephrotic syndrome
Circulatory failure

Renal
Vascular
  Haemolytic uraemic syndrome (HUS)
  Vasculitis
  Embolus
  Renal vein thrombosis
Tubular
  Acute tubular necrosis (ATN)
  Ischaemic
  Toxic
  Obstructive
Glomerular
  Glomerulonephritis
Interstitial
  Interstitial nephritis
  Pyelonephritis
Acute on chronic renal failure

Postrenal
Obstruction
  Congenital
  Acquired

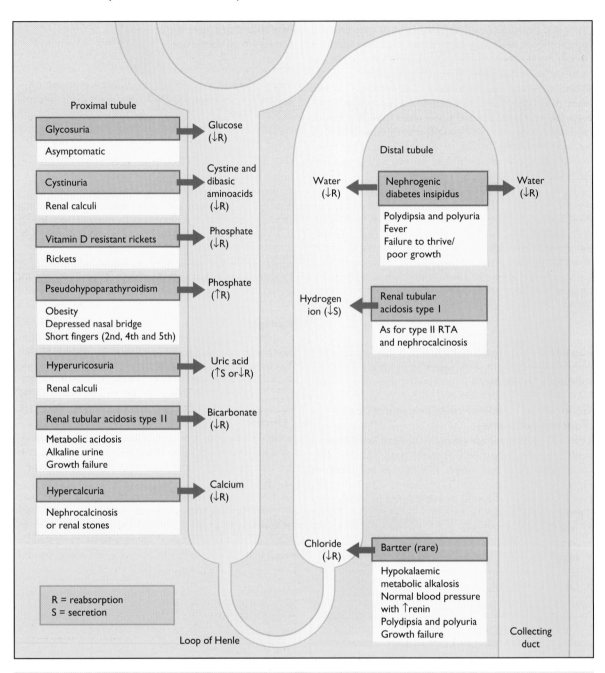

Fig. 15.26 Schematic diagram of specific transport defects in some renal tubular disorders.

urinary tract, the small kidneys of chronic renal failure or large, bright kidneys with loss of cortical medullary differentiation typical of an acute process.

Prerenal failure

This is suggested by hypovolaemia. The fractional excretion of sodium is less than 1%. The hypovolaemia needs to be corrected urgently, with fluid replacement and circulatory support, if acute tubular necrosis is to be avoided.

Renal failure

If there is circulatory overload, restriction of fluid intake and challenge with a diuretic may increase urine output sufficiently to allow gradual correction of sodium and water balance. A high-calorie, low-protein feed will decrease catabolism, uraemia and hyperkalaemia. Emergency management of metabolic acidosis, hyperkalaemia and hyperphosphataemia is shown in Figure 15.28. If the cause of renal failure is not obvious, a renal biopsy

Fig. 15.28 Metabolic abnormalities in acute renal failure and their therapy	
Metabolic abnormality	**Treatment**
Metabolic acidosis	Sodium bicarbonate
Hyperphosphataemia	Calcium carbonate
Hyperkalaemia	Calcium exchange resin
	Salbutamol
	Glucose and insulin
	Dialysis

should be performed to identify rapidly progressive glomerulonephritis, as this needs immediate treatment with immunosuppression.

Postrenal failure

Requires assessment of the site of obstruction and relief by nephrostomy or bladder catheterisation. Surgery can be performed once fluid volume and electrolyte abnormalities have been corrected.

Dialysis is indicated when there is:
- failure of conservative management
- hyperkalaemia
- severe hypo- or hypernatraemia
- pulmonary oedema or hypertension
- severe acidosis
- multisystem failure.

Peritoneal dialysis is the most common choice for children as it easier to perform than haemodialysis. If plasma exchange is part of treatment, haemodialysis is used. If there is cardiac decompensation or hypercatabolism, continuous arteriovenous or venovenous haemofiltration or dialysis provides gentle, continuous dialysis and fluid removal.

Acute renal failure in childhood generally carries a good prognosis for renal recovery unless complicating a life-threatening condition, e.g. severe infection, following cardiac surgery or multisystem failure.

Haemolytic uraemic syndrome

Haemolytic uraemic syndrome (HUS) is a triad of acute renal failure, microangiopathic haemolytic anaemia and thrombocytopenia. It is the most common renal cause of acute renal failure in childhood. The disorder is thought to be due to activation of neutrophils which damage vascular endothelium. Typical haemolytic uraemic syndrome (also called diarrhoea-associated HUS) is secondary to gastrointestinal infection with verocytotoxin producing *E. coli* O157:H7 or, less often, *Shigella*. It follows a prodrome of bloody diarrhoea. Although the platelet count is reduced, in contrast to disseminated intravascular coagulation, the clotting is normal. Other organs may also be involved, e.g. brain, pancreas and heart.

With early supportive therapy, including dialysis, typical diarrhoea-associated HUS usually has a good prognosis, although occasionally there may be persistent proteinuria or mild hypertension which needs follow-up. In contrast, atypical HUS has no diarrhoeal prodrome, may be familial and frequently relapses. It has a high risk of hypertension and chronic renal failure and a high mortality. Children with intracerebral involvement or with atypical HUS may be treated with prostacyclin or plasma exchange, but their efficacy is unproven.

 Haemolytic uraemic syndrome (HUS) – the triad of acute renal failure, haemolytic anaemia and thrombocytopenia.

Hypertension

Symptomatic hypertension in children is usually secondary and of renal origin. Most often, this is due to renal parenchymal disease from scarring following reflux nephropathy. Coarctation of the aorta is another important cause in children. Other causes (Fig. 15.29) are rare.

Presentation includes proteinuria, vomiting, headaches, facial palsy, hypertensive retinopathy and convulsions. Failure to thrive and cardiac failure are the most common features in infants. Phaeochromocytoma may cause paroxysmal palpitations and sweating. Some causes are correctable, e.g. nephrectomy for unilateral scarring, angioplasty for renal artery stenosis, surgical repair of coarctation of the aorta, resection of a phaeochromocytoma, but in most, medical treatment is necessary with antihypertensive drugs.

Preventing the development of hypertension is important. Any child with renal scarring should have their blood pressure checked twice a year throughout life. Children with a family history of essential hypertension should be encouraged to restrict their salt intake, avoid obesity and have their blood pressure checked regularly.

Fig. 15.29 Causes of hypertension
Renin-dependent
Renal parenchymal disease
Renovascular, e.g. renal artery stenosis
Renal tumours
Coarctation of the aorta
Catecholamine excess
Phaeochromocytoma
Neuroblastoma
Endocrine causes
Congenital adrenal hyperplasia
Cushing syndrome or corticosteroid therapy
Essential hypertension

Chronic renal failure

Chronic renal failure (CRF) is much less common in children than adults, with an incidence of only 10 per million child population entering end-stage renal failure each year. Congenital and familial causes are more common in childhood than acquired diseases (Fig. 15.30).

Clinical findings
CRF presents with:
- anorexia and lethargy
- polydipsia and polyuria
- failure to thrive/growth failure
- bony deformities from renal osteodystrophy (renal rickets)
- hypertension
- acute on chronic renal failure (precipitated by infection or dehydration)
- incidental finding of proteinuria or anaemia.

Many children with chronic renal failure have had their renal disease detected before birth by antenatal ultrasound or have previously identified renal disease. Symptoms rarely develop before renal function falls to less than half of normal.

Management
The aims of management are to prevent the symptoms and metabolic abnormalities of renal failure; to allow normal growth and development and to preserve residual renal function. The management of these children should be supervised by a specialist paediatric nephrology centre.

Diet
Anorexia and vomiting are common. During the first two years of life, calorie and protein requirements are 2–3 times higher per kg than in the adult. Improving nutrition using calorie supplements and nasogastric or gastrostomy feeding is often necessary to prevent growth failure. Protein intake should be reduced to be adequate for growth and maintains a normal albumin, but prevents the accumulation of toxic metabolic byproducts.

Prevention of renal osteodystrophy
Phosphate retention and hypocalcaemia due to decreased activation of vitamin D result in secondary hyperparathyroidism, osteitis fibrosa and osteomalacia. Phosphate restriction by decreasing the dietary intake of milk products, calcium carbonate as a phosphate binder, and activated vitamin D supplements help prevent renal osteodystrophy.

Control of salt and water balance and acidosis
Many children with congenital structural malformations and renal dysplasia as a cause of CRF have an obligatory loss of salt and water and need salt supplements and free access to water. Treatment with bicarbonate supplements is necessary to prevent acidosis.

Anaemia
Reduced production of erythropoietin and circulation of metabolites that are toxic to bone marrow result in anaemia. This responds well to the administration of recombinant human erythropoietin.

Hormonal abnormalities
Many hormonal abnormalities occur in CRF. Most importantly there may be growth hormone resistance with normal or high growth hormone levels but poor growth. Trials of the efficacy and safety of recombinant human growth hormone are currently underway. Many children with CRF have delayed puberty and a subnormal pubertal growth spurt.

Dialysis and transplantation
It is now possible for all children, no matter how small, to enter renal replacement therapy programmes when end-stage renal failure is reached. The optimum management is by renal transplantation. Technically this is difficult in very small children, but many centres choose 10 Kg as their lower limit. Kidneys donated by parents have a higher success rate than cadaveric donor kidneys, which are matched as far as possible to the recipient's HLA type. Patient survival is high and first-year graft survival is around 80%, although technical difficulties reduce this rate in very young recipients and with small donor kidneys. Graft losses from both acute and chronic rejection or recurrent disease mean that the five-year graft survival is reduced to 70% and some children need retransplantation. Current immunosuppression is with combinations of prednisolone, azathioprine and cyclosporin.

Ideally a child is transplanted before dialysis is required, but if this is not possible a period of dialysis may be necessary. Peritoneal dialysis, either by cycling overnight by machine (continuous cycling peritoneal dialysis) or by manual exchanges over 24 hours (continuous ambulatory peritoneal dialysis) is preferable to haemodialysis as it can be done by the parents at home and is therefore less disruptive to the family's life and the child's schooling.

Fig. 15.30 Causes of chronic renal failure	
Structural malformations	40%
Glomerulonephritis	25%
Hereditary nephropathies	20%
Systemic diseases	10%
Miscellaneous/unknown	5%

FURTHER READING
Edelmann CM Jr, (ed.) *Pediatric Kidney Disease*. Little, Brown, London, 1992. A comprehensive textbook.

Holliday MA, Barratt TM, Avner ED. *Pediatric Nephrology*. Williams & Wilkins, Baltimore, 1994. A comprehensive textbook.

Postlethwaite RJ. *Clinical Paediatric Nephrology*. 2nd edn. Butterworth-Heinemann. Oxford. 1994. Short textbook.

Smellie JM et al. Controversy in the investigation of urinary tract infection in children. *Arch Dis Child*. 1995; **72**: 247–259. Review articles.

Woolf AS, Wingard PJD. Unravelling the pathogenesis of cystic kidney diseases. *Arch Dis Child*. 1995;**72**:103–6. Review article.

CHAPTER 16

Genitalia

•Inguinoscrotal disorders • Abnormalities of the penis • Common genital disorders in female children

Most abnormalities of the genitalia in male infants are due to abnormal embryogenesis:

- failure of the testis to descend through the inguinal canal into the scrotum results in an undescended testis
- persistence of the processus vaginalis (Fig. 16.1a–e) results in an inguinal hernia, hydrocele or hydrocele of the cord
- incomplete development of the urethra results in hypospadias.

Inguinoscrotal disorders

UNDESCENDED TESTIS

At birth 2% of male infants have bilateral and 3% unilateral undescended testes. The incidence is high in preterm infants as testicular descent through the inguinal canal occurs only in the third trimester. By 3 months of age the overall rate for all male infants is 1.5%, with little change thereafter.

Classification

Retractile

The testis can be brought into the base of the scrotum with-out tension, but rapidly retracts into the inguinal region. No treatment is required. If tension is necessary to bring the testis to the base of the scrotum, a patent processus vaginalis may be present. Follow-up is indicated as occasionally the testis subsequently ascends into the inguinal canal.

Palpable

The testis can be palpated, usually in the region of the inguinal canal, but cannot be manoeuvred into the scrotum. Occasionally, testes are ectopic, when they lie outside the normal line of descent of the testis.

Impalpable

No testis can be felt on careful examination. The testis may be absent, intra-abdominal or inguinal.

Examination

Should be carried out in a warm room, with warm hands and a relaxed child. Palpate with one hand just medial to the anterior superior iliac spine and gently milk the contents of the inguinal canal towards the scrotum. Only when this hand reaches the pubic tubercle should the other hand be used to palpate the scrotum.

Investigation

Management can usually be determined following clinical examination.

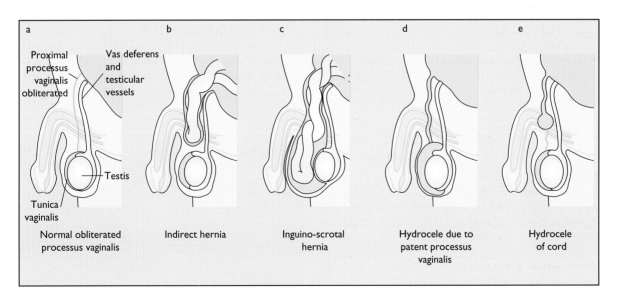

Fig. 16.1 (a) The normal testis. Following normal testicular descent, the processus vaginalis, an evagination of the parietal peritoneum between the internal inguinal ring and testis, disappears leaving only the tunica vaginalis around the testis. Persistence of the processus vaginalis results in an inguinal hernia (b,c), a hydrocele (d) or hydrocele of the cord (e).

Investigations which may be helpful are:
- ultrasound – this has a role in identifying testes in the inguinal canal in obese boys
- hormonal – for bilateral impalpable testes, the presence of testicular tissue can be confirmed using intramuscular human chorionic gonadotrophin (HCG) by showing a rise in serum testosterone level
- laparoscopy – the investigation of choice for the impalpable testis to determine if it is intra-abdominal or absent.

Management
Indications for treatment are:
- fertility – for optimal fertility, the testis should be 1°C below body temperature. Undescended testes are best corrected before two years of age to optimise fertility
- malignancy – there is an increased risk of malignancy in an undescended testis, but its magnitude is uncertain. The highest risk is for testes which are still intra-abdominal at puberty, when it may be as high as 10%. The risk is greater with bilateral than unilateral undescended testes. Early orchidopexy of a unilaterally undescended testis is thought to reduce the risk to be nearly the same as a normally descended testis, but this remains unproven
- cosmetic and psychological – if one testis proves to be absent, a prosthesis is possible, but insertion is best delayed until the adult size of the solitary testis is known.

Most children with an undescended testis are treated by orchidopexy, when the testis is mobilised and the patent processus vaginalis closed via an inguinal incision, and the testis is secured in the scrotal pouch via a scrotal incision. It should be performed at 1–2 years of age, usually as a day-case procedure. Other forms of treatment are:
- hormone therapy – intramuscular HCG or intranasal luteinising hormone releasing factor (LHRF) is given in some centres to promote testicular descent, but it is uncommon for it to prevent the need for surgery
- orchidectomy – the treatment of choice for unilateral intra-abdominal testes which cannot be corrected by simple orchidopexy, because of the increased risk of malignancy
- microvascular orchidopexy or staged orchidopexy – to preserve the testis in the rare occurrence of bilateral intra-abdominal testes, when the testicular vessels are too short to allow a single-stage procedure.

INGUINAL HERNIA
Inguinal hernias (see Fig. 16.1b,c) in children are invariably indirect and due to a patent processus vaginalis. Hernias are more frequent in preterm infants, in boys than girls and on the right side rather than left.

Inguinal hernias usually present as an intermittent swelling in the groin or scrotum on crying or straining (Fig.16.2). Unless the hernia is observed whilst the child coughs or cries, the diagnosis may depend upon the history and the identification of thickening of the spermatic cord (round ligament in girls). The groin swelling may become visible on raising the intra-abdominal pressure by gently pressing on the abdomen.

About 30% of hernias in infants under two years of age present as an irreducible lump in the inguinal region or scrotum. The lump is firm, immobile and tender and it is impossible to identify the spermatic cord above the swelling. Ninety-five per cent of 'irreducible' hernias can be reduced following analgesia with an opioid and/or gentle compression for up to about five minutes. If reduction is impossible, surgery is required urgently, because of the risk of strangulation of both bowel and testis. If complete reduction is achieved, surgery is delayed for 24–48 hours to allow resolution of oedema. Treatment is surgical, with dividing and closing the processus vaginalis. This differs from adults in whom hernias require repair of a muscular defect of the inguinal canal.

 All hernias in infants should be repaired promptly.

HYDROCELE
Hydroceles (see Fig. 16.1d) are often present at birth. They are firm or fluctuant, non-tender and transilluminate. The majority resolve spontaneously but surgery may be required in older children. Hydroceles of the cord (see Fig. 16.1e) present as unchanging, non-tender lumps associated with the spermatic cord.

VARICOCELE
Varicoceles are varicosities of the testicular veins and may occur in boys around puberty. They are almost invariably on the left side. Treatment aims to optimise fertility and consists of obliteration of the testicular vein by surgery, laparoscopy or radiological embolisation.

THE ACUTE SCROTUM
The causes of an acutely painful, swollen scrotum are listed in Figure 16.3. Torsion of the testis must be relieved within about six hours of the onset of symptoms for the testis to remain viable. Surgical exploration is required unless torsion can be excluded confidently. Fixation of the contralateral testis is usually performed at the same time.

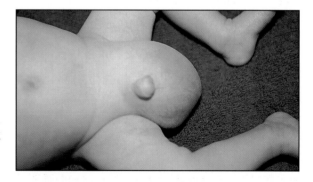

Fig. 16.2 Bilateral inguinal hernias in a preterm infant.

Fig. 16.3 Causes and clinical features of the acute swollen scrotum		
Cause	**Peak age**	**Clinical features**
Hernia (irreducible)	< 2 years	Immobile, firm. Tender and inflamed if strangulating
Hydrocele, acute presentation	1–3 years	Mobile, blue appearance, transilluminates
Torsion of testis	Neonate (uncommon)	Hard, tender testis
	Puberty	Red scrotum. Testis and spermatic cord firm and exquisitely tender
Torsion of appendage of testis	4–8 years	Scrotum swollen but not red
		Tender upper pole of testis – a 'blue spot' on transillumination
Acute idiopathic scrotal oedema	4–8 years	Erythema beyond scrotum, minimal tenderness of the testis
Epididymitis	Rare before puberty	Tender epididymis
		Requires urological investigation as associated with reflux of infected urine via vas deferens

Doppler ultrasound may allow the differentiation of torsion of the testis from epididymitis but must not delay surgery. Torsion in the neonate usually occurs before birth and the testis is usually non-viable.

 Torsion of the testis requires immediate surgery.

Abnormalities of the penis

HYPOSPADIAS

Hypospadias consists of:
- a hooded prepuce – the prepuce is formed only dorsally
- a ventral urethral meatus – in the majority of cases the urethra opens adjacent to the glans penis, but in severe cases the opening may be on the penile shaft or in the perineum (Fig. 16.4)
- chordee – a ventral curvature of the shaft of the penis, most apparent on erection. It is only present in the more severe forms of the anomaly.

Some degree of hypospadias occurs in approximately 3 per 1000 male infants.

Surgery

Correction is usually undertaken before two years of age. The aims of surgery are to produce:
- a terminal urethral meatus so that the boy can stand to micturate
- a straight erection.

It is essential that the foreskin is preserved, because it may be required for surgical correction of hypospadias.

 Infants with hypospadias must not be circumcised.

CIRCUMCISION

At birth, the foreskin is adherent to the surface of the glans penis. These adhesions separate spontaneously with time, allowing the foreskin to become more mobile and eventually retractile. Whereas, at six years of age, approximately 8% of boys have a non-retractile foreskin and 63% have preputial adhesions, by 16 years this has declined to only 1% and 3% respectively. Forcible retraction of healthy non-retractile foreskins and other manipulations for preputial adhesions should be avoided.

Indications

Circumcision is one of the most common operations performed on children. Most are performed for religious reasons or because parents believe it to be hygienic, to avoid the possibility of the operation when the child is older and to further reduce the already low risk of cancer of the penis. There are relatively few medical indications.

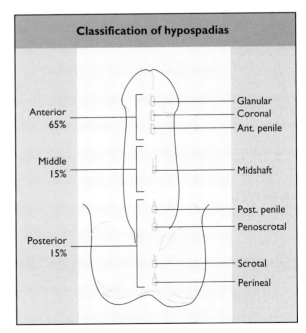

Fig. 16.4 Location of the urethral meatus in hypospadias.

1. Phimosis

Unfortunately, this term, which means muzzling, is used to describe several conditions:

- an asymptomatic, normal but non-retractile prepuce, when no action is required
- a non-retractile foreskin scarred by repeated, ill-advised attempts at retraction, when circumcision is required
- lichen sclerosis (*balanitis xerotica obliterans*, BXO) when the tip of the prepuce becomes thickened, white and fixed to the glans, often in a previously retractile foreskin. There is dysuria, soreness, poor urinary stream and bleeding. It is uncommon before five years of age. Circumcision is required, often with meatal dilatation.

2. Recurrent balanitis

There is infection under the prepuce, with inflammation and oedema, often associated with a white discharge of liquefied smegma. Treatment is with broad-spectrum antibiotics and regular baths. A single episode of balanitis often dissolves preputial adhesions, allowing the foreskin to become more retractile. Circumcision is only indicated if the balanitis is recurrent.

3. Ballooning of the prepuce

This causes concern to parents, but little to the child. It usually resolves spontaneously as the prepuce becomes more retractile.

4. Recurrent urinary tract infections

There is some evidence that the incidence of urinary tract infections (UTI) is lower in circumcised than uncircumcised boys. Circumcision may be appropriate in boys with recurrent UTI, especially if there is an associated urinary tract anomaly or established renal damage.

Surgery

Circumcision during the neonatal period is often performed on postnatal wards or at the baby's home. Unfortunately, it is not uncommon for the baby to receive little or no analgesia. Circumcision for medical indications should be performed under a general anaesthetic. While the child is anaesthetised, a local anaesthetic block can be given to reduce postoperative pain. This can be supplemented with oral analgesics given regularly for at least 48 hours. There is a general misconception that circumcision is a trivial procedure with minimal morbidity. Healing can take up to 10 days, with discomfort for several days. Damage to the glans, bleeding and infection are well-recognised complications.

PARAPHIMOSIS

The glans becomes engorged when a tight foreskin has been retracted proximal to the glans and cannot be pulled distally. The foreskin can usually be reduced following prolonged, gentle compression, with analgesia. Occasionally a general anaesthetic may be required and emergency circumcision or a dorsal slit may be appropriate. Following reduction of a paraphimosis, the prepuce will usually become retractile, so subsequent circumcision is rarely required.

Common genital disorders in female children

INGUINAL HERNIAS

These are less common than in boys. Sometimes the ovary herniates and can be difficult to reduce. Rarely, androgen insensitivity syndrome can present as a hernia in a phenotypical female who has a male genotype.

HYDROCELE

Hydroceles in the inguinal canal may be indistinguishable from an irreducible hernia and require surgery.

LABIAL ADHESIONS

These may give the appearance of absence of the vagina, except there is a characteristic translucent midline raphe partially or totally occluding the vaginal opening. Urine flow is rarely affected. Treatment with an oestrogen cream usually dissolves the adhesions. The cream should be applied sparingly and for a brief course to limit absorption. Active separation of the adhesions under anaesthesia is sometimes required.

VULVOVAGINITIS/VAGINAL DISCHARGE IN YOUNG GIRLS

Vulvovaginitis and vaginal discharge are not uncommon in young girls. They may result from poor hygiene, tight clothing such as leotards and inappropriate wiping after defaecation. It may result from bacterial or fungal infection. Obesity often contributes to the problem. Vulvovaginitis may be associated with threadworm infection. Parents should be advised about hygiene, the avoidance of bubble bath and scented soaps and the use of loose fitting cotton underwear. In some instances it results from sexual abuse, when swabs should be taken to identify any pathogens. Topical treatment of vulvovaginitis with an antifungal cream, which may be combined with a hydrocortisone cream and an antibiotic or antiseptic, may be helpful. Systemic antibiotics may be required for secondary infection. Oestrogen cream applied sparingly to the vulva, may relieve the problem in resistant cases by increasing vaginal resistance to infection. If these measures fail, an examination under anaesthesia may be needed to exclude a vaginal foreign body.

FURTHER READING

Ashcraft K W, Holder T M (eds). *Paediatric Surgery* 2nd ed, WB Saunders, Philadelphia 1993. Comprehensive textbook

MacMahon R A (ed). *An Aid to Paediatric Surgery*. Churchill Livingstone, Melbourne 1991. Short textbook.

Oster J. Further fate of the foreskin. *Archives of Disease in Childhood* 1968; 43: 200–203. Classic review article.

CHAPTER 17

Liver Disorders

• *Neonatal liver disease* • *Viral hepatitis* • *Acute liver failure* • *Chronic liver disease* • *Cirrhosis and portal hypertension* • *Management of children with liver disease* • *Liver transplantation*

In children:
- persistent neonatal jaundice is the most common presentation of liver disease in the neonatal period
- the earlier in life biliary atresia is diagnosed and treated surgically, the better the prognosis
- the transmission of hepatitis B surface antigen from mother to baby can usually be prevented by a course of hepatitis B immunisation started at birth
- chronic liver disease leads to multi-organ failure (Fig. 17.1), growth failure and developmental delay which is reversible by liver transplantation
- chronic liver disease, cirrhosis and portal hypertension should be treated in tertiary or national centres.

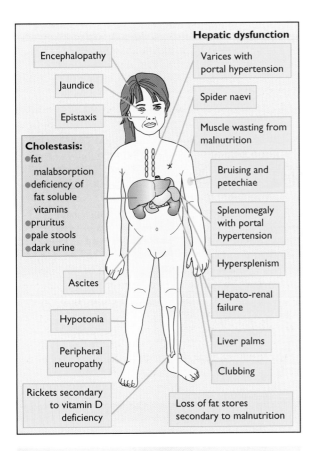

Fig 17.1 *Clinical features of liver disease. In addition, these children may have growth failure and developmental delay.*

Neonatal liver disease

Most newborn infants become clinically jaundiced. About 15% are still jaundiced at more than two weeks of age, when it is called persistent neonatal jaundice. This is usually an unconjugated hyperbilirubinaemia, which resolves shortly afterwards (Fig. 17.2) Persistent neonatal jaundice caused by liver disease is a conjugated hyperbilirubinaemia and is usually accompanied by:
- pale stools
- dark urine
- bleeding tendency
- failure to thrive.

The urgency to diagnose liver disease in the neonatal period as soon as possible is that early diagnosis and management improves the prognosis.

 Persistent neonatal jaundice- is it from liver disease?

Fig 17.2 *Causes of persistent neonatal jaundice*

Unconjugated
Physiological or breast-milk jaundice
Infection (particularly urinary tract)
Hypothyroidism
Haemolytic anaemia, e.g. G6PD deficiency
High gastrointestinal obstruction
Crigler–Najjar syndrome

Conjugated (>20% of total bilirubin)
1. Bile duct obstruction
    Biliary atresia
    Choledochal cyst
    Intrahepatic biliary hypoplasia
2. Neonatal hepatitis
    Congenital infection
    Inborn errors of metabolism
        α_1-antitrypsin deficiency
        Galactosaemia
        Tyrosinaemia
        Cystic fibrosis
        Lipid and glycogen storage disorders
        Peroxisomal disorders
    Total parenteral nutrition (TPN) cholestasis

Case history

BILIARY ATRESIA

This term infant was given oral vitamin K shortly after birth. He was breast-fed. He became mildly jaundiced on the third day of life. At five weeks of age he presented with poor feeding and vomiting and a history of a nose bleed and bruising on his forehead and shoulders. His urine had become dark and stools pale intermittently. He was pale, jaundiced, had several bruises and hepatomegaly. Investigations showed:

- Hb 8.8 g/l
- Platelets 465×10^9/l
- Prothrombin time – grossly prolonged
- Bilirubin 178 micromol/l – 80% conjugated.

The investigation of conjugated hyperbilirubinaemia is shown in Figure 17.3. The TEBIDA radionulide scan showed no excretion at 24 hours (Fig. 17.4) and a liver biopsy suggested biliary atresia (Fig. 17.5). A hepatoportoenterostomy was performed at 6 weeks of age (Fig. 17.6).

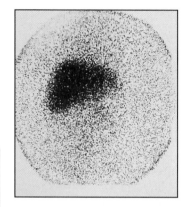

Fig 17.4 Radio-isotope scans (TEBIDA) of liver showing good hepatic uptake of isotope and no excretion into bowel. This scan suggests extrahepatic biliary obstruction or atresia or severe intrahepatic cholestasis.

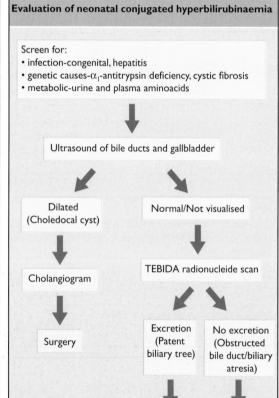

Evaluation of neonatal conjugated hyperbilirubinaemia

Screen for:
- infection-congenital, hepatitis
- genetic causes-α_1-antitrypsin deficiency, cystic fibrosis
- metabolic-urine and plasma aminoacids

↓

Ultrasound of bile ducts and gallbladder

Dilated (Choledocal cyst) → Normal/Not visualised

Dilated (Choledocal cyst) → Cholangiogram → Surgery

Normal/Not visualised → TEBIDA radionucleide scan → Excretion (Patent biliary tree) → Liver biopsy

TEBIDA radionucleide scan → No excretion (Obstructed bile duct/biliary atresia) → Liver biopsy Laparotomy

Fig 17.3 Evaluation of neonatal conjugated hyperbilirubinaemia

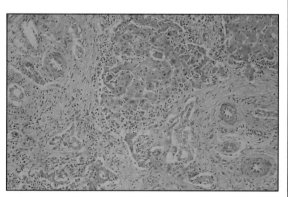

Fig 17.5 Liver biopsy of biliary atresia showing bands of fibrous tissue with bile duct proliferation.

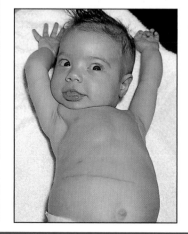

Fig 17.6 Shortly after successful bile drainage by hepatoporto-enterostomy (Kasai procedure) for biliary atresia. The infant is still jaundiced.

BILE DUCT OBSTRUCTION
Biliary atresia

Occurs in 1 in 14000 live births. There is destruction or absence of the extrahepatic biliary tree. It is a progressive disease, involving the intrahepatic biliary ducts, leading to chronic liver failure and death unless surgical intervention is performed. Babies with biliary atresia have a normal birthweight but fail to thrive as the disease progresses. Jaundice persists from the second day onwards with pale stools and dark urine, but both jaundice and stool colour may fluctuate. Hepatomegaly is present and splenomegaly develops secondary to portal hypertension and cirrhosis.

Standard liver function tests are of little value in the differential diagnosis. Abdominal ultrasound may be normal, or the gallbladder is either contracted or not seen. A fasting TEBIDA (iminodiacetic acid derivatives) radioisotope is taken up by the liver, but not excreted into the bowel. Liver biopsy demonstrates features of extrahepatic biliary obstruction, i.e. fibrosis and proliferation of bile ductules, although these may be features of neonatal hepatitis. The diagnosis is confirmed at laparotomy by operative cholangiography, which fails to outline a normal biliary tree.

Treatment consists of surgical bypass of the fibrotic ducts – hepatoportoenterostomy (Kasai procedure) – in which the jejunum is anastomosed to patent ducts in the cut surface of the porta hepatis. If surgery is performed before the age of 60 days, 80% of children will achieve bile drainage. The success rate diminishes with increasing age, hence the need for early diagnosis and treatment. Postoperative complications include cholangitis and fat malabsorption. Even when bile drainage is successful there is progression to cirrhosis and portal hypertension. If the operation is unsuccessful liver transplantation has to be considered without delay.

Choledochal cysts

These are cystic dilatations of the extrahepatic biliary system. About 25% present in infancy with cholestasis. In the older age group, choledochal cysts present with abdominal pain, a palpable mass and jaundice or cholangitis. The diagnosis is established by ultrasound or radionucleide scanning. Treatment is by surgical excision of the cyst with the formation of a roux-en-Y anastomosis to the biliary duct. Future complications include cholangitis and a 2% risk of malignancy which may develop in any part of the biliary tree.

NEONATAL HEPATITIS

Neonatal hepatitis implies hepatic inflammation from many different aetiologies. Causes are listed in Figure 17.2, but in many babies no cause is identified. In contrast to biliary atresia, these infants may have intrauterine growth retardation and hepatosplenomegaly at birth. Liver biopsy (Fig. 17.7) may be non-specific.

Alpha-1-antitrypsin deficiency

Deficiency of the protease alpha-1-antitrypsin is associated with emphysema in adults and with liver disease in infancy and childhood. It is inherited as an autosomal recessive disorder with an incidence of 1 in 2000–4000 in the UK. There are 26 phenotypes of the protease inhibitor (Pi) which are coded on chromosome 14. Liver disease is associated with the phenotype PiZZ. The defect is in the structure of the enzyme which cannot be secreted by the Golgi apparatus and is stored in the endoplasmic reticulum of the cell.

The majority of babies present with persistent neonatal jaundice, but some develop bleeding, including intracranial haemorrhage, from vitamin K deficiency. Hepatomegaly is present. Splenomegaly develops with cirrhosis and portal hypertension. The diagnosis is confirmed by estimating the level of alpha-1-antitrypsin in the plasma and identifying the phenotype. Approximately 30% of children will recover, 60% will develop cirrhosis and portal hypertension, some of whom will require liver transplantation.

There is as yet no explanation for the heterogeneous presentation or the varying prognosis, although factors such as breast-feeding may be important. Pulmonary disease is not significant in childhood. The disorder can be diagnosed antenatally.

Galactosaemia

This very rare disorder has an incidence of 1 in 40000. The infants develop poor feeding, vomiting, jaundice and hepatomegaly when fed milk. Chronic liver failure, cataracts and developmental delay are inevitable if galactosaemia is untreated. A rapidly fatal course with shock, haemorrhage and disseminated intravascular coagulation may occur.

The condition can be screened for in persistent jaundice by detecting galactose, a reducing substance, in the urine. The diagnosis is made by measuring the enzyme galactose-1-phosphate-uridyl transferase in red cells. A galactose-free diet prevents progression of liver disease.

Other causes

Neonatal hepatitis may be caused by tyrosinaemia, cystic fibrosis, lipid and glycogen storage disorders, peroxisomal

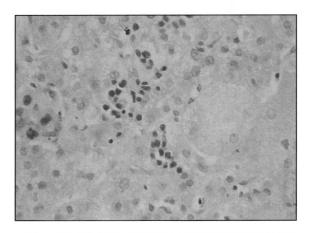

Fig 17.7 Liver biopsy in neonatal hepatitis showing inflammatory infiltrate throughout the liver, and giant cell and rosette formation of liver cells.

disorders, intrahepatic biliary hypoplasia or may be associated with parenteral nutrition.

Viral hepatitis

The clinical features of viral hepatitis include nausea, vomiting, abdominal pain, lethargy and jaundice. Thirty to fifty per cent of children do not develop jaundice. A large tender liver is common and 30% will have splenomegaly. The liver transferases are usually elevated tenfold. Coagulation is usually normal.

Hepatitis A
Hepatitis A virus (HAV) is an RNA virus which is spread by faecal–oral transmission. As socio-economic conditions improve, the incidence of hepatitis A in childhood is falling, and many adults will not be immune.

The disease may be asymptomatic, but the majority of children have a mild illness and recover both clinically and biochemically within 2–4 weeks. Some develop prolonged cholestatic hepatitis which is self-limiting, or fulminant hepatitis. Chronic liver disease does not occur

The diagnosis can be confirmed by detecting IgM antibody to the virus.

There is no treatment and no evidence that bed rest or diet is effective. Close contacts should be given prophylaxis with human normal immunoglobulin (HNIG) or vaccinated within two weeks of the onset of the illness.

Hepatitis B
Hepatitis B virus (HBV) is a DNA virus which is an important cause of acute and chronic liver disease worldwide, with the highest incidence and carrier rates in the Far East (15%) and the Mediterranean (5%). HBV is transmitted by:
- perinatal transmission from carrier mothers
- blood transfusions, needle stick injuries or biting insects
- renal dialysis
- lateral spread within families.

Children with HBV may be asymptomatic or have classical features of acute hepatitis. The majority will resolve spontaneously, but 1–2% develop fulminant hepatic failure, while 5-10% become chronic carriers. The diagnosis is made by detecting HBV antigens and antibodies. IgM antibodies to the core antigen (anti-HBc) are positive in acute infection. There is no treatment for acute HBV infection.

Chronic hepatitis B
Infants infected with HBV by vertical transmission from their mothers usually become asymptomatic carriers. Approximately 30–50% of carrier children will develop chronic HBV liver disease, which may progress to cirrhosis in 10%. There is a long-term risk of hepatocellular carcinoma (13% of cancers in children in Taiwan is HBV-related). Treatment for chronic HBV is controversial. Interferon treatment for chronic hepatitis B is successful in 50% of children infected horizontally and 30% of children infected perinatally.

Prevention
Prevention of HBV infection is important. All pregnant women should have antenatal screening for the hepatitis surface antigen (HBsAg). Babies of all HBsAg-positive mothers should receive a course of hepatitis B vaccination, with hepatitis B immunoglobulin also given if the mother is also hepatitis B e antigen (HBeAg) positive. Other members of the family should also be vaccinated.

Hepatitis C (non-A, non-B hepatitis)
Hepatitis C virus (HCV) is an RNA virus which was responsible for 90% of post-transfusion hepatitis until screening of donor blood was introduced. In the UK, about 1 in 2000 donors have HCV antibodies, but the prevalence is higher in southern Europe. The prevalence is high among intravenous drug users. Children at greatest risk are those who received unscreened blood or blood products, in particular those with haemoglobinopathies or haemophilia. Vertical transmission from infected mothers is rare unless there is co-infection with HIV. It seldom causes an acute infection, but at least 50% develop chronic liver disease, with cirrhosis and hepatocellular carcinoma after a number of years. Interferon treatment is being evaluated.

Hepatitis delta virus
Hepatitis delta virus (HDV) is a defective RNA virus which depends on hepatitis delta virus for replication. It occurs as a co-infection with hepatitis B virus or as a superinfection causing an acute exacerbation of chronic hepatitis B virus infection. Cirrhosis develops in 50–70% of those who develop chronic HDV infection.

Epstein–Barr virus
Children with Epstein–Barr virus (EBV) infection are usually asymptomatic. Forty per cent have hepatitis which may become fulminant. Less than 5% are jaundiced.

Acute liver failure

Acute liver failure in children is uncommon, but has a high mortality. The most common cause in childhood is viral hepatitis undefined or metabolic disease (Fig. 17.8). The child may present within hours or weeks with jaundice, encephalopathy, coagulopathy, hypoglycaemia and electrolyte disturbance. Early signs of encephalopathy include alternate periods of irritability and confusion with drowsiness. Older children may be aggressive and unusually difficult. Complications include encephalopathy, which may be associated with cerebral oedema, haemorrhage from gastritis or coagulopathy, sepsis and pancreatitis.

Diagnosis

Bilirubin may be normal in the early stages, particularly with metabolic disease. Transaminases are greatly elevated (10–100 × normal), alkaline phosphatase is increased, coagulation is very abnormal and plasma ammonia is elevated. It is essential to monitor the acid-base balance, blood glucose and coagulation times. An EEG will show acute hepatic encephalopathy and a CT scan may demonstrate cerebral oedema.

Management

This includes:

- maintaining the blood sugar (> 4 mmol/l) with intravenous dextrose
- preventing sepsis with broad-spectrum antibiotics
- preventing haemorrhage with intravenous vitamin K, fresh frozen plasma and H_2-blockers
- treating cerebral oedema by fluid restriction and mannitol diuresis.

A poor prognosis is likely when the liver begins to shrink in size, if there is a rising bilirubin with falling transaminases, an increasing coagulopathy or progression to coma. Without liver transplantation 70% of children who progress to coma will die.

REYE SYNDROME

Reye syndrome is an acute non-inflammatory encephalopathy of uncertain cause with microvesicular fatty infiltration of the liver. It must be differentiated from other causes of acute liver failure and from inborn errors of metabolism (fatty acid oxidation disorders).

A prodromal viral illness is followed 1–3 days later by vomiting, encephalopathy, hypoglycaemia and convulsions. Jaundice is absent and coagulation abnormalities are less than in fulminant hepatitis. The aetiology is unknown, but there has been a close association with aspirin therapy. Since 1986 the Committee on Safety of Medicines in the UK has advised that aspirin should not be given for febrile illness to children aged less than 12 years. Since then there has been a marked decline in the incidence of Reye syndrome.

The clinical presentation varies from acute hepatitis to the insidious development of hepatosplenomegaly, cirrhosis and portal hypertension with lethargy and malnutrition. The most common cause of chronic hepatitis is post-viral hepatitis (B, C or undefined), but Wilson disease should always be excluded. Histology may demonstrate chronic persistent hepatitis, when there is an inflammatory infiltrate in the liver confined to the portal tracts, or chronic active hepatitis when the inflammation has spread from the portal tract into the liver lobules.

AUTOIMMUNE CHRONIC ACTIVE HEPATITIS

The mean age of presentation is 7–10 years. It is more common in girls. It may present as an acute hepatitis, as fulminant hepatic failure or chronic liver disease with autoimmune features such as skin rash, lupus erythymatosus, arthritis, haemolytic anaemia or nephritis. Diagnosis is based on the presence of hypergammaglobulinaemia (IgG >20 g/l) and positive autoantibodies, smooth muscle antibodies (SMA), antinuclear antibodies (ANA), liver/kidney microsomal antibodies (LKM) and a low serum complement C4.

CYSTIC FIBROSIS

Overt liver disease (cirrhosis and portal hypertension) occurs in 20% of children by mid-adolescence. It may be secondary to abnormal bile acid concentration and/or biliary strictures. Attempts to detect early liver disease by ultrasound or radioisotope scanning have been unsuccessful. Histology includes fatty liver, focal nodular cirrhosis or secondary biliary cirrhosis. Standard supportive and nutritional therapy is required and liver transplantation may be considered for those with end-stage liver disease, either alone or in combination with a heart/lung transplant.

WILSON DISEASE

Wilson disease is an autosomal recessive disorder with an incidence of 1 per 200 000. There is an accumulation of copper in the liver, brain, kidney and cornea. The basic

---

Chronic liver disease

The causes of chronic liver disease are given in Figure 17.9.

Fig 17.8 Causes of acute liver failure in children

Infection	Viral hepatitis A, B, C, undefined
Poisons/drugs	Paracetamol, isoniazid, halothane, Amanita phalloides
Metabolic	Wilson disease, tyrosinaemia
Autoimmune hepatitis	
Reye syndrome	

Fig 17.9 Causes of chronic liver disease in children

Chronic hepatitis
  Post-viral hepatitis B, C, undefined
  Autoimmune hepatitis
  Drugs (nitrofurantoin, alpha-methyldopa)
  Inflammatory bowel disease
  Primary sclerosing cholangitis (± ulcerative colitis)
Wilson disease (>3 years)
Alpha-1-antitrypsin deficiency
Cystic fibrosis
Secondary to:
  Neonatal liver disease
  Bile duct lesions

genetic defect is a combination of reduced synthesis of caeruloplasmin (the copper-binding protein) and defective excretion of copper in the bile. Wilson disease has not been reported as presenting in children under the age of three years. A hepatic presentation is likely in children less than 12 years, who may present with almost any form of liver disease including acute hepatitis, fulminant hepatitis, cirrhosis and portal hypertension. Neurological features are common in the second decade and include deterioration in school performance, mood and behaviour change, and extrapyramidal signs such as incoordination, tremor and dysarthria. Renal tubular dysfunction, with vitamin D-resistant rickets, and haemolytic anaemia also occurs. Copper accumulation in the cornea (Kayser–Fleisher rings) are not seen before seven years of age.

The diagnosis is confirmed by detecting low serum caeruloplasmin, low serum copper, excess urine copper and increased hepatic copper.

Penicillamine reduces hepatic and central nervous system copper and is the drug of choice in combination with zinc to reduce copper absorption. Pyridoxine is given to prevent peripheral neuropathy. Neurological improvement may take up to 12 months of therapy. Thirty per cent of children with Wilson disease will die from hepatic complications if untreated. Liver transplantation is considered for children with acute liver failure or severe end-stage liver failure.

CONGENITAL HEPATIC FIBROSIS

Congenital hepatic fibrosis (CHF) presents in children over two years old with hepatosplenomegaly, abdominal distension and portal hypertension. Renal disease may co-exist. Congenital hepatic fibrosis differs from cirrhosis as liver function tests are always normal in the early stage. Liver histology shows large bands of hepatic fibrosis containing abnormal bile ductules. The consequent portal hypertension causes bleeding from varices.

Cirrhosis and portal hypertension

Cirrhosis is the end-stage of many forms of liver disease. It is defined pathologically as extensive fibrosis with regenerative nodules. It may be secondary to hepatocellular disease or to chronic bile duct obstruction (biliary cirrhosis). The main pathophysiological effects of cirrhosis are diminished hepatic function and portal hypertension with splenomegaly, varices and ascites (see Fig. 17.1). Hepatocellular carcinoma may develop.

Children with compensated cirrhosis may be asymptomatic if liver function is adequate. They will not be jaundiced and may have normal liver function tests. As the cirrhosis increases, however, the results of deteriorating liver function and portal hypertension are obvious (Fig. 17.10).

Physical signs include palmar and plantar erythema and spider naevi, malnutrition and hypotonia. The liver may be impalpable but dilated abdominal veins and splenomegaly suggest portal hypertension.

Investigations include:
- screening for the known causes of chronic liver disease (see Fig. 17.9)
- upper gastro-intestinal endoscopy to evaluate the presence of oesophageal varices and/or erosive gastritis
- abdominal ultrasound – may detect a shrunken liver and splenomegaly with gastric and oesophageal varices
- liver biopsy – may be difficult because of increased fibrosis but may indicate an aetiology (e.g. alpha-1-antitrypsin granules, copper storage).

As cirrhosis decompensates, biochemical tests may demonstrate an elevation of aminotransferases and alkaline phosphatase. The plasma albumin is low and the prothrombin time prolonged.

Oesophageal varices

Are an inevitable consequence of portal hypertension and may develop rapidly in children. They are best diagnosed by upper GI endoscopy as barium swallow may miss small varices. Acute bleeding is treated conservatively with blood transfusions and H_2-blockers (ranitidine, cimetidine). If bleeding persists, vasopressin analogues, sclerotherapy or endoscopic injection may be effective. Portacaval shunts may preclude liver transplantation and are not performed if transplantation is a future possibility.

Ascites (Fig. 17.11)

Is a major problem. The cause of ascites is uncertain, but contributory factors are hypoalbuminaemia, sodium retention, renal impairment and fluid redistribution. It is treated by sodium and fluid restriction and diuretics. Additional therapy for refractory ascites includes albumin infusions, paracentesis or peritoneovenous shunts.

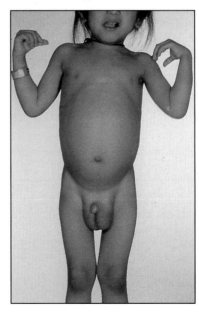

Fig 17.10 Cirrhosis and portal hypertension. This picture shows:
1. Malnutrition, with loss of fat and muscle bulk
2. Distended abdomen from hepatosplenomegaly and ascites
3. Scrotal swelling from ascites
4. No jaundice despite advanced liver disease.

Spontaneous bacterial peritonitis

Should always be considered if there is undiagnosed fever, abdominal pain, tenderness or an unexplained deterioration in hepatic or renal function. Diagnostic paracentesis should be performed and the fluid sent for white cell count and differential. Treatment is with broad-spectrum antibiotics.

Encephalopathy

Is precipitated by gastrointestinal haemorrhage, sepsis, sedatives, renal failure or electrolyte imbalance. It is difficult to diagnose in children as the level of consciousness may vary throughout the day. Infants present with irritability and sleepiness, while older children present with abnormalities in mood, sleep rhythm, intellectual performance and behaviour. Plasma ammonia may be elevated and an EEG is always abnormal.

Renal failure

May be secondary to renal tubular acidosis, acute tubular necrosis or functional renal failure.

Management of children with liver disease

The management of children with liver disease is essentially supportive, with the emphasis on correction of nutritional abnormalities, prevention of complications and intensive family support.

Nutrition

Malnutrition may be due to protein malnutrition, fat malabsorption, anorexia and fat-soluble vitamin deficiency (vitamins A, E, D and K).

Treatment is to provide a high-protein, high-carbohydrate diet with 50% more than the recommended dietary allowance. In children with cholestasis, medium-chain triglycerides, which are absorbed by the portal circulation, will provide fat, but 20% long-chain triglycerides are required to prevent essential fatty acid deficiency. Many children will require nasogastric tube feeding or parenteral nutrition (Fig. 17.12).

Fat-soluble vitamins

Vitamin A deficiency causes night blindness in adults and retinal changes in infants. It is easily prevented with oral vitamin A.

Vitamin E deficiency causes peripheral neuropathy, haemolysis and ataxia. It is very poorly absorbed in cholestatic conditions and high oral doses are required.

Vitamin D deficiency causes rickets and pathological fractures. It is prevented by using a water soluble form of vitamin D. Vitamin D resistant rickets indicates renal tubular acidosis.

Pruritis

Many children with cholestasis have severe pruritus. It is alleviated by phenobarbitone to stimulate bile flow, cholestyramine, which is a bile salt resin, or evening primrose oil (arachadonic acid) applied to the skin.

Encephalopathy

It is usually not necessary to treat encephalopathy in infants or young children. It may be managed by treating the precipitating factor (sepsis, gastrointestinal haemorrhage) or by protein restriction or oral lactulose, a nonabsorbable carbohydrate which reduces ammonia reabsorption by lowering colonic pH and increasing colonic transit.

Liver transplantation

Liver transplantation is accepted therapy for acute or chronic end-stage liver failure and has revolutionised the prognosis for these children. Transplantation for metabolic disease or hepatic malignancy is more controversial.

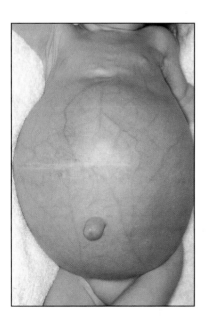

Fig 17.11 This infant has a grossly distended abdomen from ascites. There are dilated abdominal veins secondary to portal hypertension and an umbilical hernia from increased abdominal pressure. There is a surgical scar.

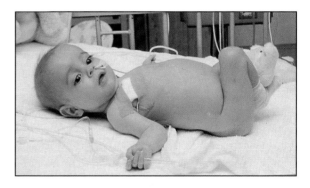

Fig 17.12 Many infants and children with liver disease need intensive nutritional supplementation. This malnourished infant is having both parenteral nutrition via a central line and continuous nasogastric feeding.

The indications for transplantation in chronic liver failure are:
- severe malnutrition unresponsive to intensive nutritional therapy
- recurrent complications (bleeding varices, resistant ascites)
- failure of growth and development
- poor quality of life.

Liver transplant evaluation includes assessment of the vascular anatomy of the liver and exclusion of irreversible disease in other systems. Absolute contraindications include untreatable cardiopulmonary disease or cerebrovascular disease.

Preparation of the family and child requires a great deal of counselling and support. The donor liver is selected to match the size and blood group of the recipient. There is coniderable difficulty in obtaining small organs for children, and many children receive part of an adult's liver, which is reduced to fit the child's abdomen (reduction hepatectomy). The complications are numerous and include:
- primary non-function of the transplanted liver (10%)
- hepatic artery thrombosis (10–20%), which is more common than in adults
- rejection (50–80%)
- sepsis, the main cause of death.

In large national centres, the overall one-year survival is approximately 90% with an overall five-year survival of 75%. Most deaths occur in the first three months. Children who survive the initial postoperative period usually do well. Long-term studies indicate normal psychosocial development and quality of life in survivors.

FURTHER READING

Booth IW Kelly DA. *Atlas of Paediatric Gastroenterology, Hepatology and Nutrition.* Times Mirror International Publishers, London, 1996.

Mowat AP. *Disease in Childhood*, 3rd ed. Butterworth-Heinemann, Oxford, 1994. Comprehensive textbook.

Tanner S. *Paediatric Hepatology.* Churchill Livingstone, Edinburgh, 1989. Textbook.

CHAPTER 18

Malignant Disease

• *Leukaemia* • *Lymphomas* • *Brain tumours* • *Neuroblastoma* • *Wilms tumour* • *Rhabdomyosarcoma*
• *Bone tumours* • *Retinoblastoma* • *Liver tumours* • *Germ cell tumours* • *Langerhans cell histiocytosis*

Cancer in children is not common:
• one child in 650 develops cancer by 15 years of age
• there are 120–140 new cases per million children aged <15 years per year, about 1400 in the UK.

The types of malignant disease (Fig. 18.1) are very different from those in adults, where carcinomas of the lung, breast, gut and skin predominate. The age at presentation varies with the differing types of disease:
• leukaemia affects children at all ages
• neuroblastoma and Wilms tumour are most frequent in the first five years of life
• Hodgkins disease and bone tumours have their peak incidence in adolescence and early adult life.

The survival rate for many tumours has increased dramatically (Fig. 18.2). Cancer used to be the second most common cause of death in children, after accidents. Now it ranks in fourth position. The overall five-year survival of children with malignant disease is over 60%, most of whom can be considered cured. This improved life expectancy can be attributed mainly to the introduction of multi-agent chemotherapy and specialist multidisciplinary care. For some children the price of survival is long-term medical or psychosocial difficulties.

 In children leukaemia is the most common malignancy followed by brain tumours.

Aetiology

In most cases the precise aetiology is unclear, but it is likely that most cancers involve structural change in the cell genome and an interaction between environmental factors (e.g. radiation, viruses) and host genetic susceptibility (e.g. gene mutation). The identification of abnormal oncogene expression in some tumours is additional evidence of the genetic influence in tumour formation. Several syndromes are associated with an increased risk of cancer in childhood, e.g. Down syndrome and leukaemia, neurofibromatosis and glioma. A few cancers show a clearly defined inheritance pattern, e.g. bilateral retinoblastoma which is associated with a deletion on chromosome 13. Modern genetic techniques show that many cancers demonstrate specific chromosomal alterations. Their identification may be of value in confirming uncertain diagnoses or providing information helpful in predicting outcome.

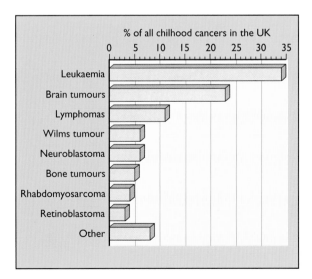

Fig. 18.1 *Relative frequency of different types of cancer in children.*

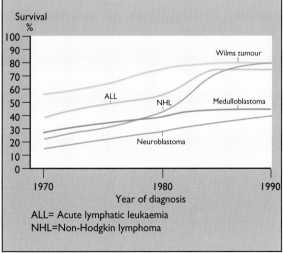

Fig. 18.2 *Five-year survival rates showing the considerable improvement over the last 20 years.*

Clinical presentation

Cancer presents with:

- a localised mass
- the consequences of disseminated disease, e.g. bone marrow infiltration systemic ill-health.

Investigations

In leukaemia the full blood count is usually abnormal but peripheral blast cells are not always present. Solid tumours are identified and localised on ultrasound, X-rays, CT and MR scans. Tumour marker studies are helpful for neuroblastoma when there is increased urinary catecholamine excretion (VMA, vanillyl mandelic acid) and for germ cell tumours and liver tumours in which there is alphafetoprotein (AFP) production. However, all diagnoses must be confirmed histologically either by biopsy or by bone marrow aspiration. This may not always be possible for brain tumours. The differentiation between some solid tumours may be difficult by standard microscopy, and further differentiation requires specialised pathology facilities such as immunohistochemistry and electron microscopy.

 All diagnoses must be confirmed histologically whenever possible.

Management

Once a tumour has been diagnosed, the parents and child need to be seen and the diagnosis explained to them in a realistic, positive way. Detailed staging to define the extent of the primary and to assess the presence of metastatic disease is essential to plan treatment. Considerable progress has been made in improving outcome by evaluating new treatment regimens through national and international collaborative studies.

Most children with cancer in the UK are treated in regional centres whose development has encouraged work by experienced multidisciplinary teams with facilities for the intensive medical and psychosocial support required. Subsequent management is often shared between the specialist centre, referral hospital and local services within the community to provide the optimum care with the least disruption to the family.

Treatment

Treatment may involve chemotherapy, surgery and radiotherapy.

Chemotherapy

Plays a more prominent role in childhood cancer than in adult disease. It is used:

- as primary curative treatment, e.g. in acute lymphoblastic leukaemia
- as adjuvant treatment to deal with residual disease and for actual or presumed micrometastases after initial local treatment with surgery, e.g. Wilms tumour
- to shrink bulky primary or metastatic disease before definitive local treatment with surgery and/or radiotherapy, e.g. sarcomas, neuroblastoma.

Radiotherapy

Retains a role in the treatment of some tumours, but the risk of damage to growth and function of normal tissue is greater in a child than in an adult. The adequate screening of sensitive normal tissues and careful positioning of the patient during treatment raises practical difficulties in children.

Surgery

Is increasingly restricted to primary biopsy for diagnosis and removal of any residual disease after chemotherapy and/or radiotherapy.

High-dose therapy with bone marrow rescue

The limitation of chemotherapy and radiotherapy is the risk of irreversible damage to normal tissues, particularly bone marrow. Bone marrow transplantation can be used as a strategy to treat patients after administering potentially lethal doses of chemotherapy and/or radiation. The source of the bone marrow may be allogeneic (from a compatible donor) or autologous (from the patient himself, harvested beforehand while the marrow is uninvolved or in remission). The use of peripheral blood stem cell harvesting may provide a more acceptable alternative to autologous bone marrow transplantation.

Side-effects of chemotherapy

Chemotherapy causes a range of side-effects (Fig. 18.3).

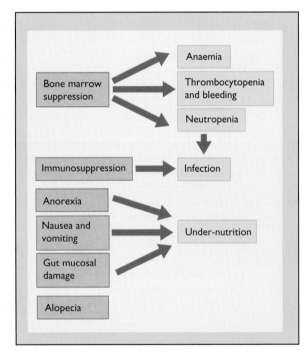

Fig. 18.3 Short-term side-effects of chemotherapy.

 Fever and neutropenia require hospital admission, cultures and intravenous antibiotics.

Infection from immunosuppression

Children receiving chemotherapy or wide-field radiation are immunocompromised. Chemotherapy induced neutropenia places children at risk of septicaemia. Children with fever and neutropenia must be admitted to hospital for cultures and broad spectrum antibiotics. Some important infections include *Pneumocystis carinii* pneumonia (especially in children with leukaemia) and disseminated fungal infection (e.g. aspergillosis and candidiasis) and coagulase negative staphylococcal infections of central venous catheters.

Most common viral infections are no worse in children with cancer than in other children, but measles and varicella/zoster may have atypical presentation and be life threatening. If non-immune, these children are at risk from contact with measles or varicella, although some protection can be afforded by prompt administration of immunoglobulin or zoster immune globulin. Acyclovir is used to treat established varicella infection but no treatment is available for measles. During the period of depressed immunity, throughout chemotherapy and from six months to a year subsequently, the use of live vaccines is contraindicated.

Bone marrow suppression

Anaemia may require blood transfusions. Thrombocytopenia presents the hazard of bleeding, and considerable blood product support may be required, particularly for children with leukaemia, those undergoing intensive therapy requiring bone marrow transplantation and the more intensive solid tumour protocols.

Gut mucosal damage

Gram-negative infections may be associated with chemotherapy-induced gut mucosal damage. Mouth ulcers are painful, often severe and can prevent the child eating adequately.

Other side-effects

Many individual drugs have very specific side-effects, for example cardiotoxicity with doxorubicin, renal failure and deafness with cisplatin, haemorrhagic cystitis with cyclophosphamide and neuropathy with vincristine. These require careful monitoring.

Supportive care

Cancer treatment produces frequent, predictable and often severe multisystem side-effects. Supportive care is an important part of management. This includes attention to infection, nutrition, nausea and vomiting. The discomfort of multiple venepunctures for blood sampling and intravenous infusions can be avoided with central venous catheters, although these do carry a risk of infection (Fig. 18.4).

Psychosocial support

The diagnosis of a potentially fatal illness has an enormous and long-lasting impact on the whole family. They need the opportunity to discuss the implications and their anxiety, fear, guilt and sadness. Most will benefit from the counselling and practical support provided by health professionals. Help with practical issues including transport, finances, accommodation and care of siblings are early priorities. The provision of detailed written material for parents will help them understand their child's disease and treatment. The children themselves and their siblings need an age-appropriate explanation of the disease. Once treatment is established and the disease appears to be under control, families should be encouraged to return to as normal a lifestyle as possible. Early return to school is important and children with cancer should not be allowed to underachieve the expectations previously held for them. It is easy to underestimate the severe stress that persists within families in relation to the uncertainty of the long-term outcome. This often manifests itself as marital problems in parents and behavioural difficulties in both the child and siblings.

Long-term survivors

It is estimated that by the end of this century 1 in 1000 young adults will be survivors of childhood cancer. Some will have residual problems as a consequence of the disease or its treatment (Fig. 18.5). All survivors need regular long-term follow-up to provide appropriate treatment or advice. Some will require specific counselling about poor growth, infertility and sexual dysfunction. The risk of second tumours is relatively small (<10%) but may rise with increasing survival rates. There is now a need to reduce, whenever possible, the toxicity of treatment to spare the children adverse short- and long-term effects.

Terminal care

When a child relapses, further treatment may be considered. A small number can still be cured and others may have a further significant remission with good quality life. However, for some children a time comes when death is inevitable and the staff and family must make the decision to concentrate on palliative care.

Most parents prefer to care for their terminally ill child at home but will need practical help and emotional

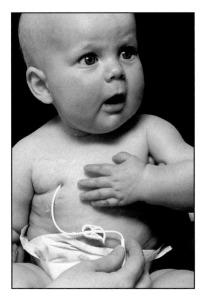

Fig. 18.4
The central venous catheter allows pain-free blood tests and injections for this child on chemotherapy, which has caused the alopecia.

18.5 Problems which may occur following cure of childhood cancer	
Problem	**Cause**
Specific organ dysfunction	Nephrectomy for Wilms tumour
	Toxicity from chemotherapy e.g. renal from cisplatin or ifosfamide, cardiac from doxorubicin or mediastinal radiotherapy
Growth/endocrine problems	Growth hormone deficiency from pituitary irradiation
	Bone growth retardation at sites of irradiation
Infertility	Gonadal irradiation
	Alkylating agent chemotherapy (cyclophosphamide, ifosfamide)
Neuropsychological problems	Cranial irradiation (particulary at age < 5yrs)
	Brain surgery
Second malignancy	Irradiation
	Alkylating agent chemotherapy
Social/educational disadvantage	Chronic ill health
	Absence from school

support. Pain control and symptom relief are a serious source of anxiety for parents but they can be achieved successfully at home. Health professionals with experience in palliative care for children can work with the family and local health care workers. After the child's death, families should be offered continuing contact with an appropriate member of the team who looked after their child, and given support through their bereavement.

Leukaemia

Acute lymphoblastic leukaemia (ALL) accounts for 80% of leukaemia in children. Most of the remainder are acute myeloid/acute non-lymphocytic (AML/ANLL) leukaemia. Chronic myeloid leukaemia and other myeloproliferative disorders are rare.

Clinical presentation
Clinical symptoms and signs result from infiltration of the bone marrow or other organs with leukaemic blast cells (Fig. 18.6).

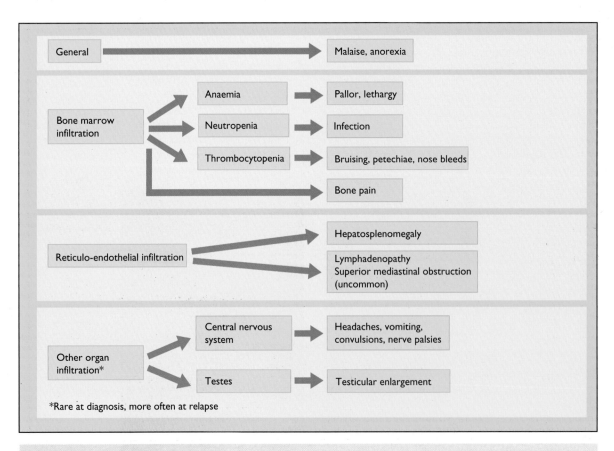

Fig. 18.6 Signs and symptoms of acute leukaemia.

In most children leukaemia presents insidiously over several weeks with some or all of:
- malaise
- infections
- pallor
- abnormal bruising
- hepatosplenomegaly
- lymphadenopathy
- bone pain.

In some children the illness progresses very rapidly.

In most but not all children the blood count is abnormal with low haemoglobin and thrombocytopenia and evidence of circulating blast cells. Bone marrow examination is essential to confirm the diagnosis and for immunological and cytogenetic information.

Both ALL and AML are classified by morphology. Immunological phenotyping further subclassifies ALL into common (75%), T cell (15%), null (10%) and B cell (1%). Prognosis and some aspects of clinical presentation vary according to different subtypes and treatment is adjusted accordingly.

The prognosis in ALL is related to tumour load. The single most significant indicator is the white cell count (WBC). A high WBC ($>50 \times 10^9$/l), bulky organomegaly, lymphadenopathy and central nervous system disease at diagnosis worsen prognosis. Boys do worse than girls and infants generally fair badly. Overall, at least 65% of patients with ALL are now expected to be cured. Although the outlook for AML was extremely poor, there has been some recent progress, but cure rates are still below 50%.

Treatment of acute lymphoblastic leukaemia
A typical treatment regimen is shown in **Figure 18.7**.
1. Remission induction
Preparation for treatment includes transfusion, treatment of infection and the use of adequate hydration and allopurinol to protect renal function against the effects of rapid cell lysis. Remission implies eradication of the leukaemic blasts and restoration of normal marrow function. Four weeks of combination chemotherapy is used and current induction schedules achieve remission rates of 95%.
2. Intensification
Subsequent blocks of intensive chemotherapy given to consolidate remission are of value despite the associated toxicity.
3. Central nervous system
Cytotoxic drugs penetrate poorly into the CNS. As leukaemic cells in this site may survive effective systemic treatment, additional treatment with intrathecal chemotherapy and cranial irradiation have been used to prevent CNS relapse. However,

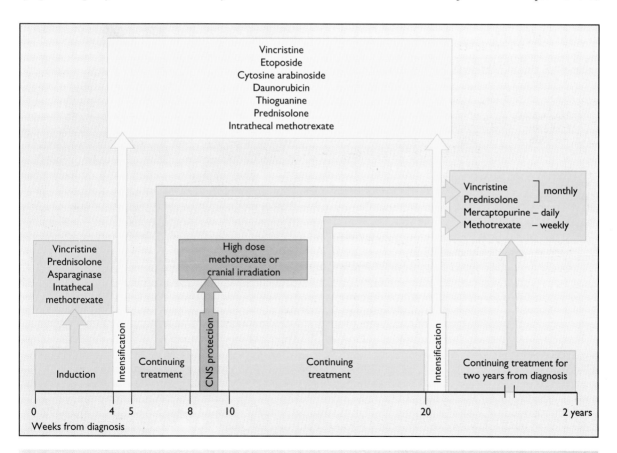

Fig. 18.7 Typical treatment regimen of acute lymphoblastic leukaemia.

these result in significant neuropsychological sequelae, especially in younger children, and alternative strategies using systemic chemotherapy with high-dose methotrexate are currently being evaluated.

4. Continuing therapy

Chemotherapy of modest intensity is continued over a relatively long period of time, usually two years from diagnosis. Cotrimoxazole is given routinely to prevent *Pneumocystis carinii* pneumonia.

Treatment of relapse

High-dose chemotherapy, usually with total body irradiation (TBI) and bone marrow transplantation, is used as an alternative to conventional chemotherapy after a relapse. In children with a very high risk of relapse (e.g. high WBC/ALL) it is introduced as primary treatment after initial induction chemotherapy.

Lymphomas

'Lymphoma can be divided into Hodgkin disease and non-Hodgkin lymphoma (NHL). NHL is more common in childhood, Hodgkin disease is seen more frequently in adolescence.

NON-HODGKIN LYMPHOMA

A firm distinction between solid and haematological lymphoid malignancy is somewhat artificial as some subtypes of ALL and NHL may represent a continuum of the same disease. In most cases of childhood NHL the clinical features and treatment reflect the immunological origin of the malignant cells involved (Fig. 18.9). T cell malignancy may present either as ALL or as NHL, both characterised by a mediastinal mass with a varying degree of bone marrow infiltration. B cell malignancies present more commonly as NHL.

HODGKIN DISEASE

This is relatively uncommon in prepubertal children. It usually presents as painless lymphadenopathy, most frequently in the neck. Lymph nodes are much larger and firmer than the benign lymphadenopathy commonly seen in children. The clinical history is often long, and systemic symptoms (sweating, pruritis, weight loss and fever – the so-called 'B' symptoms) are uncommon even in more advanced disease.

After diagnostic biopsy the disease is staged to determine treatment. Intra-abdominal disease is generally assessed radiologically, and staging laparotomy as formerly practised, with biopsies and splenectomy, is no longer performed in

---

Case history

ACUTE LYMPHOBLASTIC LEUKAEMIA

A four-year-old girl was generally unwell, feeling lethargic, looking pale and occasionally developing a fever over nine weeks. Two courses of antibiotics for recurrent sore throat failed to result in any benefit. Her parents returned to their general practitioner when she developed a rash. Examination showed pallor, petechiae, modest lymphadenopathy and mild hepatosplenomegaly. A full blood count showed:

Hb 8.3 g/dl
WBC 15.6×10^9/l
Platelets 44×10^9/l

Blast cells were seen on peripheral blood film. CSF examination was normal. Bone marrow examination confirmed acute lymphoblastic leukaemia (Fig. 18.8).

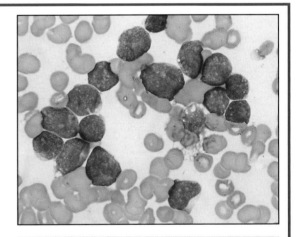

Fig. 18.8 Leukaemic blast cells on a bone marrow smear.

18.9 Principal presentation, treatment and prognosis for non-Hodgkin lymphoma

Site	Type	Treatment	Prognosis
Localised - often head and neck, e.g. cervical nodes, oropharynx	Usually of B-cell origin	Short, moderately intensive multi-agent chemotherapy	Good
Intrathoracic -anterior mediastinal mass -pleural effusion	Typical T-cell disease	As for ALL	Approaching that for ALL
Intra-abdominal disease -bulky gut or lymph node masses	Typical advanced B-cell disease	Very intensive mulitagent chemotherapy	Previously very poor; now much improved

the UK. Lymphangiography is a technically difficult examination in small children but may be useful occasionally. Combination chemotherapy (possibly with radiotherapy to sites of bulky disease) is the treatment for all except those with localised disease who receive radiotherapy alone. Overall, about 80% of all patients can be cured and the prognosis even for those with disseminated disease is about 60%.

Brain tumours

In contrast to adults, brain tumours in children are almost always primary and 60% are infratentorial. Signs and symptoms are usually of raised intracranial pressure:

- headache
- vomiting (especially mornings)
- papilloedema
- squint from VIth nerve palsy
- nystagmus
- ataxia
- personality or behaviour change.

The tumour is identified on CT or MR scan (Fig. 18.10). Lumbar puncture must not be performed in the presence of raised intracranial pressure without neurosurgical advice. Brain tumours present particular diagnostic difficulties as histological appearance may not be representative of tumour behaviour and biopsy is not always safe. The outcome of treatment is strongly influenced by the anatomical position of the tumour as well as the histological subtype (Fig. 18.11).

The implications of the tumour site, the hazard of surgery and the use of high-dose radiation all compound to place children with brain tumours at particular risk of growth, endocrine and neuropsychological problems. Survivors may present complex difficulties with varying combinations of physical disability, growth failure, sensory loss, seizures and educational problems.

Neuroblastoma

Neuroblastoma arises from neural crest tissue in the adrenal medulla and sympathetic nervous system. It is unusual in that it may regress spontaneously in very young infants, and the disease presents a spectrum of aggression from benign ganglioneuroma through ganglioneuroblastoma to malignant neuroblastoma.

It is most common before the age of five years. Most children present with an abdominal mass, but the primary can lie anywhere along the sympathetic chain from the neck to the pelvis. Classically the abdominal primary is of adrenal origin, but at presentation the tumour mass is often large and complex, crossing the midline and enveloping major blood vessels and lymph nodes (Fig. 18.12).

Paravertebral tumours may invade through the adjacent

Brain Tumours

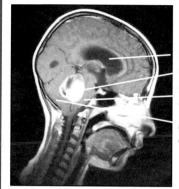

Dilated lateral ventricle

Cystic tumour mass

Invasion/compression of brain stem

Compressed cerebellar hemisphere

Fig. 18.10 Sagittal MR scan showing a medulloblastoma in the posterior fossa.

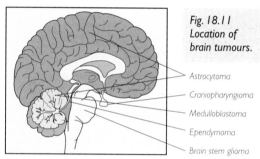

Fig. 18.11 Location of brain tumours.

Astrocytoma

Craniopharyngioma

Medulloblastoma

Ependymoma

Brain stem glioma

(a) Astrocytoma 40%. The most common brain tumour type. Juvenile cerebellar astrocytoma is cystic, often slowly growing, and the results of treatment with surgery are excellent. Non-juvenile astrocytoma occurs at all sites, but more frequently in the cerebral hemispheres. They vary from relatively benign to highly malignant (glioblastoma multiforme) and despite surgery and radiotherapy the outlook, particularly for children with high-grade tumours, is poor. The value of chemotherapy in the treatment of astrocytoma is not yet established but may be used more frequently in future.

(b) Medulloblastoma 20%. Nearly always arises in the midline of the posterior fossa. Presentation is with ataxia as well as headache and vomiting. The tumour may seed through the CNS via the CSF and up to 20% have spinal metastases at diagnosis. Treatment with whole CNS radiation after maximal surgical resection, has produced five-year survival rates of 50%. Chemotherapy has a place in the treatment of children with a higher than average risk of relapse, e.g. after incomplete surgical excision and those with intraspinal metastases.

(c) Ependymoma 8%. Mostly occurs in the posterior fossa where it behaves like medulloblastoma, but can also arise in the ventricles or spinal cord.

(d) Brain stem glioma 6%. Peak incidence is in early childhood. It presents with cranial nerve defects, ataxia and pyramidal tract signs but frequently without raised intracranial pressure. The diagnosis is often based on clinical findings and CT/MR scan, as biopsy can be hazardous. The prognosis for this group of children is particularly poor (<20% survival) and radiotherapy is usually only palliative. Chemotherapy has no established role.

(e) Craniopharyngioma 4%. A developmental tumour arising from the squamous remnant of Rathke's pouch. It is not truly malignant but is locally invasive and grows slowly in the suprasellar region. It presents with increased intracranial pressure, visual field loss and pituitary dysfunction, typically as growth failure. Surgical excision with or without subsequent radiation is required. Although prognosis for survival is good, these children may be visually impaired and often have complex endocrine deficiencies.

Fig. 18.12 Presentation of neuroblastoma	
Common	**Less common**
Pallor	Paraplegia
Weight loss	Cervical lymph-
Abdominal mass	adenopathy
Hepatomegaly	Proptosis
Bone pain	Periorbital bruising
Limp	Skin nodules

intervertebral foramen and cause spinal cord compression. Over the age of two years, clinical symptoms are mostly from metastatic disease, particularly bone pain, bone marrow suppression, weight loss and malaise (Fig. 18.12).

The diagnosis can often be made from characteristic clinical and radiological features (Fig. 18.13) and raised urinary catecholamine (VMA, HVA) levels. Confirmatory biopsy is usually obtained and evidence of metastatic disease detected with bone marrow sampling, bone scan and MIBG (metaiodobenzylguanidine) scan. MIBG is a radio-labelled tumour-specific agent, which provides a sensitive radioisotope scan to measure disease extent and monitor response to treatment (Fig. 18.14). Its therapeutic use is being explored.

The most important prognostic features are age and stage of disease at diagnosis. Unfortunately, the majority of children over one year present with advanced disease and have a poor prognosis. Increasingly, information about the biological characteristics of neuroblastoma is being used to guide therapy and prognosis. Over expression of the N-myc oncogene and evidence for deletion of material on chromosome 1 (del1p) in tumour cells are two examples associated with poorer prognosis.

The few children with localised primaries without metastatic disease can often be cured with surgery alone. For the majority with advanced disease, chemotherapy has the central role. Children showing a good initial response may benefit from consolidation with high-dose chemotherapy with autologous bone marrow rescue. Unfortunately the risk of relapse is high and the prospect for cure for children with metastatic disease is less than 30%

Screening for asymptomatic disease in infants during the first year of life is possible by detecting elevated urinary catecholamines. Most experience with this strategy has been in Japan, but its impact on overall survival remains to be established. It is possible that screening may identify some patients with spontaneously regressing disease but not detect all those who develop more aggressive disease at an older age.

Neuroblastoma

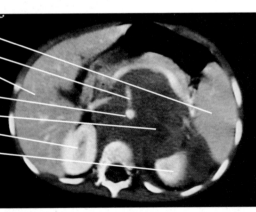

Displaced spleen
Coeliac axis
Liver
Aorta
Neuroblastoma tumour mass
Normal kidney
Displaced kidney

Fig. 18.13 A transverse CT scan of the abdomen showing a very large neuroblastoma tumour mass. Its intimate relationship with the great vessels makes it extremely difficult to resect surgically.

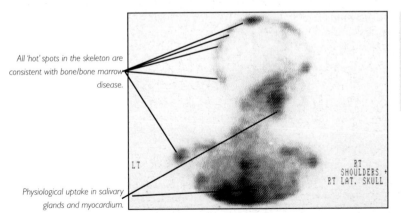

All 'hot' spots in the skeleton are consistent with bone/bone marrow disease.

Physiological uptake in salivary glands and myocardium.

LT

RT SHOULDERS + RT LAT. SKULL

Fig. 18.14 MIBG scan, a radio-labelled targeting agent specific for neuroblastoma, is used to monitor response to treatment.

Wilms tumour (nephroblastoma)

Wilms tumour originates from embryonal renal tissue. The region for the Wilms tumour susceptibility genes was identified from the rare association with sporadic aniridia and the recognition that this was associated with loss of genetic material from chromosome 11. Over 80% present before five years of age. It is very rarely seen after ten years of age. Most children present with a large abdominal mass, often found incidentally in an otherwise well child (Fig. 18.15). Occasionally, children have chronic symptoms of poor appetite and poor weight gain. Haemorrhage into the mass may cause abdominal pain and pallor. Macroscopic haematuria and hypertension are uncommon but important. About 5% have bilateral disease which is usually apparent at diagnosis.

Radiological diagnosis from ultrasound or CT (Fig. 18.16) is usually characteristic, showing an intrinsic renal mass distorting the normal structure. Information to assess distant metastases, usually in the lung, initial tumour resectability and function of the contralateral kidney is required. Primary nephrectomy is usually undertaken. Children with metastatic disease, those with very large tumours and with inferior vena cava involvement may benefit from initial chemotherapy followed by delayed nephrectomy. All children require chemotherapy but radiotherapy is restricted to those with more advanced disease.

Overall, the prognosis is good and more than 80% of all patients can be cured. The cure rate even for the patients (15%) with metastatic disease at presentation is over 60%, but salvage of children who relapse is generally not successful. Recent clinical trials have shown that it is possible to reduce the intensity of treatment for less advanced disease without compromising survival.

Fig. 18.15 Presentation of Wilms tumour	
Common	**Uncommon**
Abdominal mass	Abdominal pain
	Anorexia
	Haematuria
	Hypertension

Rhabdomyosarcoma

Rhabdomyosarcoma originates from primitive mesenchymal tissue. There are a wide variety of primary sites resulting in varying presentation and prognosis.

Head and neck sites

Are the most common, causing, for example, proptosis (Fig. 18.17), nasal obstruction and blood-stained nasal discharge.

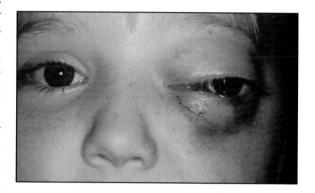

Fig. 18.17 Rhabdomyosarcoma causing proptosis.

Wilms tumour

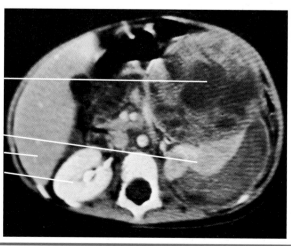

Huge tumour, showing the characteristic mixed tissue densities (cystic and solid). It arises within the kidney and envelopes a remnant of normal renal tissue.

Remnant of left kidney

Liver

Normal kidney

Fig. 18.16 Huge Wilms tumour arising within the left kidney showing characteristic cystic and solid tissue densities.

Genitourinary tumours

The next most common, cause dysuria and urinary and obstruction or blood-stained vaginal discharge.

Metastatic disease (lung, liver, bone or bone marrow)

Present in approximately 15% of patients at diagnosis and is associated with a particularly poor prognosis.

Treatment depends on the site, size and extent of disease. Staging investigations must provide a comprehensive assessment of these factors. The minority (15%) of patients with completely resected local disease require only a short course of chemotherapy to treat presumed micrometastatic disease, and no radiotherapy. The tumour margins are always deceptively ill-defined, and attempts at primary surgical excision are often unsuccessful and should be discouraged unless this can be achieved without mutilation or irreversible organ damage. The majority of patients, require aggressive combination chemotherapy and often radiotherapy.

Bone tumours

Malignant bone tumours are uncommon before puberty. Osteogenic sarcoma is more common than Ewing sarcoma, but Ewing sarcoma is seen more often in younger children. Both have a male predominance.

Limbs are the most common site. Persistent localised bone pain is a characteristic symptom, usually preceding the detection of a mass. At diagnosis most patients are well and even metastatic disease (most common in the lungs) is asymptomatic. A bone X-ray shows destruction and variable periosteal new bone formation. In Ewing sarcoma there is often a substantial soft tissue mass. Initial evaluation must include careful assessment of the primary site to define the extent of the local disease, particularly if limb salvage surgery is contemplated.

Both tumours are difficult to treat, but the prognosis has improved in recent years. In both tumours, treatment involves the use of combination chemotherapy given before surgery. There is increasing experience in avoiding amputation by using en-bloc resection of tumours with endoprosthetic resection (Fig. 18.18). In Ewing sarcoma, radiotherapy has a place in the management of local disease, especially when surgical resection is impossible or incomplete, for example in the pelvis or axial skeleton.

Retinoblastoma

Although very rare, retinoblastoma accounts for about 5% of severe visual impairment in children. It may affect one or both eyes. All bilateral tumours are thought to be hereditary, as are about 20% of unilateral cases. The retinoblastoma susceptibility gene has now been identi-

fied on chromosome 13. The pattern of inheritance is dominant but with incomplete penetrance. Most cases present within the first three years of life. Children from families with the hereditary form of the disease should be screened regularly from birth. The two most common presentations of unsuspected disease are when a white pupillary reflex is noted to replace the normal red one or with a squint (Fig. 18.19).

The aim of treatment is to cure yet preserve vision. Enucleation of the eye may be necessary for more advanced disease but treatment with radiation or, more rarely, local photocoagulation may be successful for small tumours. The role of chemotherapy is uncertain. Most

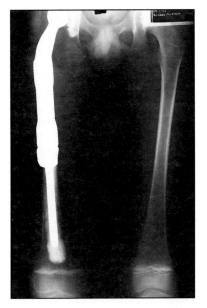

Fig. 18.18 To preserve the leg, an endo-prosthetic replacement of the proximal femur has been performed in a boy with Ewing sarcoma. The prosthesis can be extended for growth.

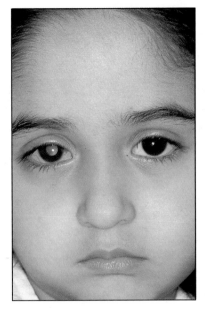

Fig. 18.19 White pupillary reflex in retinoblastoma.

patients are cured although many are visually impaired. There is a significant risk of second malignancy (especially osteogenic sarcoma) among survivors of hereditary retinoblastoma.

Liver tumours

Liver tumours are rare. Primary liver tumours in the newborn are more likely to be benign (haemangioma). Primary malignant liver tumours are mostly hepatoblastoma (65%) or hepatocellular carcinoma (25%). Hepatocellular carcinoma may arise in children with pre-existing liver disease.

Initial presentation is with abdominal distension or with a mass. Pain and jaundice are rare. Investigation with ultrasound or CT scan confirms a large intrinsic liver mass, occasionally with calcification. Elevated serum alphafetoprotein (AFP) is detected in nearly all cases of hepatoblastoma and hepatocellular carcinoma.

Most hepatoblastomas show a good response to chemotherapy (cisplatin and doxorubicin) after which surgical resection can be achieved. Liver transplantation is a possibility for a minority of patients with unresectable disease confined to the liver. That the majority of children with hepatoblastoma can now be cured. The prospects for children with hepatocellular carcinoma are less certain.

Germ cell tumours

Germ cell tumours (GCT) are rare and may be benign or malignant. They arise from the primitive germ cells which migrate from yolk sac endoderm to form gonads in the embryo. Benign tumours are most common in the sacrococcygeal region (Fig. 18.20) and most malignant germ cell tumours are found in the gonads. Serum markers (alpha-fetoprotein (AFP) and β-HCG) are invaluable in confirming the diagnosis and in monitoring response to treatment.

Malignant germ cell tumours are very chemosensitive, and a very good outcome can be expected for disease at sites other than the brain.

Langerhans cell histiocytosis

Langerhans cell histiocytosis (LCH, previously known as histiocytosis X) is a rare disorder characterised by an abnormal proliferation of histiocytes. It is no longer believed to be a truly malignant condition. However, its sometimes aggressive behaviour and its response to chemotherapy places it within the practice of oncologists.

Solitary lesions of bone (eosinophilic granuloma)
May present at any age with pain, swelling or fracture. X-ray reveals a characteristic lytic lesion with a well-defined border. Biopsy is usually necessary and full skeletal survey required to identify multiple lesions. Curettage, intracavity steroid injection or (in the past) low-dose radiotherapy are all successful forms of treatment. Asymptomatic lesions may not require any treatment.

Multiple bone lesions
Can occur at any site. When they involve the skull (Fig. 18.21) and are associated with proptosis and hypothalamic infiltration causing diabetes insipidus, this was previously known as Hand-Schüller-Christian disease. Once established, diabetes insipidus is not always reversed by successful treatment of the underlying disease and long-term replacement with desmopressin is usually required.

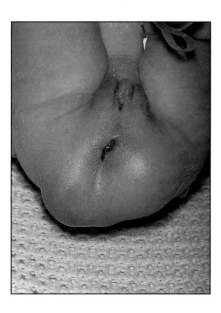

Fig. 18.20 Sacrococcygeal teratoma. These tumours are increasingly detected on antenatal ultrasound screening.

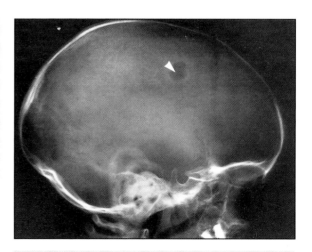

Fig. 18.21 Lytic bone lesion on a skull X-ray in Langerhans cell histiocytosis (arrow).

Systemic LCH

Most aggressive form of LCH (previously known as Letterer–Siwe disease) tends to present in infancy with a seborrhoeic rash (Fig. 18.22) and soft tissue involvement of the gums, ears, lungs, liver, spleen, lymph nodes and bone marrow. The clinical presentation may be characteristic but the diagnosis should be confirmed by biopsy, usually from skin or lymph node. Organ dysfunction is of greater adverse prognostic significance than mere involvement. This form of disease is usually progressive and requires chemotherapy although spontaneous regression may occur. The outlook is variable but most patients are cured.

 Langerhans cell histiocytosis (LCH) occurs as a spectrum from localised to systemic forms.

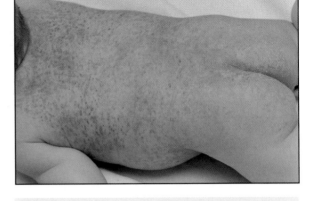

Fig. 18.22 Rash in systemic Langerhans cell histiocytosis. It is often mistaken for seborrhoeic dermatitis or eczema.

FURTHER READING

Pinkerton CR. *Paediatric Oncology.* 2nd edn. Chapman and Hall, London, 1996.

Pizzo PA, Poplack DG (eds). *Principles & Practice of Pediatric Oncology.* 2nd edn. JG Lippincott, Philadelphia 1993. Comprehensive textbook.

Schwartz CL, Hobbie WL, Constine LS, Ruccione KS. *Survivors of Childhood Cancer.* Mosby–Year Book Inc. St Louis. 1994.

Voute PA, Barrett A, Lamerle J. (eds) *Cancer in Children. Clinical Management.* 3rd edn. Springer-Verlag, Berlin. Short textbook.

CHAPTER 19

Haematological Disorders

• *Anaemia* • *Haemolytic anaemia* • *Bleeding disorders*

In children, the normal values of haemoglobin and red cell parameters vary with age (Fig. 19.1 and Appendix). Allowance for this must always be made in interpreting laboratory results.

Anaemia

In the fetus, in response to the low oxygen tension, the haemoglobin concentration is high and the fetal haemoglobin has a higher oxygen affinity than adult haemoglobin. At birth, infants born at term have a high haemoglobin concentration (14 –20 g/dl). The infant's haemoglobin and blood volume will also depend on how rapidly the umbilical cord is clamped and on the infant's position after delivery relative to the placenta. The blood volume will be increased if cord clamping is delayed and the baby is held lower than the placenta. The haemoglobin level often increases during the first day of life because of intravascular fluid loss. Thereafter, the haemoglobin concentration falls, reaching its minimum at 2–3 months of age, when the lower limit of the normal range is 9.5 g/dl. During this time there is erythroid hypoplasia of the bone marrow and a change from fetal to adult haemoglobin.

At birth, severe anaemia requiring immediate treatment is mainly from haemorrhage, either from twin to twin or feto–maternal transfusion or following placental abruption. Severe anaemia from haemolysis from rhesus isoimmunisation is now usually prevented by antenatal treatment.

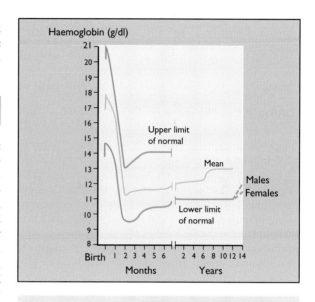

Fig. 19.1 *Changes in haemoglobin concentration with age, showing that the haemoglobin is high at birth and falls to its lowest level at 2–3 months of age.*

The main causes of anaemia after the neonatal period are shown in Figure 19.2. By far the most common cause is dietary iron deficiency, which is found in an appreciable percentage of young children in all communities, but

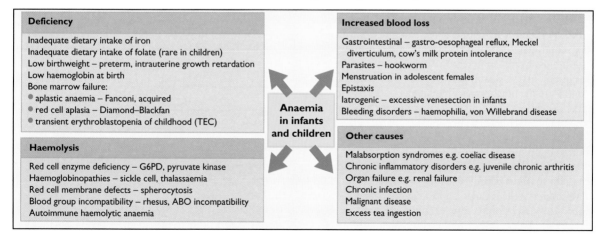

Deficiency

Inadequate dietary intake of iron
Inadequate dietary intake of folate (rare in children)
Low birthweight – preterm, intrauterine growth retardation
Low haemoglobin at birth
Bone marrow failure:
● aplastic anaemia – Fanconi, acquired
● red cell aplasia – Diamond–Blackfan
● transient erythroblastopenia of childhood (TEC)

Haemolysis

Red cell enzyme deficiency – G6PD, pyruvate kinase
Haemoglobinopathies – sickle cell, thalassaemia
Red cell membrane defects – spherocytosis
Blood group incompatibility – rhesus, ABO incompatibility
Autoimmune haemolytic anaemia

Anaemia in infants and children

Increased blood loss

Gastrointestinal – gastro-oesophageal reflux, Meckel
diverticulum, cow's milk protein intolerance
Parasites – hookworm
Menstruation in adolescent females
Epistaxis
Iatrogenic – excessive venesection in infants
Bleeding disorders – haemophilia, von Willebrand disease

Other causes

Malabsorption syndromes e.g. coeliac disease
Chronic inflammatory disorders e.g. juvenile chronic arthritis
Organ failure e.g. renal failure
Chronic infection
Malignant disease
Excess tea ingestion

Fig. 19.2 *Causes of anaemia in infants and children.*

particularly among immigrant populations in poor inner city areas or in developing countries. Iron deficiency is also seen in low birthweight infants because of their reduced iron stores combined with their greater expansion of blood volume accompanying growth than an appropriate weight term infant. Preterm infants are liable to outstrip their reserves at 4–8 weeks of age.

Blood loss is a much less common cause of anaemia in children than dietary iron deficiency, though repeated vene-section of sick newborn preterm infants often requires replacement transfusions. Hookworm is an important cause of anaemia in some countries. In adolescent girls, the onset of menarche may be complicated by the development of iron deficiency anaemia from a combination of increased demands from their growth spurt and menstrual blood loss.

IRON DEFICIENCY

The fetus absorbs iron from the mother across the placenta. At birth, the infant's iron stores are 75 mg/kg, 75% of which is circulating in the blood, the remainder is stored as ferritin and haemosiderin. The term infant has adequate reserves for the first four months of age, but during the following year is susceptible to iron deficiency. This results from a dietary iron intake which is inadequate for the increase in blood volume accompanying growth and to build iron stores. To increase the iron stores from 260 mg in a term infant at birth to 4–5 g in an adult requires about 0.8 mg of elemental iron per day. Preterm infants may require up to 2 mg/kg body weight of elemental iron per day.

Although milk has a relatively low iron content, absorption from breast milk is about 50%, whereas only 10% is absorbed from cows' milk. This is one of the main reasons why unmodified cows' milk is not recommended until one year of age. In the UK, infant formula is supplemented with iron. Iron from cereals is absorbed poorly (about 1%), and to compensate for this, cereals for infants are fortified with iron. Iron deficiency will result from undue delay in the introduction of mixed feeding beyond 3–4 months of age or a diet poor in iron-rich food (Fig. 19.3).

About 10–15% of dietary iron is absorbed. Iron absorption from food is increased when eaten in combination with food rich in vitamin C, i.e. fruit and vegetables, and is inhibited by tannin in tea. The considerable dietary iron requirements of young growing children is in marked contrast to the much smaller requirements, relative to their size, of adults, who conserve most metabolised iron. A year-old infant requires an intake of iron of about 8 mg/day. An adult male needs to have a dietary intake of about 9 mg of iron daily and menstruating females 15 mg/day.

Infants and young children are usually asymptomatic until the anaemia becomes marked, when pallor and tiredness are noted. The pallor is most readily detected on the mucosal surfaces of the tongue and mouth and conjunctivae, but clinical assessment is unreliable. Koilonychia, when the nails become spoon-shaped, is uncommon in children. Iron deficiency anaemia is associated with behavioural and intellectual deficits which may be reversible with iron therapy.

Iron deficiency anaemia in children is often found incidentally when blood tests are performed. In some communities there is routine screening.

Diagnosis

The diagnosis is confirmed from the blood count and film and the investigations listed in Figure 19.4. In iron deficiency anaemia, the haemoglobin concentration is less than 11g/dl, other than in infants when an age related chart of normal values should be used. Iron deficiency is not necessarily accompanied by anaemia. In interpreting the red cell indices, the lower MCV of infants must be taken into account. Anaemia may also be caused by β- or α-thalassaemia trait. In severe iron deficiency, it may not be possible to identify β-thalassaemia trait as the raised HbA$_2$ level may be masked. Haemoglobin electrophoresis with quantitaion of HbA$_2$ should be undertaken if the MCV remains low once the serum ferritin is normal. There is no simple laboratory test to identify α-thalassaemia trait. In populations where α-thalassaemia is common, the serum ferritin should be measured to identify iron deficiency.

Management

For the majority of children who have no symptoms, management involves improving the diet and giving iron supplements. Investigations for other causes are advisable if the history or examination suggests a non-dietary cause or if there is failure to respond to therapy.

Iron therapy is given orally. Ferrous sulphate is the most readily absorbed preparation and has fewer side-effects in children than in adults. Other preparations are associated

Fig. 19.3 Dietary sources of iron	
Good	**Average**
Red meat	Dark green vegetables
Oily fish	Poultry
Fortified breakfast cereals	Pulses
Savoury baby food	Bread, chapatti
Dried baby food	Wholegrain pasta
Rusks	Tofu (soy bean curd)

Fig. 19.4 Investigations in iron deficiency
Haemoglobin concentration – reduced
Red blood cell count – reduced
MCV – reduced
Blood film – hypochromic, microcytic
Serum ferritin – reduced
Serum iron – reduced
TIBC – increased
Serum iron:TIBC ratio – reduced
TIBC = total iron-binding capacity

with less gastrointestinal upset but contain less elemental iron or are less readily absorbed. Their use should be limited to children who are intolerant of ferrous sulphate. Parents should be advised that oral iron causes the stools to turn black and some preparations may temporarily stain the teeth. Iron supplementation should be continued for a minimum of three months, not only to correct the haemoglobin concentration but also to replenish the iron stores.

Preterm infants should only be started on iron therapy at several weeks of age. Their iron stores are not depleted until this age and they may be receiving iron in blood transfusions. In addition, the protective effect of lactoferrin from breast-feeding will be reduced by saturating the lactoferrin with iron.

 Iron deficiency in children is common and is usually dietary.

APLASTIC ANAEMIA

Aplastic anaemia is a rare condition characterised by a reduction in or absence of haemopoietic elements in all cell lines in the bone marrow leading to peripheral blood pancytopenia. It can be either inherited or more commonly is acquired.

Fanconi anaemia

Fanconi anaemia is the most common inherited cause. It is an autosomal recessive condition accompanied by constitutional malformations which include hyperpigmentation, short stature, abnormal radii and thumbs and renal malformations together with developmental delay. These are evident before the bone marrow failure, which usually occurs only at school age.

Presentation is usually with bruising and purpura from thrombocytopenia, with the gradual development of anaemia. It is a DNA repair disorder and is accompanied by an increased risk of developing acute leukaemia and other malignancies.

Acquired aplastic anaemia

Acquired aplastic anaemia is similar to that seen in adults but is uncommon in children. Usually, no cause is identified. Rarely, it may follow the ingestion of drugs, e.g. sulphonamides, chloramphenicol, gold compounds for arthritis, antithyroid drugs or infections (hepatitis and Epstein–Barr virus). The condition may occur at any age. It is usually progressive and most untreated children die within a few years. Successful allografts from sibling donors have proved curative. The efficacy of HLA-matched unrelated donor marrow is being assessed. If no donor is available, antihuman thymic globulin (ATG), either from horses or rabbits, together with cyclosporin and cytokines can produce a response that allows freedom from blood products, but is usually associated with serum sickness. If definitive treatment fails, supportive care with red cell and platelet infusion and prompt treatment of infection is necessary to maintain life. Overwhelming sepsis or haemorrhage are the main causes of death.

Haemolytic anaemia

Haemolysis is premature lysis of red blood cells. Their lifespan may be reduced from the normal 120 days to less than 5 days. The bone marrow can compensate by increasing the rate of red cell production (up to 7 times normal); anaemia only occurs when this is insufficient to keep pace with red cell destruction. Haemolytic anaemias may be inherited or acquired (Fig. 19.5). Inherited defects may be due to:
- enzyme deficiencies
- haemoglobinopathies
- disorders of the red cell membrane.

Haemolysis may lead to:
- elevated unconjugated bilirubin
- excess urinary urobilinogen
- abnormalities of blood film, e.g. spherocytes
- reduced plasma haptoglobin
- reticuloendothelial hyperplasia – hepatomegaly and splenomegaly.

Increased red cell production may lead to:
- reticulocytosis
- erythroid hyperplasia of the bone marrow, which may cause skeletal deformity of the face and skull.

RED CELL ENZYME DEFICIENCIES

I. G6PD DEFICIENCY

Glucose-6-phosphate dehydrogenase (G6PD) is the rate-limiting enzyme of the hexose monophosphate shunt by which red cells generate $NADPH_2$. This maintains glutathione in a reduced state, which is essential for preventing oxidative damage to the cell. Red cells lacking G6PD are susceptible to oxidant-induced haemolysis. The gene for G6PD is located on the X chromosome, so the deficiency mainly affects males. Heterozygous females have about half the normal G6PD activity, but may be affected due to random inactivation of one X chromosome (the Lyon hypothesis).

Women can be severely affected if homozygous or if the normal X chromosomes have been inactivated by chance, as occurs in about 2% of heterozygotes. There are many different variants with variable clinical severity. In the Mediterranean, Middle Eastern and Oriental populations, affected males have very low or absent enzyme activity in their red cells. Affected Afro-Caribbeans have 10–15% normal enzyme activity. Their young red blood cells have normal enzyme activity, while older cells are deficient. Worldwide over 100 million people are deficient in G6PD, making it the most common enzyme deficiency.

Clinical manifestations

These result from episodes of haemolysis:
- neonatal jaundice – onset is usually in the first three days of life. It is most common in the Mediterranean and Far Eastern variants. Worldwide, it is the most common cause of severe neonatal jaundice requiring exchange transfusion

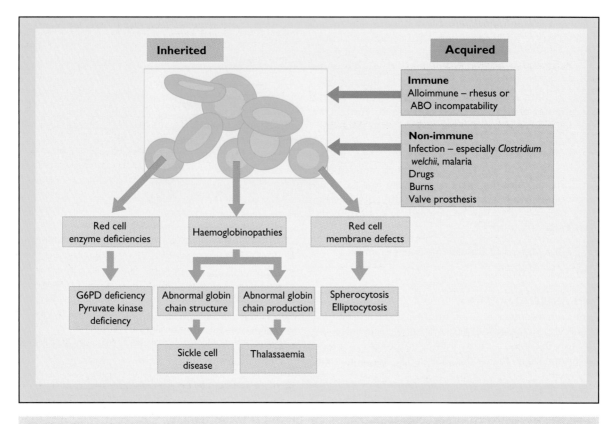

Fig. 19.5 *Causes of haemolytic anaemia.*

- drug- or infection-induced haemolysis – infections are now thought to be a more common precipitating factor than drugs. Intravascular haemolysis is associated with fever, malaise and the passage of dark urine which may contain haemoglobin as well as urobilinogen. The haemoglobin level falls rapidly. Exposure to naphthalene in mothballs may also induce haemolysis
- favism – ingestion of broad beans can cause acute haemolysis in Mediterranean and Far Eastern variants. This is not seen in Afro-Caribbeans.

Chronic haemolysis is rare.

Diagnosis
Specific enzyme assays are available for G6PD activity, but during a haemolytic crisis levels may be elevated, misleadingly, due to the higher enzyme concentration in reticulocytes. A repeat assay is then required in the steady state to confirm the diagnosis.

Management
The parents of a child with G6PD deficiency should be provided with a list of drugs to avoid (Fig. 19.6). Many drugs which were thought to induce haemolysis, e.g. aspirin, chloroquine and vitamin K, are now regarded as safe in therapeutic dosage. Eating fava beans should be avoided by affected children of Mediterranean origin. In acute haemolysis, blood transfusion may be required. In Afro-Caribbeans, haemolysis is usually self-limiting as the newly formed red cells have normal enzyme activity.

2. PYRUVATE KINASE DEFICIENCY
This is much rarer, and causes a chronic haemolytic anaemia of variable severity without spherocytes. It mainly affects north Europeans. It is inherited as an autosomal recessive disorder. The diagnosis requires a specific assay of the enzyme. Splenectomy may be required for some severely affected children.

HAEMOGLOBINOPATHIES
These are inherited disorders of haemoglobin structure or

Fig. 19.6 Drugs which may cause haemolysis in G6PD deficiency	
Antimalarials	Primaquine
Antibiotics	Some sulphonamides, e.g. cotrimoxazole
	Nitrofurantoin
	Nalidixic acid
	Ciprofloxacin
Others	Dapsone
	Naphthalene (mothballs)

(Adapted from Beutler E, *N Eng J Med* 1991;324:169–174)

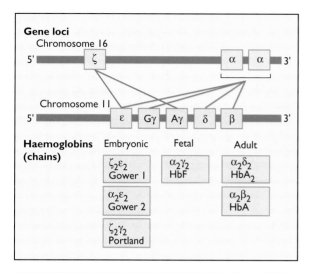

Fig 19.7 Haemoglobins according to age.

its production. The molecular defects accounting for most of these disorders have been characterised by gene analysis. Human haemoglobins are a tetrameric structure which consists of two globin chains from the α globin gene (on chromosome 16) and two globin chains from the β globin gene (on chromosome 11). The tetramer constitution varies according to age (Fig. 19.7) and follows a sequential pattern of development. In early embryonic life, haemoglobins Gower 1, Gower 2 and Portland are produced. Later in pregnancy, fetal haemoglobin (HbF) is produced and accounts for 70–90% of haemoglobin at birth. The production of β chains in adult HbA starts from the second trimester and rapidly increases after birth, when HbF production is suppressed. By one year of age HbF levels are less than 2%. As most haemoglobinopathies result from aberrations of β chain synthesis (other than α-thalassaemia), clinical manifestations are usually delayed until after six months of age.

The types of haemoglobin at birth and in adults and in some of the haemoglobinopathies are shown in Figure 19.8. Using advances in DNA analysis, antenatal diagnosis can be offered for most forms of haemoglobinopathies. Genetic counselling can enable parents to make informed decisions. As many of these conditions occur in particular ethnic groups, selective ante- and postnatal screening may offer early recognition of affected individuals. In some parts of the UK, postnatal screening for haemoglobinopathies is performed on the blood sample taken for national biochemical screening (Guthrie test). This means that the diagnosis is made before affected children develop any clinical manifestations.

1. SICKLE CELL DISEASE

Sickle cell disease (HbSS), the homozygous state, results from a single amino acid substitution (glutamine for valine) on codon 6 of the β chain. The gene mainly affects those populations originating from tropical Africa. It corresponds with the distribution of falciparum malaria as sickle trait, the heterozygous state, is thought to offer protection. It is therefore most common in black Africans or Americans, or Afro-Caribbeans, but is also seen in the Mediterranean, Middle East and parts of India.

Pathogenesis

In sickle cell disease the haemoglobin molecule becomes deformed in the deoxygenated state. Rigid tubular spiral bodies are formed which deform the red cells into a sickle shape. Irreversibly sickled red cells have a reduced life span and are trapped in the microcirculation causing ischaemia. This is exacerbated by low oxygen tension, dehydration and cold.

Clinical manifestations

These are listed in Figure 19.9.

Management

Acute

Adequate hydration, oxygenation and warmth need to be ensured. Infection may precipitate painful or haemolytic crises and needs to be treated vigorously. Analgesia is

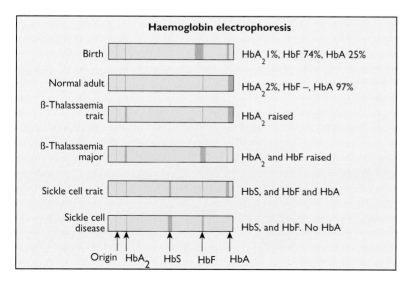

Fig. 19.8 Patterns of haemoglobin electrophoresis showing the types of haemoglobin at birth, in adults and in a range of haemoglobinopathies.

Fig. 19. 9 Clinical manifestations of sickle cell disease

Anaemia

Moderate (usually Hb 6–8 g/dl) with clinically detectable jaundice from chronic haemolysis

---

Painful crises

Vaso-occlusive crises causing pain may affect all organs of the body with varying frequency and severity. A common mode of presentation in late infancy is the hand–foot syndrome, in which there is dactylitis with swelling and pain of the fingers and feet from vaso-occlusion (Fig. 19. 10). The bones of the limbs and spine are common sites, whereas cerebral and pulmonary infarction are uncommon but more serious. The commonest presentation of cerebral infarction is acute hemiparesis from blockage of the medium to large arteries, unlike vaso-occlusion in the small vessels elsewhere in the body. Vascular necrosis of the femoral heads may also occur

---

Haemolytic crises

Associated with a further drop in the haemoglobin level

1. Aplastic crises, where the haemoglobin can fall precipitously, are most often caused by parvovirus infection
2. Sequestration crises, with accumulation of sickled cells, can cause marked, sudden splenic enlargement, abdominal pain and circulatory collapse

---

Infection

Autosplenectomy, due to usually asymptomatic splenic infarction during infancy, markedly increases the susceptibility to infection from encapsulated organisms, such as pneumococci and *Haemophilus influenzae*. There is also an increased incidence of osteomyelitis caused by *Salmonella* and other organisms. The risk of overwhelming sepsis is more common in early childhood

---

Priapism

Needs to be treated promptly with exchange transfusion as it may lead to fibrosis of the corpora cavernosa and subsequent erectile impotence

---

Splenomegaly

Common in young children, but becomes less frequent in older children

---

Cardiac enlargement

From chronic anaemia

Long-term problems

Short stature and delayed puberty

Adenotonsillar hypertrophy causing sleep apnoea syndrome leading to nocturnal hypoxaemia, which can cause vaso-occlusive crises

Renal dysfunction – may exacerbate enuresis because of failure to concentrate urine

Pigmented gallstones – due to excessive bilirubin production

Leg ulcers

Heart failure from uncorrected anaemia

---

required for pain. When severe, opioid analgesics are required. These can be given most effectively using a patient-controlled infusion in older children or a nurse-controlled infusion for younger children. Blood transfusions may be required during an aplastic, sequestration or haemolytic crisis for a sudden, marked fall in haemoglobin. Exchange transfusion reduces the proportion of sickle cells without unduly raising the haemoglobin level and is indicated for neurological and pulmonary infarction and priapism.

Long term

HbS is a low-affinity haemoglobin, efficient in delivering oxygen, so chronic steady state anaemia is not an indication for giving blood transfusions. Vaso-occlusive crises will be prevented if the proportion of HbS is less than 30%. Regular blood transfusion is often associated with allo-immunisation and is only used following a neurological complication or for multiple severe crises. Blood or exchange transfusion may be required before major surgery. Allogeneic bone marrow transplantation has been performed for a few patients with severe disease. However, there is controversy about this form of therapy and to whom it should be offered. Suitable candidates would be those who experience multiple painful crises or have an abnormal cerebral circulation. Treatment with hydroxy-urea, which increases HbF, is being assessed.

Penicillin (twice a day) should be taken throughout life to prevent pneumococcal infection. Children should receive the standard course of Haemophilus influenzae type b (Hib) vaccine. Pneumococcal and meningococcal vaccine should be given at about two years of age, to obtain a good antibody response. Affected children should also

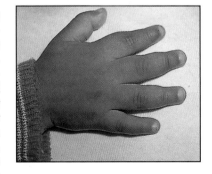

Fig. 19.10 Swelling of the fingers from dactylitis, the hand–foot syndrome, is a common mode of presentation of sickle cell disease in children.

be given daily folic acid to compensate for the increased demands due to red blood cell breakdown.

About 85% of those affected survive to the age of 20 years. The main risk of death is in the first three years of life, mainly from infection. An advantage of screening antenatally or in the neonatal period is that prophylaxis against infection can be started immediately and the parents informed about the disease.

 Sickle cell disease carries a greatly increased risk of pneumococcal infection

2. SICKLE CELL TRAIT

The heterozygote with sickle cell trait (HbAS) is asymptomatic and rarely has problems except under conditions of low oxygen tension. General anaesthesia does not constitute a risk in this population as long as they have been identified and hypoxia avoided.

3. SICKLE CELL–HAEMOGLOBIN C (SC) DISEASE

Affected children usually have a nearly normal haemoglobin level and fewer painful crises than those with sickle cell disease, but they may develop proliferative retinopathy. Their eyes should be checked periodically.

4. THALASSAEMIA

Thalassaemia syndromes are due to inherited defects of globin chain synthesis. There are two main types of thalassaemia:
- α-thalassaemia in which there is a reduced rate of α chain synthesis
- β-thalassaemias which are associated with a deficiency of β chains.

Alteration in the genes controlling globin chain synthesis leads to a reduction in or absence of the particular globin.

This results in an excess of the other chain which precipitates within the red cell membrane, bringing about its cell death within the bone marrow (ineffective erythropoiesis) and premature removal of circulating red cells by the spleen.

β-thalassaemia occurs most often in people from the Mediterranean and Middle East. Over 150 million people carry the b-thalassaemia gene. In the UK, thalassaemia is seen predominantly in those of Greek Cypriot or Bangladeshi origin.

As there is reduced production of β chains, γ chain synthesis continues beyond the neonatal period producing an increased proportion of HbF and HbA_2. The disease severity of β-thalassaemia depends on the amount of HbA and HbF present:
- thalassaemia major (homozygous for abnormal β genes) - anaemia is severe and regular blood transfusions are required.
- thalassaemia intermedia – homozygous, but, as can be predicted from the site and nature of the mutation, anaemia is only moderate. Blood transfusions may be required to prevent skeletal deformities but not for the anaemia alone.
- thalassaemia minor (heterozygous for abnormal β gene) – asymptomatic carrier.

β-Thalassaemia major
Clinical features
These are:
- severe anaemia and jaundice from six months of age
- failure to thrive/growth failure
- extramedullary haemopoiesis causing bone marrow expansion which leads to the classical facies with maxillary overgrowth (Fig. 19.12) and skull bossing. There is marked hepatosplenomegaly.

Case history

ACUTE SICKLE CHEST SYNDROME

A nine-year-old girl with known homozygous sickle cell disease presented with increasing chest pain for six hours. She had a non-productive cough. On examination she had a fever of 39.7°C. Her breathing was laboured and respiratory rate increased, and there was reduced air entry at both bases.

Investigations

Haemoglobin 6g/dl, WBC 14×10^9/l, Platelets 350×10^9/l
Chest X-ray (Fig. 19.11)
SaO_2 89% in air
Arterial PO_2 9.3 kPa (70 mmHg) breathing face mask oxygen
Blood and sputum cultures and viral titres taken.

A diagnosis of acute sickle chest syndrome was made, a potentially fatal condition. She was given oxygen by continuous positive airways pressure (CPAP). An exchange transfusion was performed. Broad-spectrum antibiotics were commenced. She responded well to treatment.

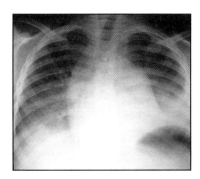

Fig. 19.11 Chest X-ray in acute sickle chest syndrome showing bilateral lower zone consolidation. (Courtesy of Dr Parviz Habibi.)

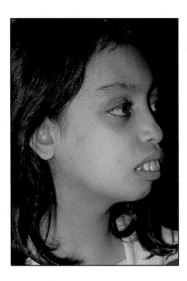

Fig. 19.12 Facies in β-thalassaemia major showing maxillary over-growth and skull bossing.

Management

The condition is uniformly fatal without regular blood transfusions. The aim is to maintain the haemoglobin concentration above 10 g/dl in order to reduce growth retardation and prevent bone deformation. Leucocyte-poor blood is used to minimise transfusion reactions. However, repeated blood transfusion causes chronic iron overload and consequent tissue damage. Chelation therapy with subcutaneous desferrioxamine, given regularly overnight, promotes urinary iron excretion. Negative iron balance is rarely achieved and compliance can be a problem. The complications of multiple transfusions and particularly iron deposition in young adults are shown in Figure 19.13. Small doses of vitamin C daily increase urinary iron excretion.

Bone marrow transplantation has successfully restored haemopoietic function. It is limited to those children who have an HLA-matched compatible sibling donor. Other areas of research are the development of oral chelating agents and the possibility of gene modulation.

β-thalassaemia trait

Heterozygotes are usually asymptomatic. The red cells may be hypochromic and microcytic. Anaemia is mild or absent with a disproportionate reduction in MCH (18–22 fl) and MCV (60–70 fl). The red blood cell count is therefore usually increased ($>5.5 \times 10^{12}$/l). The most important diagnostic feature is the raised HbA_2 and in about half there is a mild elevation of HbF level of 1–3%, on haemoglobin electrophoresis. β-Thalassaemia trait may be confused with mild iron deficiency and lead to unnecessary iron therapy. Detection should lead to genetic counselling.

α-thalassaemia

There are normally four α globin genes. The manifestation of the α-thalassaemia syndromes depends on the number of remaining functional genes. The most severe form (four-gene deletion) leads to Hb Barts which causes fetal hydrops and is incompatible with life. Hb H (three-gene deletion) leads in later life to moderate chronic haemolysis. One or two gene deletions do not cause clinical manifestations but may give rise to hypochromic and microcytic red cells. As with all haemoglobinopathies, genetic counselling is important.

OTHER DEFECTS OF HAEMOGLOBIN STRUCTURE OR PRODUCTION

There are many haemoglobin variants caused by structural globin chain defects, e.g. HbE, the most common variant in South-east Asia, which causes a mild microcytic anaemia. The haemoglobin variants may occur in combination with thalassaemia. Sickle cell trait together with β-thalassaemia trait clinically resembles sickle cell disease.

 β-thalassaemia major is fatal without regular blood transfusions.

DISORDERS OF THE RED CELL MEMBRANE

SPHEROCYTOSIS

This is an autosomal dominant disorder with variable penetrance caused by abnormalities in proteins of the red cell membrane. About 25% are new mutations. It affects about 1 in 5000 Caucasians. It results in the red cell losing its membrane as it passes through the spleen. The surface to volume ratio is reduced and the cells become spheroidal.

Clinical features

The disorder is often suspected because of a positive family history. Even within the same family the clinical manifestations are highly variable. The clinical features include:
- jaundice – usually develops during childhood but may cause severe haemolytic jaundice in the first few days of life
- anaemia – presents in childhood with mild anaemia (haemoglobin 9–11 g/dl), but the haemoglobin level may fall with an intercurrent infection
- mild to moderate splenomegaly – depends on the rate of haemolysis. This may be the mode of presentation in the first year of life

Fig. 19.13 Complications of multiple blood transfusions	
Iron deposition	Heart – cardiomyopathy
	Liver – cirrhosis
	Pancreas – diabetes
	Endocrine – hormone failure, especially parathyroid – hypocalcaemia
	Skin – hyperpigmentation
Antibody formation	Red cell antibodies
	HLA antibodies
Infection	Hepatitis (blood is now screened for hepatitis B and C)
	HIV infection (blood is now screened)
	Malaria
Venous access	Multiple infusions and blood samples

- aplastic crisis – associated with parvovirus infection, but is uncommon
- gallstones – pigmented gallstones due to increased bilirubin excretion.

Diagnosis

The diagnosis is confirmed by demonstrating an increased osmotic fragility when red blood cells are placed in increasingly hypotonic solutions. This is a test for the presence of spherocytes. In the absence of a positive family history, immune causes of haemolysis must be excluded by a direct antiglobulin test.

Management

No treatment is required if the disease is mild. Folic acid is given to compensate for increased demands due to ongoing haemolysis. Occasional blood transfusions may be required for aplastic crises. Splenectomy improves red cell survival and should be considered for excessive transfusion requirements or episodes of aplasia or recurrent anaemia or jaundice. It is preferable to defer this until after two years of age because of the risk of overwhelming infection. Before splenectomy, the child should be given Hib, meningococcal and pneumococcal vaccine. Prophylactic daily penicillin administration is recommended post-splenectomy but patients may not comply. How long to continue with prophylaxis remains uncertain, but many believe it should be lifelong.

Bleeding disorders

Normal clotting relies on the complex interaction between the vessel wall, platelets, and coagulation factors (Fig. 19.14) which are involved not only in pro-coagulant activity but also in fibrinolysis. When evaluating a child with a bleeding disorder, helpful features are shown in Figure 19.15.

Haemophilia A and B and von Willebrand disease account for more than 90% of all inherited bleeding disorders. Laboratory screening tests help determine the most likely causes (Fig. 19.16), while specialist investigations will characterise the deficiency.

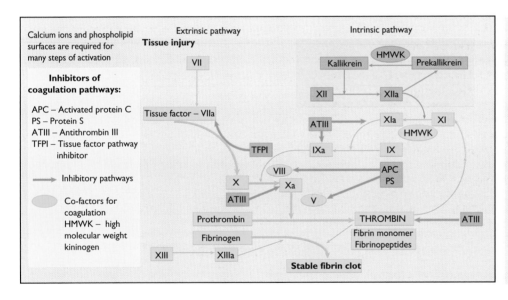

Fig. 19.14 The main physiological pathway of activation is via the extrinsic system. The intrinsic pathway is probably recruited by thrombin-activation of factor XI. The traditional contact factor system, shown in the purple box, is not part of the mechanism. (Courtesy Dr Paula Bolton–Maggs.)

Fig. 19.15 Helpful clinical features in the evaluating bleeding disorders

Age of onset

Uncomplicated previous surgery or dental extraction suggests the bleeding tendency is acquired rather than inherited

Positive family history

Some congenital bleeding disorders have a sex-linked inheritance. A detailed family tree including the sex of affected family members needs to be determined

Site and type of bleeding

Mucous membrane bleeding and skin haemorrhage	Characteristic of platelet disorders or von Willebrand disease
Bleeding into muscles or joints	Characteristic of severe clotting factor deficiencies
Scarring and delayed healing	Suggestive of disorders of connective tissue, e.g. Marfan syndrome, osteogenesis imperfecta or Factor XIII deficiency

The tests usually performed in a bleeding disorder are:
- platelet count – may be reduced
- prothrombin time (PT) – measures the extrinsic pathway and the final common pathway (factors II, V and X and the conversion of fibrinogen to fibrin)
- activated partial thromboplastin time (APTT) – tests the intrinsic pathway as well as the final common pathway
- thrombin time and fibrinogen – to exclude afibrinogenaemia and dysfibrinogenaemia.
- bleeding time, if required – to identify intrinsic platelet dysfunction in the presence of a normal platelet count.

HAEMOPHILIA

Haemophilia A is a sex-linked recessive disorder which is characterised by reduced or absent factor VIII activity (Fig. 19.17). Haemophilia B (Christmas disease) is similar but is due to reduced or absent factor IX activity. Haemophilia A occurs in about 1 in 5000–10 000 males whereas haemophilia B is six times less common. In about 30% there is no family history. Identifying female carriers requires a detailed family history, analysis of coagulation factors and DNA analysis. Antenatal diagnosis is available using DNA analysis.

The disorder is graded as severe, moderate or mild depending on the factor VIIIc level (Fig. 19.18). The severity tends to remain constant within a family.

Clinical features

In severe haemophilia, there are usually few problems in the first year of life. It is only when the child starts to walk and falls over that abnormal bleeding is first noted. This can occur at any site but is frequently into joints and muscles. Where there is no family history, non-accidental injury may initially be suspected. Mild haemophilia is likely to remain undetected until excessive bleeding after a haemostatic challenge e.g. oozing for 1–2 weeks after dental extraction in a young adult.

Management

Bleeding in severe haemophilia is treated by the prompt and adequate replacement with intravenous infusion of factor VIII concentrate. The quantity required depends on the site and nature of the bleed. In general, raising the circulating level to 30% is sufficient to control haemorrhage. Major surgery or life-threatening bleeds requires the level to be raised to 100%, and then maintained at 30–50% for up to two weeks to prevent secondary haemorrhage. This can only be achieved by regular infusions of factor concentrate and monitoring of levels by assaying plasma samples. Complications of treatment are shown in Figure 19.19.

Repeated bleeding into the joints can cause progressive arthropathy. Prompt and adequate therapy helps avoid such damage. Parents can be taught to give replacement

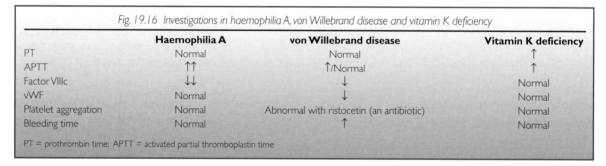

Fig. 19.16 Investigations in haemophilia A, von Willebrand disease and vitamin K deficiency

	Haemophilia A	von Willebrand disease	Vitamin K deficiency
PT	Normal	Normal	↑
APTT	↑↑	↑/Normal	↑
Factor VIIIc	↓↓	↓	Normal
vWF	Normal	↓	Normal
Platelet aggregation	Normal	Abnormal with ristocetin (an antibiotic)	Normal
Bleeding time	Normal	↑	Normal

PT = prothrombin time; APTT = activated partial thromboplastin time

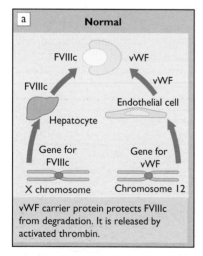
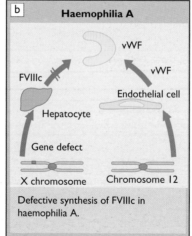
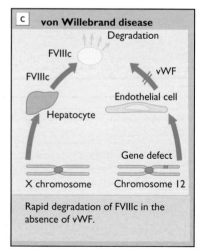

Fig. 19.17 Factor VIIIc and vWF synthesis – (a) normal relationship between Factor VIIIc and vWF, (b) haemophilia A, (c) von Willebrand disease.

therapy at home. Eventually patients will administer their treatment themselves. This avoids delay and minimises inconvenience to the family. Regular prophylactic therapy is under assessment and is likely to be the treatment of choice to avoid long-term joint damage.

Mild haemophilia can often be successfully managed without the use of blood products, by using infusions of desmopressin which results in endogenous release of factor VIII. It allows minor surgery and dental extraction to be carried out without blood products.

Management should be supervised by a haemophilia comprehensive care centre. These provide medical, nursing and psychosocial expertise for the children and their families. These centres are also supported by specialised laboratory facilities to undertake specific assays to diagnose and monitor therapy. Physiotherapy is needed to preserve muscle strength and avoid damage from immobilisation. Many families receive considerable support from self-help groups, e.g. the Haemophilia Society.

VON WILLEBRAND DISEASE (vWD)

The von Willebrand factor (vWF) has two major roles:
- it facilitates platelet adhesion to the damaged endothelium
- it acts as the carrier protein for Factor VIIIc, protecting it from breakdown.

In von Willebrand disease there is a reduction of both Factor VIIIc and vWF together with platelet dysfunction. It is a heterogeneous disorder which demonstrates considerable genetic variation. The most common subtype has an autosomal dominant inheritance. The hallmark of the disorder is mucocutaneous bleeding, often of the gums or nose, and causing menorrhagia in adolescent females or ready or excessive skin bruising.

Treatment depends on the type and severity of the disorder. Desmopressin, factor VIII or specific vWF concentrates may be given. Cryoprecipitate, which contains the entire vWF complex is no longer used as, in contrast to the concentrates, it has not undergone viral inactivation. Whenever possible, desmopressin is given rather than plasma products to reduce the risk of viral transmission. Tranexamic acid, an antifibrinolytic agent, can be used for mucous membrane bleeding as an adjunct to therapy but should be avoided in patients with haematuria due to a risk of clot retention.

 In bleeding disorders, avoid intramuscular injections and the use of aspirin and other nonsteroidal anti-inflammatory drugs.

INHIBITORS OF COAGULATION

Antithrombin III and activated protein-C (APC) are the most important naturally occurring inhibitors of coagulation and play a central role in localising fibrin at the site of tissue damage. Any imbalance between the activators and inhibitors of coagulation or fibrinolysis, e.g. from activated protein-C resistance, may predispose to thrombosis.

Protein C and S deficiencies can be inherited or acquired. Heterozygotes for protein C and S deficiency are at risk of thromboses beyond the second decade of life. Acquired deficiencies may follow varicella infection, liver disease and sickle cell disease. Treatment is by replacement with fresh frozen plasma or factor concentrate with subsequent anticoagulation with warfarin.

THROMBOCYTOPENIA

Purpura from thrombocytopenia will usually develop when the platelet count falls below 20×10^9/l, with haemorrhage liable to occur if the level falls below 10×10^9/l. The causes of purpura in children are listed in Figure 19.20.

Immune-mediated thrombocytopenic purpura

Immune-mediated thrombocytopenic purpura (ITP) is the most common cause of thrombocytopenia in childhood. The reduced platelet count is accompanied by an increase in megakaryocytes within the bone marrow. It is now known

Fig. 19.18 Severity of haemophilia		
Factor VIIIc level	**Severity**	**Bleeding tendency**
<2%	Severe	Spontaneous joint/muscle bleeds
2–10%	Moderate	Bleed after minor trauma
>10%	Mild	Bleed after surgery

Fig. 19.19 Complications of treatment

Inhibitors

5–20% develop antibodies to Factor VIIIc. Low inhibitor levels may be overcome by increasing the dose of factor VIII. High levels require a period of desensitisation with very high-dose factor VIII, to which about 75% respond, but at considerable financial cost. Alternatively, porcine factor VIII or activated prothrombin complex concentrates may be helpful. Recently, recombinant activated factor VIIa has been shown to help but it is very expensive.

Hepatitis

Hepatitis B and C can be transmitted by blood products. Donor blood is now screened. The virus should be inactivated by heat treatment of blood products, but recombinant products are inherently safer. All children with haemophilia should receive hepatitis A and B immunisation.

HIV infection

Contamination of blood products in the late 1970s and early 1980s resulted in a significant number of patients with haemophilia becoming HIV positive. In the UK, 41% of those with haemophilia A, 6% with haemophilia B and 3.5% with von Willebrand disease became HIV infected. The management of HIV-related illness has become a major component of the care provided by haemophilia centres.

Fig. 19.20 Causes of purpura in children

Thrombocytopenic

Impaired production	Leukaemia
	Aplastic anaemia
Excessive destruction	Immune –ITP
	Secondary – SLE, drugs, viral infections
	Alloimmune neonatal thrombocytopenia
Consumptive	DIC
coagulopathies	Haemolytic uraemic syndrome
	Thrombotic thrombocytopenic purpura
Congenital	Giant haemangioma
	Wiskott–Aldrich syndrome

Vascular disorders (non-thrombocytopenic)

Congenital	Connective tissue disorders
	(osteogenesis imperfecta, Ehlers–Danlos,
	Marfan syndromes)
Acquired	Meningococcal and other severe infections
Immune	HSP
	Connective tissue disorders (SLE)
Drugs	

ITP = immune-mediated thrombocytopenic purpura
SLE = systemic lupus erythematosis
DIC = disseminated intravascular coagulation
HSP = Henoch–Schönlein purpura

to result from an immune-mediated response directed against circulating platelets. The platelets are destroyed within the reticuloendothelial system, mainly in the spleen.

It mainly affects children between two and ten years of age. Its onset is often 1–2 weeks after a viral infection. Affected children develop purpura and superficial bruising (see Fig.19.21). They may have epistaxis and other mucosal bleeding. Intracranial bleeding is serious but rare, affecting less than 0.5%. The risk is present whilst the child has profound thrombocytopenia.

In about 90% of children the disease is acute and self-limiting. Most will require only assessment or a brief admission to hospital to confirm the diagnosis and assess its severity. There has been much debate about the need to perform bone marrow aspiration to exclude malignant infiltration or aplasia. If the clinical features are characteristic, there is no pancytopenia on the blood film and no treatment with corticosteroids is planned, bone marrow aspiration is not necessary.

Treatment is controversial. Many children require no therapy. Corticosteroids or high-dose immunoglobulin infusion have potential side-effects; they should be given only to ameliorate frank haemorrhage and not solely on the basis of the platelet count. The main mode of action of corticosteroids appears to be inhibition of phagocytosis of sensitised platelets and reduction of capillary fragility. Only a short course of corticosteroids, over 2–3 weeks, should be given and then discontinued irrespective of the platelet count, as a response after this time is unlikely. A low dose of prednisolone (0.25 mg/kg/day) appears to be as effective as higher doses. More recently, immunoglobulin infusions have been used as they often result in a rapid rise in the platelet count, but this therapy is invasive, carries a risk of transmission of infection and is expensive. Platelets given by infusion are rapidly destroyed and play little role in management other than in acute life-threatening haemorrhage. It is advisable to protect the child from trauma, but this may not be possible. Splenectomy is reserved for those who fail to remit and are symptomatic in spite of therapy. Most children with ITP will remit within three years from onset.

The contrast between ITP in children and in teenagers and adults is shown in Figure 19.21. If ITP in a child becomes chronic (lasts >6 months), regular screening for anti-nuclear factor and antiphospholipid antibodies should be performed as the thrombocytopenia may predate the development of autoimmune disorders.

DISSEMINATED INTRAVASCULAR COAGULATION

Acute disseminated intravascular coagulation (DIC) causes bruising and bleeding in severely ill children. A more chronic form may present with low platelets, reduced fibrinogen and only mild bleeding. Treatment relies on correcting the underlying cause while providing intensive care. Supportive care may be provided using fresh frozen plasma to replace clotting factors, and platelets. Therapy with heparin and antithrombin III remains controversial.

Fig. 19.21 Classification of acute and chronic thrombocytopenia

Age	Childhood	Adolescence and adulthood
Onset	Sudden	Insidious
Female : male	1 : 1	3 : 1
History of viral infection	Yes	No
Duration	Weeks–months	Many months–years
		Exclude auto-immune disorders

FURTHER READING

Alter B, ed. *Perinatal Hematology*. Churchill Livingstone, Edinburgh, 1989. A short book.

Hann IM, Gibson BES, Letsky EA, eds. *Fetal and Neonatal Haematology*. Baillière Tindall, London, 1994. A short textbook.

Lilleyman JS, Hann IM, eds. *Paediatric Haematology*. Churchill Livingstone, Edinburgh, 1992. A short textbook.

Nathan DG, Oski FA, eds. *Haematology of Infancy and Childhood*. Saunders, Philadelphia, 1992. Comprehensive two-volume textbook.

CHAPTER 20

Emotions and Behaviour

> • *Principles of normal development* • *Adversities in the family* • *Problems of the pre-school years* • *Problems of middle childhood* • *Adolescence* • *Management of emotional and behavioural problems*

Knowledge of children's emotions and behaviour is important in order to:
• know what is the normal range
• understand common, innocent minor deviations and responses to stress, physical illness and injuries
• recognise and manage emotional and behavioural disorders.

Principles of normal development

NORMAL PARENTING
A child's behaviour, emotional responses and personality are the end result of an interplay between genetic predisposition and environmental influences. Environment provides experience from which stems knowledge, learned behaviour and emotional responses, and attitudes to oneself and the world. Personal relationships are the major environmental factor in promoting psychosocial development and the child's family is the principal source of these. Within the family, the child should be protected, nurtured, educated and civilised so that his development is supported optimally. With the rising number of single parents and divorces, the form of the family is no longer predictable, but it is possible to make statements about what constitutes competent parenting (Fig. 20.1). Beyond this, there are qualitative aspects, and it is what attitudes parents have and how they handle their individual children which help shape their development in terms of personality.

NORMAL EARLY RELATIONSHIPS
A baby's first relationship is nearly always with his mother. He will be especially responsive to her from very soon after birth but will tolerate separations from her until, at about six months, he will start to demand or seek her physical presence and show tearful separation anxiety if she is not there. If tired, fearful, unhappy or in pain he will cling to her and be comforted by her presence as an attachment figure. This close attachment relationship derives from social interaction and the mother's sensitive responsiveness to the baby's needs, not from any blood tie. It need not be with the biological mother, though it usually is. Its importance lies in it being:
• a particularly close relationship within which the child's

development of trust, empathy, conscience and ideals is promoted, forming a prototype for future close relationships
• the child's primary source of comfort, providing his principal method of coping with stress (fear, anxiety, pain etc.).

This underscores the importance of having a young child's parent 'rooming in' if he has to be admitted to hospital. He would otherwise be doubly distressed both by the parent's absence and by the threat of strange surroundings.

If a young child is placed in strange impersonal surroundings and separated from his mother for more than a few hours a triphasic acute separation reaction sets in (Fig. 20.2):
• mounting anxiety about the fact that his mother fails to reappear produces distressed, irritable tearfulness (protest) which is hard to comfort
• after a day or two this turns into a withdrawn state with no play, no interest in food and little speech or willingness for personal contact (despair)
• the child gradually cheers up from this but the close contact with his mother has been lost and he is relatively indifferent to her when she reappears (detachment).

Recreating the original closeness takes weeks and is accompanied by a phase of irritability, misbehaviour and clinging.

Children who have never had the opportunity for a close, secure attachment relationship in their early years are at risk of growing up as selfish, shallow individuals who seek the affection of others but have difficulty with close

---

Fig. 20.1 Competent parents

Are there when needed
Protect their children from harm
Love their children
Provide affection, support, comfort, food and shelter
Use their authority so that they are in charge of their children (rather than vice versa)
Respect their children's immature status and judge it accurately
Keep adult business (sex, marital conflict, etc) away from their children
Set reasonable limits of tolerance on their children's behaviour
Establish a moderate amount of justifiable household rules
Have their own lives and do not live through their children
Maintain their own self-esteem and personal development

Fig. 20.2 Acute separation response in young children	
Protest	Crying
	Angry refusal to be comforted
	Asking for mummy
Despair	Moping
	Not playing
	Not eating
Detachment	Apparent cheering up and recovery
	Indifferent to parents on return to them

The above sequence develops over a period of days, but with considerable variation between children.

personal relationships and learning conformity with social rules of conduct.

The selective clinging of early attachment behaviour diminishes over time so that in the second year of life the child extends his emotional attachments to his father or other family members. By the age of four or five years the child can tolerate separations from his parents for several hours and, for instance, attend school. Children vary in their ability to do this: a child who is constitutionally apprehensive, who has an exceptionally anxious mother, or who has parents who fight and utter threats of abandonment will continue to cling to his mother for protection and comfort. A series of frightening events will also perpetuate clinging which may persist well into middle childhood (age 5–12). This interferes with the child's capacity to learn how to cope with anxiety on his own.

With entry into school, the importance of teachers and other children in shaping psychosocial development increases, and their influence must be taken into account in understanding any schoolchild's development.

TEMPERAMENT

Children differ from each other in personality from birth, just as they do in physical appearance. This individuality in behavioural style – how they go about things – is partly genetically determined. It is not fixed but changes slowly in the light of experience. It affects how other people deal with them. A child with a difficult temperament is prone to:
- predominantly negative mood; whingeing, moaning, crying
- intense emotional reactions; screaming rather than whimpering, jumping for joy rather than smiling
- irregular biological functions; a lack of rhythm in sleeping, hunger or elimination
- negative initial responses to novel situations, e.g. pushing a new toy away
- protracted adjustment to new situations; taking weeks or months to settle into a new playgroup.

It may be hard for parents to maintain an affectionate relationship with such children and their self-confidence falters, becoming guilty that they have failed as parents. They need support to maintain a positive, loving relationship with their child who will, if this can be done, soften

and become easier to handle over a period of months. If they lapse into irritable intolerance themselves this is likely to maintain the child's grouchy and unsatisfied manner and lead eventually to low self-esteem or the development of behaviour problems.

COGNITIVE STYLE

Below the age of five, the young child thinks in a way quite different from adults. In the term devised by Piaget this is 'pre-operational thought', the characteristics of which are summarised in Figure 20.3. In talking with and explaining things to small children, an appreciation of this is crucial. During middle childhood the dominant mode of thought is practical and orderly (operational thought) but tied to immediate circumstances and specific experiences rather than hypothetical possibilities or metaphors. Not until the mid-teens does the adult style of abstract thought (formal operational thought) begin to appear.

COPING

Children under stress use a number of mental mechanisms to handle their response or to address the source of stress itself. Many of the emotional and behavioural difficulties of childhood can be seen as misplaced and maladaptive coping. Young children tend to regress and behave as younger than they actually are. In particular they cling, using the attachment relationship as a source of comfort. It is common for children to minimise or deny a problem as a way of cutting it down to manageable size. With increasing maturity, children learn a repertoire of coping skills so that they become more flexible in their response to adversities. Less intelligent children are slower to learn a broad repertoire and deploy it selectively, which is probably the main reason for their increased vulnerability to emotional and behavioural problems. It may also be true that the susceptibility of children with chronic physical illnesses to psychological problems derives from their having a narrower range of experiences, particularly with other children, from which they can learn and practise new ways of coping.

Many responses to adversity, including injury and the onset of serious illness in childhood, show a sequence of phases over a period of weeks:
- an initial impact phase of tearfulness

Fig. 20.3 The quality of pre-school thought
The child is at the centre of his world ('I'm tired so it's getting dark')
Everything has a purpose ('The sea is there for us to swim in')
Inanimate objects are alive ('Naughty table hurt me') and have feelings and motives
Poor categorisation (all men are Daddies)
Use of magical thinking ('If I close my eyes, she'll go away')
Use of sequences or routines rather than a sense of time
The use of toys and other aspects of imaginative play as aids to thought (particularly in making sense of experience and social relationships)

- subsequent 'brave' acceptance of injury with psychological denial of the seriousness of the adversity
- recoil, characterised by difficult behaviour or overt unhappiness, perhaps with some regression
- gradual adjustment to altered circumstances.

 Children whose behaviour presents a problem are often trying to solve a problem of their own, albeit in a poorly thought-out or maladaptive way.

Adversities in the family

Family relationships are for most children the source of their most powerful emotions. Similarly, parents have more effect than anyone else on children's social learning and behaviour. It follows that families are generally the most potent environmental influence on a child's mental health. They are not all-powerful, since a predisposition to particular childhood emotional and behavioural problems can be inherited, but family influences interact with this so that overt disorder may or may not emerge. Not all disorders have their origin in family adversities: hyperkinetic disorder, tics and autism arise independent of them. Nevertheless, the non-genetic contribution of family interactions to emotional and behavioural disorders is often substantial and the mechanisms whereby they produce disorder are various. The following are some of the known risk factors:

- angry discord between family members
- parental mental ill-health, especially maternal depression
- divorce (Figs 20.4 and 20.5) and bereavement
- intrusive overprotection
- lack of parental authority
- physical and sexual abuse
- emotional rejection or unremitting criticism
- use of violence, terror, threats of abandonment or excessive guilt as disciplinary devices
- taunting or belittlement of the child
- inconsistent, unpredictable discipline
- using the child to fulfil the personal emotional needs of a parent
- inappropriate responsibilities or expectations for the child's level of maturity.

Many of these can be aggravated by a difficult or unrewarding child who thus creates an adverse environment for himself. It is wrong to blame the parents for causing their child's problem without examining how much the child contributes to the situation.

Problems of the pre-school years

MEAL REFUSAL

A common scenario is a mother complaining that her child refuses to eat any or much of what she provides; mealtimes have become a battleground. Examination reveals a healthy, well-nourished child whose height and weight are securely within normal limits on a centile growth chart, or a small and thin child with a normal growth velocity.

An account of what goes on at a typical mealtime may reveal:

- irregular meals so that the child is not predictably hungry
- unsuitable meals
- unreasonably large portions
- multiple opportunities for distraction.

Most important, how much does the child eat between meals? A well-nourished child is getting food from somewhere. Not all parents regard sweets and crisps as having any nutritional value. Many mothers, while concerned about their child's apparently poor food intake are very restrictive

---

Fig. 20.4 *Reactions to parental divorce*

Pre-school

Fear of further abandonment:
  intensified clinging at threatened separations
  sleep disturbances
  tearful, irritable and demanding
  desultory play

Middle childhood

Miserable at loss of father, pining for restitution of family
Self-blame in younger (age 6–8)
Angry blaming of one parent for divorce in older (age 9–12)
Loyalty conflicts
Anxiety and jealousy at parents' new partners
Educational underachievement

Adolescence

Wide variation in response
Various attempts to master the situation:
  detachment from family
  rapid maturation
  moral idealism
  critical of parents
Educational underachievement
Depression in some

Fig. 20.5 *Adjustment tasks facing children of divorced parents*

1. Acknowledgement of parental separation
2. Regaining sense of direction in life activities
3. Dealing with sense of loss and rejection
4. Forgiving parents for break-up
5. Accepting permanence of divorce, relinquishing wish for the previously intact family
6. Feeling able to enter into new emotional relationships

in the child's diet. One needs to ascertain what the mother is most concerned about: nutrition or lack of discipline? The former can be dealt with by discussion of the child's growth, referring to a growth chart and commenting that he has lots of energy. If the mother remains unconvinced, ask her to complete a food diary, recording all her child's intake over a few days. Many young children prefer to eat small, frequent snacks rather than larger, infrequent meals. So long as they are offered wholesome food, children have been shown to be remarkably good at maintaining a constant energy intake when allowed a free choice. Not uncommonly, the child's refusal to eat at mealtimes is bound up with a struggle for autonomy from his parent. The parent cannot win directly as it is impossible to force a child to eat. If the parents wish their child to have regular mealtimes they can use other strategies as listed in Figure 20.6.

SLEEP-RELATED PROBLEMS
Difficulty in settling to sleep at bedtime
This is a common problem in the toddler years. The child will not go to sleep unless his parent is present. Most instances are normal expressions of separation anxiety, but there may be other obvious reasons for it which can be explored in taking a history (Fig. 20.7), supplemented if necessary by the parents keeping a prospective sleep diary. Many cases will respond to common sense advice:
- creating a bedtime and a bedtime routine which cues in the child to what is required
- telling the child to lie quietly in bed until he falls asleep (children cannot fall asleep to order though that is what everyone tells them to do).

More refractory cases may merit a couple of nights of respite sedation (e.g. with trimeprazine) to enable parents to catch up on lost sleep themselves. Once they are feeling more on top of things, they can impose a graded pattern of lengthening periods between tucking their child up in bed and coming back after a few minutes to visit him,

but leaving the room before the child falls asleep. The object is to provide the opportunity for the child to learn how to fall sleep alone; a skill he has not yet developed.

Waking at night
This is normal, but some children cry because they cannot settle themselves back to sleep without their parent's presence. This is commonly associated with difficulty settling in the evenings which should be treated first. Some children who can settle in the evening may be unable to settle when they wake in the night because the circumstances are different – it is quieter, darker etc. The graded approach described above for evening settling can be used in the middle of the night. Parents will find it helpful to take alternate nights on duty to share the burden. Sedative medication is less likely to be effective than with evening settling, but problems may be sufficient to obtain a couple of nights' respite before the parents tackle the problem directly.

Nightmares
These are bad dreams which can be recalled by the child. They are common and normal among children and do not require professional attention unless they occur more than about twice a week over several weeks or are stereotyped in content, indicating a morbid preoccupation. Reassuring the child will usually suffice.

Night (sleep) terrors
These are different. The child cries out about one and a half hours after settling. His parents find him sitting up in bed, eyes open, seemingly awake but obviously disorientated, confused and distressed and unresponsive to their questions and reassurances. He settles back to sleep after a few minutes and has no recollection of the episode in the morning. A night terror is a parasomnia, a disturbance of the structure of sleep wherein a very rapid emergence from the first period of deep slow-wave sleep produces a state of high arousal and confusion. Sleepwalking has similar origins and the two may be combined. Most night terrors need little more than reassurance directed towards the parents, but they can sometimes be stopped by keeping a record of their

---

Fig. 20.6   Strategy for meal refusal
Mealtime history
What is the parent most concerned about?
Nutrition
Growth chart
Discipline
Family history
What others say
Part of a broader problem?
How much food is eaten between meals?
Food diary
Advice
Avoid confrontation at mealtimes
Develop a relaxed atmosphere; no pressure or bargaining
Use favourite foods as a reward for eating other foods
Limit duration of mealtime, remove uneaten food at end
Reduce eating between meals if necessary

Fig. 20.7   Reasons for a child not settling at night
Too much sleep in the late afternoon
Displaced sleep/wake cycle – not waking child in the morning because he did not settle until late on the previous night
Separation anxiety
Overstimulated or overwrought in evening
Kept awake by siblings or noisy neighbours or TV in the bedroom
Erratic parental practices: no bedtime or routine to cue child into sleep readiness, sudden removal from play to go to bed without prior warning
Use of bedroom as punishment
Dislike of darkness and silence – night light and playing story tapes can be helpful

timing and then briefly waking the child 15 minutes before the terror is expected each night for about a week.

DISOBEDIENCE, DEFIANCE AND TANTRUMS

Toddlers commonly and normally go through a phase of refusing to comply with parents' demands, sometimes angrily ('the terrible twos'). This is an understandable reaction to the discovery that the world is not organised around them. They also become confused and angered by the fact that the parent who provides them with comfort is also the person who is making them do things they do not wish to do; it seems unfair to them. That is why children play their parents up but may be fine with others. All this can exhaust and demoralise parents, not least because everyone offers advice or criticism (everyone thinks themselves an expert in the area of children's development and behaviour). The points listed in Figure 20.8 can be made.

Temper tantrums are ordinarily responses to frustration, especially at not being allowed to have or to do something. They are common and normal in young pre-school children. If asked for advice, a sensible first move is to take a history, analysing a couple of tantrums according to the ABC paradigm (Fig. 20.9). Next, examine the child to identify potential medical or psychological factors. Medical factors include global or language delay, hearing impairment (e.g. glue ear) and medication with bronchodilators or anticonvulsants. If none are present, some management strategies are shown in Figure 20.10.

The easiest course of action is to let the tantrum burn itself out while the parent leaves the room, returning when things quieten. Obviously this should be done in a calm, neutral manner and certainly not accompanied by threats of abandonment. Tantrums which are essentially coercive (when a child is demanding something from a parent) must be met by a refusal to give in. They can often be forestalled by the simple expedient of making rules which the child can be reminded of before the situation presents itself. An alternative course is to use 'time-out' which is a form of structured ignoring. The child in a tantrum is placed somewhere such as the hallway where no one will talk to him for a short time, e.g. one minute per year of age. During this period he is ignored completely. Parents often expect this manoeuvre to produce a contrite child, complaining if it does not do so immediately. In fact it works according to different principles and often takes several weeks to effect a gradual improvement. It may help to ask the mother to keep records to document this.

BREATH-HOLDING ATTACKS

Two kinds of attack can be recognised. In the more common 'blue' variety, frustration leads to tears and holding the breath in expiration at the end of a wail of rage. This is an innocent practice which will not harm the child and could theoretically be ignored by the parents except that to do so requires nerves of steel. All grow out of it before the age of five years.

Less common are the 'white' breath-holding attacks which are precipitated by pain or shock rather than frustration. The child slumps to the floor, pale and not breathing. A seizure may follow secondary to cerebral hypoxia (reflex anoxic seizures). Explanation and reassurance are indicated, not anticonvulsants (which do not help). Later in childhood many of these children are prone to faints.

AGGRESSIVE BEHAVIOUR

Small children can be aggressive for a host of reasons ranging from spite to exuberance. Much aggressive behaviour is learned, either by being rewarded (often inadvertently) or by copying parents or siblings. For example, many instances of aggressive demanding behaviour are provoked or intensified by a parent shouting at or hitting the child. In such cases it is the parent's behaviour which needs to change. In most instances the same principles as apply to tantrums are valid: make rules, stick to them, keep cool, don't give in and use time out if necessary. The latter can often be used on a 1–2–3 principle (Fig. 20.11). Optimistic reassurance that the child will grow out of it is mistaken; once established, an aggressive behavioural style is remarkably persistent over a period of years.

Fig. 20.8 Managing toddler disobedience

Ensure your demand is reasonable for the developmental stage of the child

Tell the child what you want him to do rather than nagging about what you don't want him to do

Praise compliance, especially when spontaneous (catch him doing the right thing)

Use simple incentives to reward good behaviour

Frame deals along the lines of 'If you (do this or that) – then we/I can do such and such' (not the other way round)

Avoid threats that cannot be carried out

Carry out threats that are made

Ignore defiance as much as possible

Fig. 20.9 Analysing a tantrum

Antecedents – what happened in the minutes before the episode
Behaviour – exactly what the episode consisted of
Consequences - what happened as a result

Fig. 20.10 Tantrums: management strategies

Affection and attention
Avoiding antecedents
Ignoring:
    Effective but can be difficult
    No surrender
Time out from positive reinforcement:
    Walk away
    Separate from siblings
    Put on a 'naughty chair'
Holding

Fig. 20.11   The 1–2–3 principle for
tantrums or aggressive behaviour

1. Stop doing that because...
2. If you don't stop that, you must go to your room (or wherever)
3. Go to your room

AUTISM

This developmental condition is rare, with a prevalence rate of approximately 3 per 10 000. It is more common in boys and presents in early childhood but is a lifelong handicap. Autistic children all have a triad of difficulties evident before the age of three years.

1. A severe language disorder
Half will never speak at all; the others show a widespread disorder of language with delayed and abnormal speech, poor comprehension of what is said to them, and no imaginative play. In the early years there is a tendency to echo questions, repeat instructions and to refer to themselves as 'you'.

2. A profound difficulty relating to other people
There is extreme indifference to others and failure to meet their eye in social encounters. They do not show normal attachment behaviour, do not come for comfort when hurt or distressed and do not form close relationships or make friends. They prefer their own company and share neither emotions nor play activities with others. It is as though they do not appreciate that other people have their own thoughts and feelings.

3. Marked routines and rituals associated with a poverty of imagination
Examples are insistence on the same foods or ways of doing things or on sameness in the environment (e.g. the arrangement of furniture in the home). Some carry round odd items such as pieces of wire to which they become very attached. Imposing change or disrupting the child's rituals precipitates violent temper tantrums.

In addition to this triad of features, odd motor patterns such as flapping hands and walking on tiptoe are common. Autistic children seem to be in their own world which they cannot and do not wish to share with others. About two-thirds have a severe learning disability. When describing an autistic child it is essential to specify his level of intelligence. In addition, epileptic seizures occur in about one-quarter of autistic children, though sometimes not until adolescence.

Autism is a behavioural syndrome, most cases of which are probably genetic though it can occasionally follow cerebral disorders such as infantile spasms or encephalitis. Most cases have no identifiable underlying condition. It is certainly not the result of any emotional trauma or deviant parenting.

There is no specific treatment for autism, though new claims for curative interventions surface regularly. The parents are often keen to try these though none have stood the test of replicated controlled evaluation. Parents need as much support as can be provided; it is a devastating handicap to deal with. Some children will require behaviour modification to reduce unwelcome or dangerous

behaviours. An appropriate special school is probably the most important positive influence on development. In the long term only a minority (probably less than 10%) will be able to live independently; most adults with autism will need care in special communities or stay with their parents, attending local day centres and remaining solitary individuals with no interest in social activities or marriage.

Other developmental conditions may share characteristics with autism. Some children with severe general learning disability have the social impairments of autism but without marked rigidity and obsessionality so they are described as having autistic features. Asperger syndrome refers to a mild form of the social impairments of autism in the presence of near-normal speech development. Such children have grave difficulties with the give-and-take of ordinary social encounters, a stilted way of speaking and develop narrow, strange interests which they do not share with others. Some children with developmental language disorders show a limitation of sociability and imagination. All these conditions can be placed on a continuum which ranges from ordinary eccentricity to severe autism and may be referred to as autistic spectrum disorders or pervasive developmental disorders.

Autistic children have:
- *a severe language disorder*
- *profound difficulty relating to other people*
- *marked routines and rituals.*

Problems of middle childhood

NOCTURNAL ENURESIS

Children can wet themselves by day or night, but in colloquial speech 'enuresis' is synonymous with bedwetting. It is quite common: about 15% of five year olds and 3% of ten year olds will wet the bed once a week or more. Boys outnumber girls by nearly two to one. There is a genetically determined delay in acquiring sphincter competence, with two-thirds of children with enuresis having a first-degree relative who was affected. There may also be interference in learning to become dry at night. Small children need reasonable freedom from stress and a measure of parental approval in order to learn night time continence. It is well recognised that emotional stress can interfere and cause secondary enuresis (relapse after a period of dryness). Most children with enuresis are psychologically normal and the treatment of secondary enuresis still relies on the symptomatic approach detailed below, though it often needs to be coupled with attempts to alleviate stress or emotional disorder.

Organic causes of enuresis are uncommon but include:
- urinary tract infection
- faecal retention severe enough to reduce bladder volume and cause bladder neck dysfunction

- polyuria from diabetes or chronic renal failure.

The management of enuresis is straightforward but needs to be painstaking to succeed. Many doctors wait until the child is seven years old before treating, but some younger children are amenable to treatment. After the age of four years enuresis resolves spontaneously in only 5% of affected children each year. Urine is tested for protein and sugar and sent for culture. In an otherwise asymptomatic child it is likely to be normal so treatment can start immediately.

The first step is to explain to both child and parent that the problem is common and beyond conscious control. The parents should stop punitive procedures; these are counterproductive.

Next the child is put on a star chart whereby he earns praise and a star each morning if his bed is dry. Wet beds are treated in a matter-of-fact way and he is not blamed for them.

A child who does not respond to a star chart will usually become dry if it is continued and he uses an enuresis alarm most nights. This is a device which, in its most modern guise, uses a sensor inside a pad inside the child's pants. If this becomes wet, an electrical circuit is completed, sounding an alarm which is attached to his pyjama jacket. In order to be effective, this must wake the child, who gets out of bed, goes to pass urine, returns and helps remake a wet bed before going back to sleep. It is not necessary to re-set the alarm that night. Parental help can be enlisted in the night if a baby alarm is used to transmit the noise of the alarm to the parents' bedroom.

The alarm method takes several weeks to achieve dryness but is effective in most cases so long as the child has the procedure carefully explained to him (or else he will sabotage it). About one-third of cases relapse after a few months in which case retreatment with the alarm usually produces lasting dryness.

Short-term relief from bedwetting can be achieved by the use of the synthetic analogue of antidiuretic hormone, desmopressin, taken as tablets or a nasal spray. This achieves a suppressant effect rather than a lasting cure, something which is also true of imipramine. The latter is best avoided because of the risks to the child and his siblings of accidental overdose which can prove fatal.

 Most children with enuresis are psychologically and physically normal.

FAECAL SOILING

It is abnormal for a child to soil himself after the age of four years. Thereafter, soilers fall into two broad groups – those with and without a rectum loaded with faeces. Because of this, it is important to ascertain whether there is faecal retention by abdominal palpation and by digital ano-rectal examination if required. Faeces in the rectum are always an abnormal finding. The reasons why a child's rectum should become loaded are various and commonly involve an interplay between constitutional factors and experience. Some children have a rectum that only empties occasionally, perhaps because of poor coordination with anal sphincter

relaxation, and are thus more prone to developing retention. Superimposed upon this are a number of other factors:

- constipation, possibly following dehydration during an illness
- inhibition of defaecation because of pain from a fissure
- inhibition because of fear of punishment for incontinence
- anxieties about using the lavatory.

Once established, a huge bolus of hard faeces may be beyond the capacity of the child to shift. Furthermore, a rectum loaded with hard or soft faeces (both are found) dilates and habituates to distension so that the child becomes unaware of the need to empty it. The loaded rectum inhibits the anus via the rectoanal reflex and stool seeps out with spontaneous rectal contractions beyond the child's control. Soiling occurs in the child's pants which may then be removed and hidden out of shame.

Ascertaining the reasons for faecal retention is important because they may need dealing with independently, as in the case of a fissure, but in general the most important thing is to empty the rectum as soon as possible. The child and parents need to understand that retention is present and how it leads to incontinence.

A stool softener (docusate or lactulose) and laxative (sodium picosulphate or senna) will work in most cases but some children will require the addition of a micro-enema if there has been no emptying within a few days. Stronger stimulant laxatives such as sodium picosulphate may be more acceptable than enemas. Once the child has an empty rectum, he can be encouraged to defaecate regularly in the lavatory, which earns stars on a star chart. Such retraining may take a number of weeks while the distended rectum shrinks to normal size. Throughout this period a regular laxative is usually needed. The stars may therefore need to be cashed in for tangible rewards such as extra pocket money in order to maintain the incentive.

In some cases, repeated soiling will have been such a humiliating experience for the child that he psychologically denies there is a problem and his cooperation is doubtful. Others find that their involuntary soiling allows them a measure of revenge against hostile parents and are reluctant to surrender a useful weapon. Such cases will need psychiatric referral. So will children who defaecate intentionally as a hostile act – depositing a stool in the parents' bed for instance. Children in this latter group are not retaining; they have an empty rectum on examination and the discovered stool looks normal. They are entrenched in distorted relationships with their parents.

Soiling may occur in conjunction with an empty rectum on examination for various other uncommon reasons. Some children have an urgency of defaecation for apparently constitutional reasons and can only postpone defaecation for a few minutes; they can be taken by surprise. Some children have a neuropathic bowel secondary to occult spinal abnormality usually associated with urinary incontinence. Similarly, diarrhoea can overwhelm bowel control. Lastly, the child may have a general learning disability with a mental age below four years, so that expectations of social bowel control need to be revised accordingly.

 Most children who soil have faecal retention.

RECURRENT ABDOMINAL PAIN

Recurrent central abdominal pain, often sharp and colicky, affects about 10% of school-age children. The causes are considered in Chapter 11. In the vast majority of cases no organic cause can be objectively demonstrated yet the child is obviously in pain. Some will have an emotional cause for their pain but in many no aetiology, physical or psychological, can be demonstrated.

The history must attend to possible sources of stress and the child should be interviewed about school, friends and family, noting the child's general level of anxiety and ability to communicate. This should be an integral part of the interview and not done as an afterthought when organic causes have been excluded. A thorough physical examination is important to reassure the child and family that there is no underlying organic cause, and provides an opportunity to gain further information about the nature of the pain and the child's reaction to it. When examining the child it is sensible to ask them to point to where the pain is and apply Apley's rule that the further the pain from the umbilicus, the more likely is organic pathology.

A short interview with the child on his own can reveal sources of stress which are otherwise unrecognised by a parent or which the child is wary of mentioning in front of his parents. Problems at school, particularly bullying and teasing or difficulties with a teacher or classwork, may only be known by the child. A report from the school may be helpful. A joint interview with both parents and the child is a good arena for explaining to child and family how organic disease has been ruled out and, if appropriate, how tension can give rise to pain, using familiar examples such as headache. It is often necessary to promote communication between family members to avoid any tendency for somatic symptoms to replace verbal communication. Referral to child psychiatry or psychology is indicated if any identified stressors cannot be relieved by straightforward means, if there is serious family dysfunction, or if the pain impairs the child's general functioning at home or school.

 Although most children with recurrent abdominal pain have no demonstrable organic pathology, this does not necessarily mean it is psychogenic.

TICS

A tic is a quick, sudden, coordinated movement which is apparently purposeful, recurs in the same part of the child's body and can often be reproduced by the child on request. It is not entirely involuntary in that it can be voluntarily suppressed but only at the expense of mounting discomfort. About one in ten children develop a tic at some stage, typically around the face and head – blinking, frowning, head-flicking, sniffing, throat-clearing and grunting being the most common. They are most likely to occur when the child is inactive (watching TV or on long car journeys) and often disappear when he is actively concentrating. They may worsen with anxiety but they are not themselves an emotional reaction. In most cases there is a family history. These simple transient childhood tics clear up over the next few months though they may recur from time to time. They should be treated with reassurance in the first place.

Less commonly the child has tics from which he is hardly ever free. They may be multiple, though there is a fluctuation in the predominance of any particular tic and in overall severity. This is the chronic tic disorder which, if it includes both multiple motor tics and vocal tics such as hooting, yelping or swearing, is known as Gilles de la Tourette syndrome. These conditions tend to be persistent and require medication, usually haloperidol or sulpiride and specialist supervision.

HYPERACTIVITY

Young children are characteristically lively, some more than others by virtue of their temperament. When their level of motor activity exceeds that regarded as normal they may be termed 'hyperactive' by their parents. This is a judgement which depends upon the parents' standards and expectation. The term can thus be used incorrectly as a complaint about a child who is normally active in overall terms but who can be cheeky and boisterous at bedtime, at meals or in class. Such a child is not hyperactive but the parents may need advice about how to handle unwanted behaviour.

In the true hyperkinetic disorder, the child is undoubtedly overactive in most situations and has impaired concentration, with a short attention span or distractibility. Because of the latter, the American terms attention deficit hyperactivity disorder (ADHD) or attention deficit disorder (ADD) are preferred by some. Differences in diagnostic criteria between these labels mean that prevalence rates among prepubertal schoolchildren are variously estimated as between 10 and 50 per 1000 children.

Affected children have disorganised, poorly regulated and excessive activity which has been evident since early childhood. They are typically reckless and impulsive, socially disinhibited, do not finish tasks they are set and have poor relationships with other children. Not uncommonly they have general or specific cognitive impairments as a result of developmental delays, but there is no specific association with brain damage. They do poorly in school and lose self-esteem. They may drift into antisocial activities in their teens, rejecting family relationships and eliciting harsh or inconsistent parental discipline.

First-line management, particularly in pre-school children, is the active promotion of behavioural and educational progress by specific advice to parents and teachers to build concentration skills, encourage quiet self-occupation, increase self-esteem and moderate extreme behaviour. Hyperactivity responds symptomatically to several types of medication though this is usually reserved for children older than about seven years of age. So-called stimulants such as methyl-phenidate channel attention and promote on-task, focused behaviour. However, disorganised attention and overactivity supervene if they are discontinued unless new skills in concentration and self-control are learned during their application. The usual approach is to put the child on medication for 1–2 years while behavioural and educational progress is actively promoted by the specific measures mentioned above. This should be supervised by a child psychiatrist.

The role of diet in the cause and management of hyper-activity is controversial. Current evidence indicates that the sort of diet which aims to reduce sugar, artificial additives or colourants has no effect. A few children display an idio-syncratic behavioural reaction such as excitability or irri-tability to particular foods. If this seems likely, putting the child on a diet restricted to a very few foods may confirm it. Individual foods can be re-introduced while examining for a worsening of behaviour, so that incriminated foods can subsequently be excluded from the child's diet. This is an arduous activity, best implemented by a specialist clinic with careful supervision from a dietician.

ANTISOCIAL BEHAVIOUR

Children steal, lie, disobey, light fires, destroy things and pick fights for various reasons:

- they may not have learned when to exercise social restraint
- they may lack social skills such as the ability to nego-tiate a disagreement
- they may be torn between the challenges of their peers and their parents' prohibitions
- they may be chronically angry and resentful
- they may find their own notions of good behaviour over-whelmed by emotion or temptation.

When serious antisocial behaviour is the dominant feature of the clinical picture and is so severe as to represent a handicap to general functioning or is associated with significant distress, a diagnosis of conduct disorder is made. Children with conduct disorder have not necessarily broken the law though their behaviour excites social disapproval. They typically come from homes in which there is consid-erable discord between family members, especially between the child and his parents. There may be an underlying hyperactivity disorder.

Treating conduct disorder is extremely difficult, not least because parental cooperation is often minimal. It involves a combination of training techniques for parents, family therapy and behaviour therapy and is a task for a mental health professional.

ANXIETY IN MIDDLE CHILDHOOD

Pathological anxiety exist in two forms. In phobias there is fear of an object or situation which is excessive, handicap-ping and cannot be dealt with by reassurance. Most children have a number of irrational fears (the dark, ghosts, kidnap-pers, dogs, spiders, bats, snakes) which are common and do not usually handicap the child's ordinary life. Some of these

persist into adulthood. If they are so severe that the child's ability to lead an ordinary life is affected, then a phobia exists. A clinical psychologist can carry out a behaviour ther-apy programme which is usually successful. Separation anxiety is an instance of a normal developmental fear which can be perpetuated beyond toddlerhood and represents a clinical problem in a schoolchild who has insecure attach-ment. It can also be a symptom of depression or general anx-iety, when it appears to have an onset after a period of secure attachment.

More diffuse anxiety presents indirectly in childhood, and it is rare for a child to complain directly about anxiety. Often it is first manifest as physical complaints: nausea, headache or pain. It may take the form of hypochondriasis and the child repeatedly asks for reassurance that he is not going to die. Some children with generalised anxiety are strikingly manipulative, attempting to gain control over their parents and the world in general so that they can feel less fearful. It may be a justifiable reaction to an event or situation or be disproportionate. If the condition follows a recognisable precipitant, such as a parental illness and the parents can be directed to provide comfort and support, prognosis is good, but if it arises insidiously, specialist referral is indicated.

 Children rarely say they are anxious – instead they complain of aches and pains or behave manipulatively.

SCHOOL REFUSAL

During the years of compulsory school attendance a child may be absent from school because of illness, because his parents keep him off school or because of truancy where the child chooses to do something else rather than attend school. A few non-attenders at school suffer from school refusal, an inabil-ity to attend school on account of overwhelming anxiety. Such children may not complain of anxiety but of its physical concomitants or the consequences of hyperventilation. Thus anxiety may present as complaints of nausea, headache or otherwise not being well, but only on weekday term-time mornings and clearing up by midday. It may be rational, as when the child is being bullied. If it is disproportionate to stresses at school it is termed school refusal, an anxiety prob-lem with two common causes – separation anxiety persisting beyond the toddler years, and anxiety provoked by some aspect of school, true school phobia. These can co-exist.

School refusal based on separation anxiety is typical of children under the age of about 11 years. It may be provoked by an adverse life event such as a death in the family or a move of house. The child is unable to tolerate separation from his attachment figure, without whom he cannot go anywhere, including school. Treatment is aimed at gently promoting increasing separations from the parents (e.g. staying overnight with relatives or friends) while insisting on an early return to school on an agreed date with school authorities, and the child's doctor supporting the parents, who will be under-standably anxious if the child is upset.

True school phobia is seen in slightly older anxious children who are frequently uncommunicative and stubborn. Some adolescents with school refusal are depressed, but more often there is an interaction between an anxiety disorder and longstanding personality issues such as an intolerance of uncertainty. The cornerstone of treatment is an early, graded return to school at a pace the child can stand while support is provided for their parents. Any underlying emotional disorder is treated simultaneously. Close liaison with the education service (teachers, educational welfare officers, educational psychologists) is crucial.

EDUCATIONAL UNDER-ACHIEVEMENT

Children who achieve less well in school than expected are sometimes brought to doctors. It is important to evaluate parents' and teachers' expectations and ensure the child is actually able to rise to them. The services of an educational psychologist are indispensable. Core medical responsibilities include testing sight and hearing and attempting to elicit the cause of under-achievement according to the list in Figure 20.12.

A particular issue arises with respect to dyslexia, a difficulty in learning to read in spite of adequate intelligence and teaching. Dyslexia is a statement of a problem not a complete diagnosis; otherwise competent children may find the complex task of learning to read difficult for a number of reasons, such as a developmental language disorder or visual perceptual problems. Post-mortem and cerebral imaging studies have shown some to have various abnormalities of brain structure, but this is not universal. A number of children with dyslexia have other developmental problems, such as motor dyspraxia or hyperactivity. A very small number have poorly established eye dominance, cannot follow lines of print on the page and seem to benefit from manoeuvres such as occluding one eye for several

months. The whole subject of dyslexia is controversial and there is no agreed classification. There is no medical treatment; affected children need special reading tuition from a skilled teacher. The child easily becomes demoralised and prone to develop bad classroom behaviour. Ultimately, many learn to read adequately, but spelling difficulties usually persist.

Adolescence

Although a popular image of adolescence is one of angry, rebellious teenagers, alienated from their parents and embroiled in emotional turmoil, studies show that most adolescents maintain good relationships with their parents, though they tend to bicker with them about minor domestic matters and what they are allowed to do. Minor psychological symptoms, such as moodiness or social sensitivity, are quite common (as they are in adults), but serious psychiatric problems are no more prevalent than in adult life. Family relationships are often influenced by the teenager's negotiation of their own autonomy, the emergence of their own sense of themselves and the first moves towards a personal identity. At the same time parents may themselves be experiencing mid-life crises of confidence in career, physical appearance or sexuality so that parental and teenage preoccupations coincide, not always helpfully.

COGNITIVE STYLE

The style of thought specifically associated with adolescence is formal operational thought (Fig. 20.13), but this is acquired at various ages by different individuals during the teenage years, and a substantial minority seem never to develop it at all. Doctors are at a disadvantage here, as they have been selected by a series of examinations for excellence of their ability to manipulate abstractions and compare hypothetical predictions; they have often forgotten what it is like to think otherwise. They communicate poorly with patients who still think concretely and practically (school-age children, about half of all teenagers and perhaps one in five adults). When interviewing adolescents, the skill is to avoid being patronising while being tentative as to whether abstract and reflective thought is solidly achieved. Using practical examples (not metaphors) and checking whether you have been understood will help avoid the common problem of being faced with an adolescent who responds to questions with a sullen 'don't know'.

Fig. 20.12   Causes of under-achievement at school

Long-standing problem

Visual problems

Hearing problems

Unrecognised general learning disability

Dyslexia

Other specific learning problems (rare)

Hyperactivity

Anti-education family back-ground

Chaotic family background

Recent onset of problem

Preoccupations (parental divorce, bullying etc)

Fatigue

Depression

Rebellion against teacher, parents or 'swot' label

Unsuspected poor attendance at school

Sexual abuse

Drug abuse

Schizophrenia (rare)

Degenerative brain condition (rare but important)

Fig. 20.13   Formal operational thought

The ability to form abstract thoughts

Comparing implications of hypotheses

Thinking about one's own thinking

Testing the logic that links propositions

Manipulating interactive abstract concepts

ANOREXIA NERVOSA

Dieting to slim is endemic among teenage girls. Part of the reason for this is the contemporary equation between thinness and attractiveness, an assumption prevalent in advertising and fashion. Resonant with this is the finding that most teenage girls (but very few boys) overestimate their body width and depth, perceiving and judging themselves as fatter than they actually are.

Slimming through self-imposed calorie restriction is usually self-limiting because the goal is achieved or because the girl gives up; hunger wins through. In some girls, however, the slimming process takes over and there supervenes what has been called a 'relentless pursuit of thinness' typically with a phobic horror of normal body weight and shape. This is anorexia nervosa. Features are:

- a distorted perception of the body which increases with weight loss
- when body weight falls below about 48 kg, pubertal development is halted and reversed so that menstruation ceases and the girl effectively becomes a pre-pubertal child. This may spare her some of the challenges of adolescence, particularly those related to sexuality
- the discovery by a girl who has felt powerless, that through self-starvation she can control her shape and development
- preoccupations and dreams of food and cooking which come to dominate mental life as a response to starvation. There ensues a tremendous mental struggle not to give in and eat, which assumes prime importance in the girl's mental life. It becomes a way of pursuing a purposeful but simple life by condensing or displacing other more complex concerns, so that thinness becomes the absolute standard and other issues are secondary
- the dramatic and visible effects of self-starvation on the girl, which can unite some parents in caring for their daughter and save a discordant marriage from divorce, something which she may fear is imminent.

An affected girl will often deny hunger, reassure everyone that she is in the peak of health, exercise to lose weight and disagree fervently that she is too thin. She will be careless of her own emaciation and seem unconcerned that she is starving herself to death. To the bewilderment of her parents she may cook for others and read cookery books avidly. She may well be deceitful to anyone she perceives as thwarting her in her quest. Thus she will conceal her poor eating by secretly disposing of her meals or lying about her weight. Both before and during her illness she will show obsessional, perfectionistic character traits; without these she would not have the capacity to establish herself as a persistent dieter. Indeed, she is likely to be described as having been quiet, compliant and hard-working, 'the last person to develop anorexia nervosa'. Her parents will often present as nice people who avoid conflict.

As a result of starvation her body develops a low metabolic rate with slow-to-relax tendon reflexes, reduced peripheral circulation, bradycardia and amenorrhoea. Fine lanugo hair appears over the trunk and limbs. She does not lose pubic or axillary hair, though incompletely established puberty is delayed. Serum T3 may be low, giving rise to a false suspicion of hypothyroidism. Plasma proteins are sometimes low and ankle oedema not uncommon. Blood and urine levels of LH and FSH are low and non-cyclical.

Some girls discover that self-restraint in carbohydrate intake can be bypassed by self-induced vomiting and that weight can be lost through diuretics. Some take laxatives in the belief that these will remove the food they have eaten. This can cause wide fluctuations in weight and metabolic abnormalities such as hypokalaemia and alkalosis. This is bulimia, which can occur at normal body weight or as an ominous complication of anorexia nervosa. It tends to affect older rather than younger teenagers. Bulimia at normal body weight can be managed by encouraging a regular diet, monitoring this by a diary and providing individual or group psychotherapy.

The prevalence rate among teenagers for anorexia nervosa is a little less than 1%, but the incidence rate has been increasing over the last 50 years. The peak age of onset is 14 years and girls outnumber boys by about 20 to 1. Bulimia is more common, though prevalence rates vary widely depending on the degree of severity. It similarly shows a markedly female preponderance and may also be becoming more frequent.

Management

The initial management of anorexia nervosa is to restore near normal body weight by refeeding. If possible this should first be done as an outpatient and will need a series of meetings with the girl and her parents in which the seriousness of the situation is explained. The girl's weight, not her eating, is monitored and a gain of about 500 g a week is required. Failure to meet this target results in admission to hospital for refeeding with no appeal or bargaining accepted. Good nursing is the key to this but there are a very small number who continue to lose weight in hospital and tube-feeding may be required. An initial daily dietary intake of about 2000 calories is adopted, as trying to enforce large meals is usually unsuccessful. A more psychotherapeutic approach may be introduced when weight has reached the level it was before dieting started. It is aimed at counselling the girl and her family in more constructive ways of confronting developmental demands including handling conflict, personal autonomy and relationships.

The prognosis is reasonably good, but about a quarter of the most intransigent who have needed treatment in specialist units develop a chronic relapsing course. Rather less than 5% die by suicide, malnutrition or infection, though usually not until later in life. Most recover their weight permanently, though they often remain wary of eating and minor psychosexual problems affect about one-third of them.

 Girls with anorexia nervosa seldom agree that they are too thin and may deceive everyone by pretending to eat.

CHRONIC FATIGUE SYNDROME

Chronic fatigue syndrome (CFS) refers to persisting high levels of subjective fatigue leading to rapid exhaustion on physical or mental exertion. The term is broader and more neutral than the specific pathology or aetiology implied by myalgic encephalomyelitis (ME) or post-viral fatigue syndrome, which follows an apparently viral febrile illness. There is sometimes serological evidence of recent infection with Coxsackie B or Epstein–Barr virus (EBV) or a hepatitis virus. Some cases have no history or evidence of a precipitating infection and there are no specific diagnostic tests. The clinical picture is somewhat diffuse and there are no pathognomonic symptoms. Myalgia, migratory arthralgia, headache, difficulty getting off to sleep, poor concentration and irritability are virtually universal. Stomach pains, scalp tenderness, eye pain and photophobia, and tender cervical lymphadenopathy are frequently encountered. Depressive symptoms are common and there is continuing debate as to how much of the clinical picture is physical and how much psychological. Usually parents insist on there being a physical cause, and there is a risk that the doctor will be pressurised into excessive unprofitable investigations. Most experienced doctors now regard the final clinical picture as resulting from both physical and psychological factors.

The majority of cases will remit spontaneously with time but this takes months or sometimes years. Earlier recommendations of continuous rest have been shown to be unhelpful and can lead to secondary complications. The preferred approach is to adopt a gentle rehabilitative approach, possibly involving physiotherapy, so that exercise tolerance is gradually increased. If too much pressure is put upon the child, tantrums or mute withdrawal can occur. Argument about how much of the condition is physical, how much psychological are unhelpful. Parents and child need continuing support to maintain as much of a normal life, including school attendance, as possible. The mood of children with depressive symptoms may respond to antidepressant medication but this is a partial treatment and it is unlikely that this will result in alleviation of the fatiguability.

DEPRESSION

Low mood can arise secondary to adverse circumstances or sometimes spontaneously. Depression as a clinical condition is more than sadness and misery, it extends to affect motivation and the ability to experience pleasure and provokes inner ideas of guilt and despair. It may disturb sleep, appetite and weight. It leads to social withdrawal, an important sign. Such a state is well recognised among adolescents but occasionally affects prepubertal children. The general picture is comparable to depression in adults, but there are differences (Fig. 20.14).

A diagnosis of depression depends crucially upon interviewing the adolescent on his own as well as taking a history from the parents. Teenagers will, out of loyalty, often pretend to their parents that things are all right. It is necessary to ask about feelings directly and ask specifically about suicidal ideas and plans.

Treatment depends upon the relationship between low mood and causal circumstances. Adversity such as bullying should be reversed if possible. If this cannot be done, as in the case of impending parental divorce, then counselling support is required. If it seems as though environmental factors are an insufficient explanation, then an antidepressant which is reasonably safe in overdose, is indicated. Suicidal teenagers need admission to a psychiatric unit but an intentional overdose is not good evidence of suicidal intent. Like adults, teenagers who take overdoses do so for a variety of motives of which suicide is only one. For a good proportion, the overdose is a way of expressing revenge, or a blind and desperate gesture which may draw attention to a predicament perceived by them as irresolvable. Most teenagers who overdose are not clinically depressed.

 Most adolescents who take an overdose are not clinically depressed.

DRUG MISUSE

Most teenagers are exposed to illicit drugs at some stage. A number will then experiment with them, some of these become habitual users. Usually this is for recreational purposes, but a few use them to avoid unpleasant feelings or memories. A very small number become dependent, psychologically or physically. What is taken varies with culture and opportunity but alcohol and cannabis are common; solvents, LSD and amphetamine derivatives a little less so, and cocaine or heroin currently least prevalent. The addictive potential of the last two is the greatest and their dangers are well known.

Abuse implies heavy misuse. The signs vary with the agent but include:

*   intoxication
*   unexplained absences from home or school
*   mixing with known users
*   high rates of spending or stealing money
*   possession of the equipment required for ingestion
*   medical complications associated with use.

Doctors may be asked by worried parents whether an

Fig. 20.14 Features of depression in adolescents

More common than adults

Apathy, boredom and an inability to enjoy oneself rather than depressed mood

Separation anxiety which reappears having resolved in earlier life

Decline in school performance

Running away from home

Hypochondriacal ideas and complaints of pain in chest, abdomen and head

Irritable mood or frank anti-social behaviour

Less common than adults

Loss of appetite and weight

Loss of sleep

Loss of libido

Slowing of thought and movement

Delusional ideas

adolescent is abusing and the question can often only be resolved by interviewing the adolescent (and quite often not then). Medical input is predominantly focused on solitary users who usually have other psychopathology including depression, or with the physical consequences of intoxication or injection when these threaten health. Solvent abuse (mainly glue and aerosol sniffing) is quite widespread as a group activity in some areas and is usually of no more consequence than under-age drinking. It can ocassionally give rise to cardiac dysrhythmias, bone marrow suppression or renal failure, and any of these can cause death, as may a fall when intoxicated. Cannabis and LSD use are usually not dangerous but in occasional adolescents trigger anxiety or psychotic disorders. Ecstasy taken at dances or raves can cause dangerous hyperthermia and dehydration.

Doctors need to ensure that any adolescent known to them who is thought to be using drugs knows the specific risks to health. Dependence is rare among teenagers and most likely to be to alcohol. The few who are using illicit drugs for respite from psychological distress need referral to a psychiatrist.

general practitioners and paediatricians in particular, are good generalists in child mental health issues and the psychiatrist or psychologist should be seen as a specialist extension of their expertise.

In general, the management of children's emotional and behavioural problems:
- is psychological rather than pharmacological
- does not need the child to be admitted to hospital
- involves parents as key participants
- may involve a variety of health and social service professionals.

Often more than one intervention is required, so that treatments are combined and several professionals become involved. The main treatment interventions employed are described in Figure 20.16.

Medication plays a comparatively small role though particular instances are the use of stimulant drugs in hyperkinetic disorder and antidepressants with depressed adolescents. There is a temptation to sedate a child who is causing a problem, but this is rarely effective or ethical.

Management of emotional and behavioural problems

ASSESSMENT

It is best to interview both parents if possible. While doing so, consider the quality of their marriage and the parents' mental state. Ask open questions where possible and feel able to ask directly about feelings. Assess the attitudes of the parents to the child. Obtain examples of the problem and estimate its frequency, severity, duration and the impact it has on both child and family.

Interview the child alone if it seems appropriate. Explain to the parents that you always like to have a few words with children on their own as you are their doctor, too. Assess the extent of the child's suffering (he may be somewhat brazen and minimise this). Keep your questions very simple and specific, making sure the child understands what it is you want to know. This also applies to teenagers. Consider whether reports from school or other involved agencies might help. In many instances it is worth asking the parents to keep a prospective record of the problem by means of a diary or chart which you can inspect in a few days time. Tell them what headings you want (such as Antecedents, Behaviour and Consequences for temper tantrums).

MANAGEMENT

Figure 20.15 shows an approach to managing a child displaying an emotional or behavioural problem. The process of making a referral to a psychiatric or psychological service is most likely to succeed if the referrer has already taken some of the history and engaged the parents and child in an attempt to alleviate the problem. Many doctors,

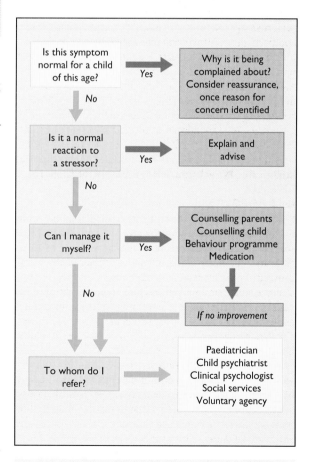

Fig. 20.15 An approach to children's psychological problems.

Fig. 20.16 *Main treatment interventions employed for emotional and behaviour problems*

Explanation and reassurance

Suitable for mild problems with a good prognosis arising in children from supportive families who can work out with some help a sensible way of managing the problem until it subsides.

Counselling of child or parents

Used to modify attitudes and habits of thought. A child with a difficult temperament would be an indication for parental counselling, an adolescent who is anxiously hypochondriacal could be counselled himself.

Individual or group dynamic psychotherapy

More structured and intense extension of counselling which can help children who, for example, have emotional conflicts which are manifest as relationship difficulties with a parent. It requires a number of sessions, usually one a week, carried out in privacy. Once the mainstay of child psychiatry it is now more sparingly used, especially with children with a distorted inner mental world.

Behaviour therapy

Uses a pragmatic approach to problems which alters the environmental factors which trigger or maintain behaviours. It is particularly effective in the management of behaviour problems in young children.

Family therapy

Has become widely used by child mental health professionals. It uses a series of interviews with the entire household to alter dysfunctional patterns of relationships between family members on the basis that many children's problems are perpetuated by the ways in which family members live with and deal with each other.

MENTAL HEALTH PROFESSIONALS IN THE UK

Many emotional and behaviour problems which do not resolve with sensible parenting are managed by the various non-medical professions involved with children. Thus health visitors, teachers, educational welfare officers (educational social workers) and school nurses see a number of problems and can offer advice or direct help.

If necessary, troubled children may then be referred by the above to educational psychologists or community paediatricians who see a number of children in a school setting, and social workers will become involved with problematic children from poorly functioning families, particularly when there are child protection issues.

General practitioners and community paediatricians also see a large number of problems at a primary care level, particularly among pre-school children and can manage these themselves or refer them accordingly to secondary care services. Hospital paediatricians also see a number of children with emotional and behavioural problems. They may manage them themselves or refer on to specialised children's mental health services. These include a number of different professionals, and although they have a number of interviewing and simple treatment skills in common, each mental health profession has particular skills and responsibilities.

Specialist child mental health professionals commonly work together in a multidisciplinary team when managing complex cases. Such teams may work in child guidance units or be placed in the community or in hospital child and adolescent psychiatry outpatient clinics.

Inpatient psychiatric units and day units for children and adolescents are specialist resources for the most severe cases and are often shared by several clinics and hospitals.

Clinical psychologists work with child and adolescent psychiatrists or operate independently, accepting referrals directly from general practitioners and paediatricians. This is useful for those psychological issues which can be separated out from physical concerns, e.g. phobias, or for a specific psychological task, e.g. the behavioural management of enuresis. Specifically educational problems should be addressed by educational psychologists and referral to these is usually made directly by the child's school.

The more complex cases, especially those where there are physical symptoms or coexisting physical conditions, or when signs of mental illness are present, will need specialist medical expertise and should be referred to a child and adolescent psychiatrist. In a good, integrated child mental health service there should be dialogue and cross-referral between general practitioners, paediatricians, child clinical psychologists, child psychotherapist, psychiatric social workers and child psychiatrists. Mental ill-health in children and teenagers is too pervasive a problem to be only a specialist concern.

FURTHER READING

Black D, Cottrell D. (eds) *Seminars in Child and Adolescent Psychiatry,.* Gaskell, London, 1993. General textbook.

Garralda M E. (ed) *Managing Children with Psychiatric Problems.* BMJ Publishing Group, London, 1993. Short book on approaches to treatment.

Graham P. *Child Psychiatry: A Developmental Approach.* 2nd edn. Oxford University Press, Oxford, 1991. General textbook.

Hall D, Hill P, Elliman D. *The Child Surveillance Handbook.* 2nd edn. Radcliffe Medical Press, Oxford, 1994. Book on young children from a general practice viewpoint.

Rutter M, Taylor E, Hersov L. (eds) *Child and Adolescent Psychiatry: Modern Approaches.* 3rd edn. Blackwell Scientific, Oxford, 1994. Authoritative comprehensive textbook.

Skin

Skin conditions are immediately apparent, leading to prompt medical consultation. In the neonatal period, skin lesions are common. While most are transient or treatable, some naevae are permanent and disfiguring, causing anguish for parents and subsequently for the child. Fortunately, some of these lesions can now be removed by laser therapy when the child is older. Many skin conditions in children are chronic and can lead to psychological problems from teasing and ill-informed, critical comments from doctors and peers. In teenagers, any chronic skin disorder, such as even relatively mild acne, can cause considerable upset.

The newborn

The skin at birth is covered with *vernix caseosa*, a bactericidal greasy coat produced by epithelial cell breakdown. In the preterm infant the skin is thin and poorly keratinised and subcutaneous fat is lacking. Transepidermal water loss is markedly increased when compared to a term infant. The preterm infant is also unable to sweat until a few weeks of age, in contrast with the term infant who is able to sweat from a few days of age.

Common birth marks and rashes in the newborn period are described under the examination of the newborn infant (see Chapter 7). Some rare skin conditions which present in the newborn period are described in this chapter.

COLLODION BABY

This is a rare manifestation of the inherited ichthyotic skin diseases, where the skin is dry and scaly. Infants are born with a taut parchment of collodion-like membrane (Fig. 21.1). The membrane becomes fissured and desquamates, leaving normal or ichthyotic skin.

EPIDERMOLYSIS BULLOSA

This is a rare group of conditions with blistering of the skin and mucous membranes. Autosomal dominant varieties tend to be milder, autosomal recessive varieties may be very severe and fatal. Blisters occur spontaneously and following minor trauma (Fig. 21.2). They need to be differentiated from scalds. Management is mainly supportive to avoid injury from even minor trauma and secondary infection. In the severe forms, the fingers and toes may become fused, and contractures of the limbs develop from repeated blistering and healing. Mucous membrane involvement may result in oral ulceration and stenosis from oesophageal erosions. Management should be by a team including a paediatric dermatologist, paediatrician, plastic surgeon and dietician.

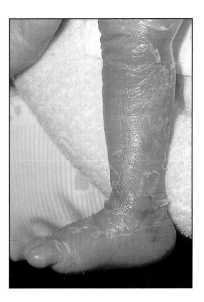

Fig. 21.1
Collodion skin in a newborn infant.

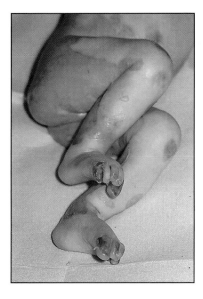

Fig. 21.2
Severe, autosomal recessive form of epidermolysis bullosa.

MELANOCYTIC NAEVI

Congenital pigmented naevi involving extensive areas of skin (Fig. 21.3) are rare but disfiguring and carry a risk of subsequent malignant melanoma. Such lesions require referral to a specialist promptly after birth for removal.

Acquired small melanocytic naevi become increasingly common as children grow older, particularly in those with fair skin and on sun-exposed sites. Most of the lesions are benign. However, the incidence of malignant melanoma in adults has increased dramatically. Between 1974 and 1988 the number of new cases of malignant melanoma in the UK rose from 1732 to 4438, an increase of 156%. Risk factors include having a large number of melanocytic naevi, fair skin, repeated episodes of sunburn, living in a hot climate with chronic skin exposure to the sun and a family history of melanoma. Sun block should be applied to the skin before exposure to intense sunshine.

 Parents should prevent their children becoming sunburnt.

Rashes of infancy

NAPKIN RASHES

Napkin rashes are common, although they appear to have become less of a problem since the widespread use of disposable napkins. The causes are shown in Figure 21.4. Chemical irritant dermatitis is the most common form of napkin rash. It is due to the irritant effect of urine and faeces on the skin. Urea-splitting organisms in urine increase the alkalinity, aggravating the problem. Napkin rashes will occur if napkins are not changed frequently enough or if the baby has diarrhoea. However, they occur even when the napkin area is cleaned regularly.

The rash affects the convex surfaces of the buttocks, perineal region, lower abdomen and top of the thighs. Characteristically, the flexures are spared, which differentiates it from other causes of napkin rash. The rash is erythematous and may have a scalded appearance. More severe forms are associated with erosions and ulcer formation. Mild cases respond to the use of a barrier cream, such as zinc and castor oil or metanium. Napkins need to be changed regularly. More severe cases respond to mild topical corticosteroids. While leaving the child without a napkin will accelerate resolution it is rarely practical at home.

Candida infection often complicates napkin rashes. The rash is erythematous, includes the skin flexures and there may be satellite lesions (Fig. 21.5). Treatment is with a topical antifungal agent.

SEBORRHOEIC DERMATITIS

This rash of unknown cause presents in the first two months of life. It starts on the scalp as an erythematous scaly eruption. The scales become heaped to form a thick yellow adherent layer, commonly called cradle-cap. The scaly rash may spread to the face, behind the ears and then extend to the flexures and napkin area (Fig. 21.6). In contrast with atopic eczema it is not itchy and the child is unperturbed by it. Mild cases will resolve with emollients. The scalp scales need to be cleared with a mild topical steroid or, if the scaling is very thick, with an emulsifying ointment containing a mixture of sulphur and salicylic acid applied to the scalp daily for a few hours and then washed off. The rash on the body will clear with a mild topical corticosteroid, either alone or mixed with an antibacterial and antifungal agent if appropriate.

Fig. 21.4 Causes of napkin rashes	
Common	**Rare**
Chemical irritant dermatitis	Acrodermatitis enteropathica
Seborrhoeic dermatitis	(see Chapter 11)
Candida infection	Langerhans cell histiocytosis
Atopic eczema	(Letterer-Siwe disease)
	(see Chapter 18)
	Wiskott-Aldrich syndrome
	(see Chapter 12)

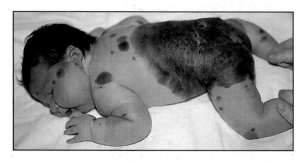

Fig. 21.3 A large congenital pigmented hairy naevus.

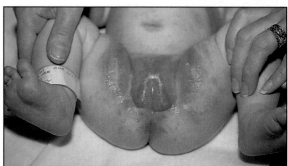

Fig. 21.5 Napkin rash from Candida *infection. The skin flexures are involved and there may be satellite lesions.*

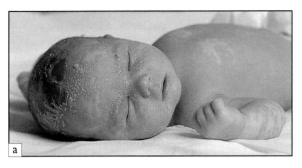
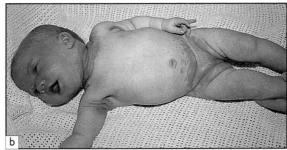

Fig. 21.6   Seborrhoeic dermatitis. a) Cradle cap. b) Distribution on the scalp and face, behind the ears, flexures and nappy area.

ATOPIC ECZEMA

Atopic eczema affects 5–10% of all children. Its onset is usually in the first two years of life. It is however rare in the first two months when seborrhoeic dermatitis is common. There is usually a family history of atopic disorders – eczema, asthma and hayfever. Up to half the children with atopic eczema will develop asthma or hayfever. Exclusive breast-feeding may delay the onset of eczema in predisposed children. Atopic eczema is mainly a disease of childhood with about 50% resolving by five years of age and a further 30% by the early teens.

Diagnosis

The diagnosis is made clinically. Most affected children are atopic. If performed, most affected children have an elevated plasma IgE concentration and positive skin and radioallergosorbent (RAST) tests to do a wide range of allergens. If the disease is unusually severe, atypical or associated with unusual infections or failure to thrive,

an immune deficiency disorder should be excluded.

Clinical features

Itching is the main symptom (Figs 21.7 and 21.8). The excoriated areas become erythematous, weeping and crusted. The change in distribution of the rash with age is shown in Figure 21.9. The skin is dry, and prolonged scratching and rubbing of the skin may lead to lichenification (Fig. 21. 10).

Complications

The reasons for exacerbations of eczema are listed in Figure 21.11. Infection can occur readily, as the natural barrier of the skin is damaged, and is most often bacterial, usually staphylococcal or streptococcal. Herpes simplex virus infection is potentially very serious as it can spread rapidly on damaged eczematous skin causing an extensive vesicular reaction, eczema herpeticum or Kaposi varicelliform eruption (see Chapter 12). Lymphadenopathy is common and usually resolves when the skin improves.

Itching

Fig. 21.7   Itchy rashes
Atopic eczema
Chicken pox
Urticaria/allergic reactions
Contact dermatitis
Scabies
Insect bites
Fungal infections
Dermatitis herpetiformis
Pityriasis rosea

 No itch? – then it's not eczema

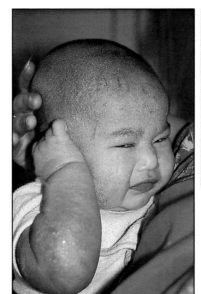

Fig. 21.8 Excoriation of the skin from scratching. Itch is the key clinical feature in eczema at all ages, leading to an 'itch–scratch–itch' cycle.

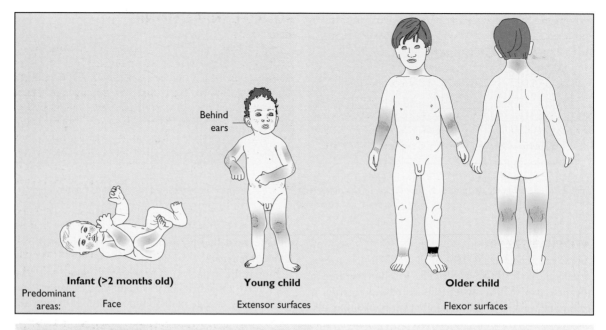

Behind
ears

Infant (>2 months old)

Predominant
areas: Face

Young child

Extensor surfaces

Older child

Flexor surfaces

Fig. 21.9 Distribution of atopic eczema. The distribution of eczema changes with age. In infants the face and sometimes the trunk and napkin area are affected. In young children the lesions affect the extensor surfaces of the limbs, while in older children the skin flexures are characteristically involved.

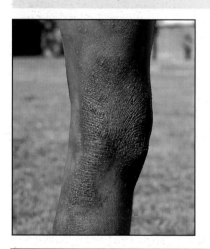

Fig. 21.10
Lichenifica-
tion, thicken-
ing of the skin
and accent-
uation of skin
creases from
persistent
scratching.

Fig. 21.11   Causes of exacerbation of eczema

Bacterial infection:

staphylococcus

streptococcus

Viral infection:

herpes simplex

Fungal infection

Contact with an allergen

Environmental – heat, humidity

Change or reduction in medication

Psychological stress

Unexplained

Management

In most children the condition is mild and can be well contained. However, some children suffer severe disease which can affect the child's whole outlook on life. The parents become distressed seeing their child's uncontrolled scratching resulting in skin damage. The parents and child need considerable advice, help and support from health professionals, other affected families or fellow sufferers.

Avoiding irritants

It is advisable to avoid soap and biological detergents. Clothing next to the skin should be of pure cotton where possible, avoiding nylon and pure woollen garments. Nails need to be cut short and mittens at night may be helpful.

Emollients

These, e.g. hydrous ointment and aqueous cream, should be used frequently, two or three times daily, when the skin is very dry. Ointments are preferable to creams when the skin is dry. A daily bath using oil and emulsifying ointment as a soap substitute is also beneficial.

Topical corticosteroids

This is the most effective treatment for eczema, but must be used with care. Mild corticosteroids, such as 1% hydrocortisone ointment, can be applied to the eczematous areas twice daily. Moderately potent topical steroids play a pivotal role in the management of acute exacerbations, but their use must be kept to a minimum since they may cause thinning of the skin as well as systemic side-effects.

Occlusive bandages

These are helpful when scratching and lichenification are

a problem. These may be impregnated with tar paste or dilute corticosteroid creams. The bandages are worn at night until the skin has improved.

Antibiotics or antibacterial agents
Can be applied topically with hydrocortisone for mild infections. They may occasionally cause a sensitivity reaction and should only be used for short periods. Systemic antibiotics are required for more serious infections. The antiviral agent acyclovir is given for eczema herpeticum.

H_1 histamine antagonists
Itch suppression is with H_1 histamine antagonists given at night. They are not helpful during the day as they are sedative in the dose required to suppress itch.

Dietary elimination
Can be considered in those who do not respond to topical treatment. The main food allergens are cow's milk, egg, soy and wheat. However, any food may be implicated. Three to four weeks of dietary elimination is usually sufficient to detect a response. This should be carried out under the supervision of a dietician to ensure complete avoidance of specific food constituents and that the diet remains nutritionally adequate. As interpreting the result of dietary elimination is problematic, a double-blind placebo-controlled food challenge is required to be fully objective. Children often become able to tolerate the offending foods as they become older.

Infections and infestations

Acute bacterial and viral infections of the skin are considered in Chapter 12.

VIRAL WARTS
These are caused by the human papilloma virus. Warts are common in older children, usually on the fingers and soles of the feet (veruccae). Most disappear spontaneously over a few months or years and treatment is only indicated if the lesions are painful or are a cosmetic problem. They can be treated by the daily application of salicylic acid and lactic acid paint or glutaraldehyde lotion. Cryotherapy with liquid nitrogen or with carbon dioxide snow is an effective treatment but can be painful and often needs to be repeated.

MOLLUSCUM CONTAGIOSUM
This is caused by a DNA virus of the pox group. The lesions are small, skin-coloured, pearly papules with central umbilication (Fig. 21.12). They may be single but are usually multiple. Lesions will disappear spontaneously within a year but may spread to other sites. If necessary, they can be treated by pricking the centre with a sharpened stick dipped in liquid phenol or, more often, with cryotherapy.

FUNGAL INFECTIONS
Ringworm
Dermatophyte fungi invade dead keratinous structures, such as the horny layer of skin, nails and hair. The term ringworm is commonly used because of the lesion's annular appearance. Tinea capitis (scalp ringworm), usually transmitted from dogs and cats, causes a scaling and patchy alopecia, with the hairs broken just above the scalp. When there is a severe inflammatory pustular patch, this is called a kerion (Fig. 21.13). Examination under ultraviolet (Wood's) light shows bright greenish/yellow fluorescence of the infected hairs with some fungal species.

Rapid diagnosis can be made by microscopic examination of skin scrapings for fungal hyphae. Definitive identification of the fungus can be undertaken by culture. Treatment of mild infections is with topical antifungal preparations, but more severe infections require systemic treatment with griseofulvin for several weeks. The animal source of infection also needs to be treated.

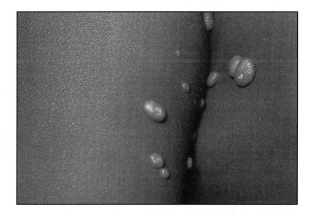

Fig. 21.12 *Molluscum contagiosum on the chest and upper arm showing the pearly papules with central umbilication through which the infectious central core is eventually shed.*

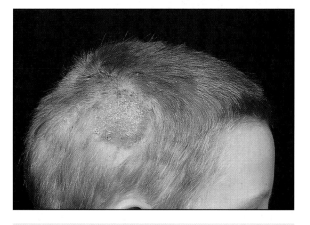

Fig. 21.13 *Ringworm of the scalp.*

PARASITIC INFESTATIONS
Scabies

Scabies is caused by an infestation with the mite, *Sarcoptes scabiei*, which burrows several millimetres to a few centimetres into the stratum corneum, causing a papular and vesicular rash. Severe itching occurs 2–6 weeks after infestation and is worse in warm conditions. In older children, lesions involve the skin between the fingers and toes, axillae, flexor aspects of the wrists, belt line and areas around the nipples, genitalia and buttocks. In infants and young children, the distribution often includes the palms, soles and trunk (Fig. 21.14). The head, neck and face can be involved in babies but is uncommon.

Diagnosis is made on clinical grounds with the history of itching and characteristic lesions. Although burrows are considered pathognomonic in adults, they are frequently absent in children. Itching in other family members is a helpful clinical indicator. Confirmation can be made by microscopic examination of skin scrapings from the lesions to identify the adult mite, ova or larvae. It is often negative in children.

Complications

The skin becomes excoriated due to scratching and may look like eczema, masking the true diagnosis. Secondary bacterial infection is common, giving crusted, pustular and sometimes nodular lesions.

Treatment

As it is spread by close family contact, the child and whole family should be treated whether or not they have evidence of infestation. Monosulfiram or gammabenzene hexachloride (1% lindane) should be applied twice below the neck on two consecutive nights. In babies, the face and scalp should be included, avoiding the eyes. Gammabenzene hexachloride should not be used repeatedly in young children as possible central nervous system toxicity has been reported. Benzylbenzoate emulsion is best avoided in children as it is highly irritant.

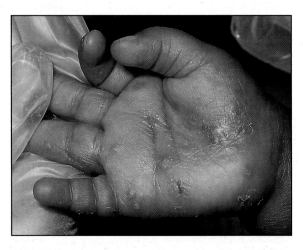

Fig. 21.14 *Scabies in a young child affecting the palm of the hand.*

Pediculosis

Pediculosis capitis is the most common form of louse infestation in children. It is widespread and troublesome among school children. Presentation may be with itching of the scalp or from identifying nits (egg capsules), which are small whitish oval capsules, approximately 0.5 mm long attached to the hair shafts near the scalp. The lice may sometimes be seen when combing the hair. Involvement of the eyelashes may cause conjunctivitis. There may be secondary bacterial infection leading to a misdiagnosis of impetigo of the scalp. Postoccipital lymphadenopathy is common.

The diagnosis is usually made on identification of the nits and lice, or on microscopic examination of the affected hair shaft. The nits fluoresce under ultraviolet light. Treatment is by applying a solution of 0.5% malathion to the hair for 12 hours. The hair is then washed and the dead nits removed with a fine-tooth comb.

Other childhood rashes

PSORIASIS

This disorder, which is often familial, rarely presents before the age of two years. In children the most common type is guttate psoriasis (Fig. 21.15), which often follows a streptococcal throat infection. Lesions are small, round or oval erythematous scaly papules, approximately 0.5–1 cm in diameter, on the trunk and upper limbs, which resolve over several weeks. Chronic psoriasis with plaques or annular lesions is less common. Fine pitting of the nails may be seen in chronic disease but is unusual in children. Children may develop juvenile psoriatic arthritis.

PITYRIASIS ROSEA

This acute benign self-limiting condition is thought to be of viral origin. It usually begins with a single round or oval scaly macule 2–5 cm in diameter, the herald patch, on the trunk, upper arm, neck or thigh. After a few days numer-

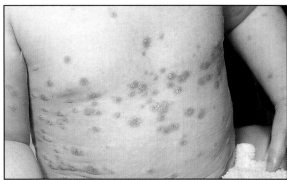

Fig. 21.15 *Guttate psoriasis.*

ous smaller dull pink macules develop on the trunk, upper arms and thighs. The rash tends to follow the line of the ribs posteriorly, described as the 'Christmas tree pattern'. Sometimes the lesions are itchy. No treatment is required as the rash resolves within 6–8 weeks.

ACNE VULGARIS

Acne may begin 1–2 years before the onset of puberty following androgenic stimulation of the sebaceous glands and increased sebum production. Obstruction to the flow of sebum in the sebaceous follicle initiates the process of acne. There is a variety of lesions, initially open comedones (blackheads) or closed comedones (whiteheads) progressing to papules, pustules, nodules and cysts. Lesions occur mainly on the face, back, chest and shoulders. They resolve, leaving temporary post-inflammatory redness and hyperpigmentation. The more severe cystic and nodular lesions often produce scarring. Menstruation and emotional stress are associated with exacerbations. The condition usually resolves in the late teens, although it persists in a few.

Topical treatment is directed at removing keratin plugs using a keratolytic agent, such as benzoxyl peroxide, applied daily after washing. Sunshine or ultraviolet light, topical antibiotics or topical retinoic acid may be helpful. For more severe pustular acne, low-dose, long-term antibiotic therapy with erythromycin or else oxytetracycline or minocycline in the older adolescent is indicated to suppress the lipolytic bacteria. The vitamin A analogue, 13-cis retinoic acid, is reserved for severe acne unresponsive to other treatments.

Rashes and systemic disease

Skin rashes may be a sign of systemic disease, such as the facial rashes in systemic lupus erythematosus or dermatomyositis. Erythema nodosum (Figs 21.16 and 21.17) and erythema multiforme (Figs 21.18 and 21.19) may be associated with a systemic disorder, but often the cause is not identified. In the more severe bullous form of erythema multiforme, Stevens-Johnson syndrome, the mucous membranes are affected (Fig. 21.20). Eye involvement may include conjunctivitis, corneal ulceration and uveitis and ophthalmological assessment is required. Morbidity and mortality in Stevens-Johnson syndrome are from dehydration and secondary infection, either bacterial or from the herpes simplex virus.

Urticaria (hives) (Fig. 21.21) is the result of a mast-cell degranulation in which histamine and other vasoactive substances such as prostaglandins and kinins are released. A cause may be identified from the history, but most are idiopathic (Fig. 21.22). In children, urticaria is usually acute. It may be accompanied by subcutaneous fluid around the lips and eyes (angioedema) and anaphylaxis (Fig. 21.23). Acute urticaria usually resolves within a few hours. If itchy, it can be treated with an H_1 histamine

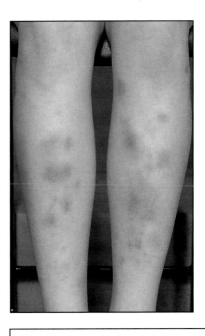

Fig. 21.16 Erythema nodosum. There are discrete tender red nodules on the shins. Fever and arthralgia may be present.

Fig. 21.17 Causes of erythema nodosum
Streptococcal infection
Primary tuberculosis
Inflammatory bowel disease
Drug reaction
Idiopathic
Sarcoidosis, the most common association in adults, is rare in children.

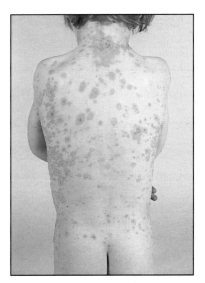

Fig. 21.18 Erythema multiforme. There are target lesions with a central papule surrounded by an erythematous ring. Lesions may also be vesicular or bullous.

Fig. 21.19 Causes of erythema multiforme
Herpes simplex infection
Mycoplasma pneumoniae infection
Other infections
Drug reaction, particularly sulphonamides
Idiopathic

antagonist. Hereditary angioedema is a rare autosomal dominant disorder caused by a deficiency of C1-esterase inhibitor. It results in recurrent urticaria and abdominal pain, with trauma often acting as a trigger. Angioedema may cause respiratory obstruction. Treatment of a severe acute attack is with fresh frozen plasma.

Urticaria

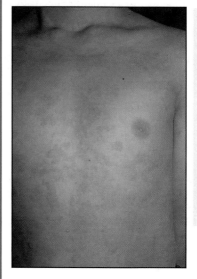

Fig. 21.21 Urticaria. There are raised oedematous lesions with a central area of pallor surrounded by a variable ring of erythema. These weals may coalesce to cover the whole body.

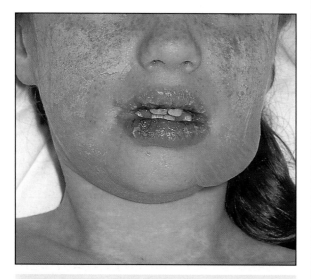

Fig. 21.20 Stevens–Johnson syndrome showing severe ulceration of the mouth.

Fig. 21.22 Causes of urticaria
Idiopathic (common)
IgE mediated
Specific food – peanuts, strawberries, shellfish, cow's milk, eggs
Animal danders – horses, cats
Physical agents – pressure, cold, heat
Complement mediated
Hereditary angioedema
Blood transfusion reactions
Mast-cell releasing agents
Drugs – opiates, penicillin etc
Prostacyclin inhibitors
Aspirin, non-steroidal anti-inflammatory drugs

Fig. 21.23 Treatment of anaphylaxis.
Adrenaline (10 microg/kg iv or 100 microg/kg via tracheal tube)
Hydrocortisone (4 mg/kg iv)
An H₁ histamine antagonist (e.g. chlorpheniramine 0.2 mg/kg iv)
Volume expansion with colloid, artificial ventilation and further dose of adrenaline if necessary

FURTHER READING

Hurwitz S. *Clinical Pediatric Dermatology*. 2nd edn. W B Saunders, 1994. Short textbook.
Verbov J. *Diagnostic Picture Tests in Pediatric Dermatology*. 1994. Mosby-Wolfe, London.

CHAPTER 22

Endocrine and Metabolic Disorders

• *Diabetes mellitus* • *Hypoglycaemia* • *Hypothyroidism* • *Hyperthyroidism* • *Parathyroid disorders*
• *Adrenal cortical insufficiency* • *Cushing syndrome* • *Inborn errors of metabolism* • *Hyperlipidaemia*

Features of endocrine and metabolic disorders in children are:
- almost all those with diabetes mellitus are insulin dependent
- hypoglycaemia must be excluded whenever they become critically ill
- congenital hypothyroidism is relatively common and is detected on routine neonatal biochemical screening
- inborn errors of metabolism are individually rare but considered in a wide range of differential diagnoses
- inherited causes of hyperlipidaemia markedly increase their risk of premature coronary heart disease.

Diabetes mellitus

The incidence of diabetes in children has increased steadily over the last 20 years and diabetes now affects 2 per 1000 children by 16 years of age. The condition is more common in northern countries, with the highest incidence in Finland. Almost all children are insulin dependent (IDDM or Type 1 diabetes). Maturity onset diabetes of the young (MODY) without ketosis can occur but is very uncommon.

 Almost all children with diabetes mellitus are insulin dependent

Aetiology
Both genetic predisposition and environmental precipitants play a role. Inherited susceptibility is demonstrated by:
- an identical twin of a diabetic having a 30–50% chance of developing the disease
- the increased risk of a child developing diabetes if a parent has insulin-dependent diabetes (1 in 20–40 if the father is affected, 1 in 40–80 if it is the mother)
- an eight to tenfold increase in the risk of diabetes among those who are HLA-DR3 or HLA-DR4 or both.

Molecular mimicry occurs between an environmental trigger and an antigen on the surface of β cells of the pancreas (which is probably GAD, glutamic acid decarboxylase). Triggers which may contribute are viral infections, accounting for the more frequent presentation in spring and autumn, and dietary, from cow's milk proteins (Fig. 22.1). An autoimmune process is thought to cause pancreatic β cell damage leading to an absolute insulin deficiency and increasing derangement of carbohydrate metabolism. There is an association with other autoimmune disorders such as hypothyroidism, Graves disease, alopecia and vitiligo.

Clinical features
The age at presentation is shown in Figure 22.2. Diabetes is increasingly diagnosed at an early stage of the illness (Fig. 22.3);

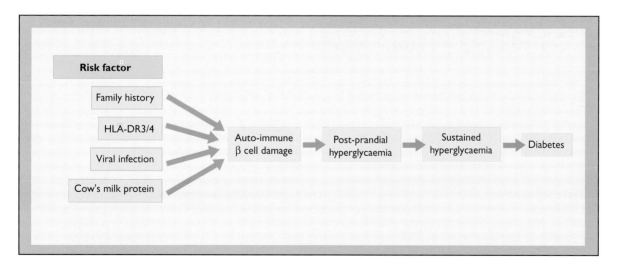

Fig. 22.1 *Stages in the development of diabetes.*

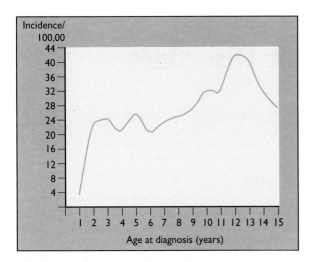

**Fig. 22.2   Age at presentation. Diabetes occurs even in young
children, but its incidence increases with age. (Data from
Metcalfe MA, Baum JD. Incidence of insulin dependent
diabetes in children aged under 15 years in the British Isles
during 1988. BMJ 1991; 302;443–447)**

Fig. 22.3 Symptoms and signs of diabetes	
Early	**Late**
Excessive drinking (polydypsia)	Vomiting
Polyuria	Dehydration
Weight loss	Abdominal pain
Enuresis (secondary)	Hypovolaemic shock
	Hyperventilation due to acidosis
	Drowsiness
	Coma

advanced diabetic ketoacidosis has become an uncommon
presentation but requires urgent recognition and treatment
(see Chapter 4). Diagnostic traps in failing to recognise diabetic ketoacidosis include mistaking the abdominal pain
for appendicitis and the hyperventilation for pneumonia.

Diagnosis

The diagnosis is usually confirmed in a symptomatic child
by finding a markedly raised random plasma glucose
(>11.1 mmol/l), glycosuria and ketonuria. Where there is
any doubt, a fasting plasma glucose (>7.8 mmol/l) or a
raised glycosylated haemoglobin (HbA$_{1C}$) is helpful. A glucose tolerance test is rarely needed in children.

Initial management

The initial management will depend on the child's clinical
condition. Those in advanced diabetic ketoacidosis require
urgent hospital admission and treatment. Most newly presenting children can be managed on subcutaneous insulin
alone, but intravenous fluid and an insulin infusion is
required if the child is vomiting or is dehydrated. In a few

centres, some of the newly presenting children not requiring intravenous therapy are not admitted to hospital, but
are managed entirely at home. An intensive educational
programme is needed for the parents and child to cover:

- a basic understanding of diabetes
- injection of insulin – technique and sites
- diet – regular meals and snacks, reduced refined
  carbohydrates, healthy diet
- matching of food intake with insulin
- adjustments for exercise and illness
- blood glucose (finger-prick) monitoring
- hypoglycaemia, its recognition and treatment
- the need to wear a Medicalert bracelet or necklace, identifying that they have diabetes
- help available from voluntary groups (British Diabetic
  Association, local groups)
- the psychological impact of a life-long condition with
  potentially serious short- and long-term complications.

A considerable period of time needs to be spent with the
family to provide this information and psychological support.

Insulin

In young children, insulin is usually given twice a day, before
breakfast and evening meals, as a mixture of short- and
medium-acting insulin. In general, about two-thirds of the
daily dose is given before breakfast and one-third before the
evening meal. Approximately one-third of each injection is
given as short-acting insulin. Each insulin can be drawn
up separately, allowing greater flexibility, or as a fixed mixture containing from 10% to 50% short-acting insulin. The
insulin can be given in a syringe with a standard needle or
using an insulin pen. The pens are readily portable and
easier to use but can be awkward for small children because
of their size. Pens may include autoinjection and are useful
in young or needle-phobic children. Older children and
teenagers may use a three or four injections a day regimen,
which allows greater flexibility by relating the insulin more
closely to food intake and exercise. A short acting insulin
is given before each meal and some long acting insulin in
the late evening to provide insulin overnight. Children are
usually started on a human insulin.

Injections can be given in the upper arms, outer thighs
or abdomen. The site needs to be rotated, otherwise fat
hypertrophy will develop, making insulin absorption erratic.
Shallow intradermal injections can also cause scarring and
should be avoided. The use of a shorter (8mm) needle in
young or thin children reduces the risk of intramuscular
injection. New synthetic insulins are being developed with
different absorption characteristics.

Diet

The diet and insulin regimen need to be matched. Food
intake is divided into three main meals with snacks between
meals and before going to bed. A high-fibre diet, which will
provide a sustained release of glucose, is encouraged, rather
than one high in refined carbohydrates which causes rapid
swings in glucose levels. A healthy diet is recommended, with
a high complex carbohydrate and relatively low fat content.
Dividing meals and snacks into portions of carbohydrate can

be done by using 10g carbohydrate 'exchanges' or approximate portions.

Blood glucose monitoring

Regular home blood glucose monitoring is useful to check and adjust the insulin regimen and for 'trouble-shooting', when a low or high level is suspected. Urine glucose testing is useful when there is difficulty with blood glucose monitoring, and urinary ketones should also be checked during intercurrent infections or when control is poor. The measurement of glycosylated haemoglobin (HbA_{1C}) is particularly helpful as a guide to overall control over the previous six weeks and should be checked every 2–3 months. Interpretation of the HbA_{1C} results is misleading if the red blood cell life span is reduced, as in sickle cell trait. As children usually dislike having finger-pricks for blood-glucose monitoring, realistic goals need to be agreed, with compromises reached about frequency of monitoring. Children can never have a 'holiday' from their diabetes so they need a great deal of encouragement to maintain continuous good control. Educational programmes for children need to be matched to their level of understanding, and award schemes for knowledge about diabetes are useful. Special courses and holiday camps are available; in the UK they are organised by the British Diabetic Association and local groups.

Hypoglycaemia

Most children develop well-defined symptoms when the blood glucose falls below about 4 mmol/l. The symptoms are highly individual, but most complain of sweatiness, feeling faint or dizzy or of a 'wobbly feeling' in their legs. If unrecognised or untreated, hypoglycaemia may progress to seizures and coma. Parents can often detect hypoglycaemia in young children by their pallor and irritability, sometimes presenting as unreasonable behaviour. If there is any doubt, the blood glucose concentration should be checked.

Treating a 'hypo' at an early stage requires the administration of easily absorbed glucose in the form of sweets (glucose tablets or similar) or a sugary drink. Children should always have easy access to their hypo remedy. Oral glucose polymers, given as a gel, are also helpful if the child is unwilling or unable to cooperate to eat. The glucose gel is easily and quickly absorbed from the buccal mucosa and can be administered by teachers or other helpers. Parents should be provided with a glucagon kit for the treatment of severe hypoglycaemia and taught how to use it. The best management of hypoglycaemia is anticipation and prevention.

Long-term management

The aims of long-term management are:
* normal growth and development
* maintaining as normal a home and school life as possible
* good diabetic control through knowledge, good technique and self-reliance
* avoidance of hypoglycaemia
* prevention of long-term complications.
These aims are not easy to achieve!

Problems in diabetic control

The aim is to maintain blood glucose as near to normal for as much of the time as possible. Shortly after presentation, insulin requirements often become minimal, the so-called 'honeymoon period', but subsequently increase. Good blood glucose control is particularly difficult in the following circumstances:
* eating too many sugary foods, sweets taken at odd times, parties, etc.
* infrequent or unreliable blood glucose testing, the most common cause of poor diabetic control. 'Perfect' results may be fabricated
* illness – although it is usually stated that infections cause insulin requirements to increase, in practice the insulin dose required is variable, partly because of reduced food intake. The dose of insulin should be adjusted according to regular blood glucose monitoring. Insulin *must* be continued during times of illness, otherwise diabetic ketoacidosis will occur.
* exercise – vigorous or prolonged exercise (cross-country running, long-distance hiking, skiing) requires reduction of the insulin dose and a considerable increase in dietary intake. Late hypoglycaemia may occur during the night, but can be avoided by taking an extra bedtime snack, including a slow-acting carbohydrate such as cereal or bread. Less vigorous exercise, such as sports lessons in school, can be managed with an extra snack before the exercise.
* onset of puberty – the rapid growth spurt in early puberty is governed by a complex interaction of hormonal changes, some of which involve insulin and insulin-like growth factors There is an increase in the insulin requirement from the conventional 0.7–1.0 U/kg/day of early childhood to 1–1.5 U/kg/day.
* family disturbance such as divorce or separation
* inadequate family motivation or understanding.

Prevention of long-term complications

It has been shown that good diabetic control delays or prevents diabetic retinopathy and nephropathy and slows the progression of retinopathy (American Multicentre Diabetes Control and Complications trial). This has only been achieved with intensive management, consisting of at least three injections of insulin daily, four or more blood glucose estimations each day and regular clinic visits. However, this regimen has a threefold increase in risk of severe hypoglycaemia and a significant increase in weight. Tight control of blood glucose which is consistent with a reasonably normal life should be encouraged. However, the intensive regimen is probably not suitable for many children because of the increased risk of hypoglycaemia and the unpopularity of multiple injections and blood tests. In particular, hypoglycaemia should be avoided in children under 5 years old as they are at increased risk of it resulting in brain damage.

 Good diabetic control in childhood reduces the risk of long-term complications.

Adolescence

Normal adolescent physical, psychosexual and developmental maturation is affected by a chronic disease such as diabetes (Fig. 22.4). Some adolescents go through a period of denial, indifference or depression about their illness and there may be conflict at home or with health professionals. Insulin injections may be omitted, diet and blood glucose monitoring ignored or falsified or the insulin regimen manipulated, causing hypoglycaemia. Diabetic teenagers know that they are not ill immediately if they cheat with their diet or miss an injection. Some will inevitably test the degree to which the rules can be broken, choosing to ignore the uncomfortable facts of diabetes provided that they 'feel OK'. This usually results in avoidance of blood testing and a tendency to work on the false assumption that feeling well equates with good control. Many teenage girls experiment with crash diets at some time, which is likely to cause major problems in diabetic control.

Battles with parents tend to concentrate on diabetic management instead of the more usual teenage concerns. Conflict may also extend to involve the professionals of the diabetic team because of intense anger against the disease, which marks them out as different from their peers. Many parents become over protective at this time, while the young person should be encouraged to take increasing responsibility for their diabetes. Health education about smoking, alcohol and contraception may need to be provided. Liason with a child psychiatrist or psychologist may be helpful.

The professionals of the diabetic team may need to encourage diabetic teenagers to take better care of themselves. It is usually unhelpful to give lectures about the long-term risks to health, as these are likely to be seen as irrelevant. However, they may be helped if:

- there are clear short-term goals
- their efforts to improve their diabetic control, e.g. an improved or satisfactory HbA_{1C}, is communicated promptly and enthusiastically
- there is a united team approach, with agreement between professionals of the essentials they wish to promote and clear, unambiguous guidelines for health and diabetic management
- peer group pressure is used to promote health. Activities, holidays etc, which allow teenagers to participate while learning about their diabetic management are encouraged
- they are used as teachers for younger members.

Organising medical care

Diabetes requires multidisciplinary care involving:

- a paediatrician with a special interest in diabetes, who needs to liaise closely with the general practitioner
- specialist diabetic nurses or paediatric community nurses trained in diabetes who are able to play a key role in both practical education and help in dealing with problems. Direct telephone access to the specialist team is invaluable. Visits to affected children's school and primary care team maintain awareness and good communication
- a dietitian who is directly involved with the team
- psychological support as required
- joint management with adult diabetologists for adolescents and young adults.

In addition to short-term problems in diabetic control, the children need to be reviewed periodically for long-term complications:

- growth and pubertal development. Some delay in the onset of puberty may occur
- blood pressure – needs to be checked for evidence of hypertension
- eyes – retinopathy or cataracts requiring treatment are rare in children but should be monitored annually
- renal disease – the detection of microalbuminuria is an early sign of nephropathy
- feet – children should be encouraged to take good care of their feet from an early age, to avoid tight shoes and treat any infections early.

 Successful long-term diabetic management depends on education and increasing self-reliance and responsibility.

Fig. 22.4 How diabetes interferes with normal adolescence	
Aims and problems of normal adolescence	**How diabetes interferes**
Physical and sexual maturation	Delayed sexual maturation
	Invasion of privacy with frequent medical examinations
Conformity with peer group	Meals must be eaten on time
	Frequent injections and blood tests
Self-image	Hypoglycaemic attacks show that they are different
Self-esteem	Impaired body image
Independence from parents	Parental over protection and reluctance to allow their child to be away from home
	Battles over diabetes
Economic independence	Loading of insurance premiums
	Discrimination by employers

Hypoglycaemia

Hypoglycaemia is a common problem in neonates (*see* Chapter 8) but is seen much less often beyond this period. It is often defined as a blood glucose of less than 2.6 mmol/l, though the development of clinical features will depend on whether other energy substrates can be utilised. Clinical features include:

- sweating
- pallor
- central nervous system signs of irritability, headache, seizures and coma.

The neurological sequelae may be permanent if hypoglycaemia persists, and include epilepsy and severe learning difficulties.

Infants have high energy requirements and relatively poor reserves of glucose from gluconeogenesis and glycogenesis. They are at risk of hypoglycaemia with fasting. Infants should never be starved for more than four hours' duration, for example preoperatively.

Fig. 22.5 Causes of hypoglycaemia beyond the neonatal period

Metabolic
Ketotic hypoglycaemia
Liver disease
   Reye syndrome
   Acute liver failure
Inborn errors of metabolism
   Glycogen storage disorders
   Galactosaemia
   Fatty acid metabolism – medium chain acyl-CoA
      deficiency (MCAD)
   Organic acidaemia
   Tyrosinaemia
   Hereditary fructose intolerance
Poisoning
   Alcohol
   Aspirin

Hormonal
Hormone Deficiency
Growth hormone – Growth hormone deficiency
ACTH – Panhypopituitarism
Cortisol – Addison disease
     – Congenital adrenal hyperplasia
Hormone Excess
Insulin – Nesidioblastosis
   Beckwith syndrome
   Administered insulin in diabetes or poisoning
   Insulinomas

Blood glucose should be checked in any child who:

- becomes septicaemic or appears seriously ill
- has a prolonged seizure
- develops an altered state of consciousness.

This is done at the bedside using glucose sensitive strips, whose accuracy is improved by use of a reflectance meter. Low results must always be confirmed by laboratory measurement. If the cause of the hypoglycaemia is unknown, measurement at the same time of the plasma insulin, growth hormone, cortisol, betahydroxybutyrate, lactic acid and urine ketones are invaluable in its investigation.

Causes

These are listed in Figure 22.5.

Ketotic hypoglycaemia is a poorly defined entity in which young children readily become hypoglycaemic following a short period of starvation, probably due to limited reserves for gluconeogenesis. The child is often short and thin and the insulin levels are low. Regular snacks and extra glucose drinks when ill will usually prevent hypoglycaemia. The condition resolves spontaneously in later life.

A number of rare endocrine and metabolic disorders may present with hypoglycaemia at almost any age in childhood. Hepatomegaly would suggest the possibility of an inherited glycogen storage disorder, in which hypoglycaemia can be profound.

Treatment

Hypoglycaemia can usually be corrected with an intravenous infusion of glucose (2–4 ml/kg of 10–15% dextrose). Great care must be taken to avoid giving an excess volume as the solution is hypertonic. If there is delay in establishing an infusion or failure to respond, glucagon is given intramuscularly (0.5–1 mg). Corticosteroids may also be used. The correction of hypoglycaemia must always be documented with satisfactory laboratory glucose measurements.

Nesidioblastosis, a rare problem of infancy where there is overdevelopment of the islet cells of the pancreas leading to hyperinsulinism, can be treated with diazoxide and somatostatin analogues, but partial pancreatectomy is often required.

 Low blood glucose on stix testing must be confirmed by laboratory measurement.

Hypothyroidism

There is minimal thyroxine transfer from the mother to the fetus. The fetal thyroid predominantly produces 'reverse T3', a derivative of T3 which is largely inactive. After birth, there is a surge in the level of TSH which is accompanied by a marked rise in T4 and T3 levels. The TSH declines to the normal adult range within a week. Preterm infants may have low levels of T3 or T4 for the first few weeks of life while their TSH is within the normal range. Indications for giving additional thyroxine during this period have not been determined.

CONGENITAL HYPOTHYROIDISM

Detection of congenital hypothyroidism is important as it is:
- relatively common, occurring in 1 in 4000 births
- one of the few preventable causes of severe learning difficulties.

Causes of congenital hypothyroidism are:
- athyrosis – the thyroid fails to develop
- maldescent of the thyroid – the most common cause of sporadic congenital hypothyroidism. In early fetal life the thyroid migrates from a position at the base of the tongue (sublingual) to its normal site below the larynx. In maldescent, the thyroid remains as a lingual mass or a thyroglossal cyst. The reason for this failure of migration is not well understood but there is an increased incidence of other congenital defects
- dyshormonogenesis, an inborn error of thyroid hormone synthesis, in about 15%
- iodine deficiency, the most common cause of congenital hypothyroidism worldwide. It can be prevented by iodination of salt in the maternal diet
- hypothyroidism due to TSH deficiency – usually associated with panhypopituitarism, but is very rare.

The clinical features (Fig. 22.6) are difficult to differentiate from normal in the early stages. Fortunately, most affected infants are now identified by neonatal biochemical screening. Most laboratories in the UK test for raised levels of TSH, though in some areas both TSH and T4 are measured.

Early treatment is essential to prevent learning difficulties. With neonatal screening, the results of long-term intellectual development have been very satisfactory and intelligence should be in the normal range. Treatment is life long with oral replacement of thyroxine, titrating the dose to maintain normal growth and T4 levels in the upper normal range.

 Although congenital hypothyroidism is present antenatally, treatment started soon after birth prevents most learning difficulties.

Fig. 22.6 Clinical features of hypothyroidism	
Infants	**Children**
Feeding problems	Cold intolerance
Prolonged jaundice	Dry skin
Constipation	Cold peripheries
Pale cold mottled dry skin	Bradycardia
Coarse facies	Thin dry hair
Large tongue	Pale puffy eyes with loss of eyebrows
Hoarse cry	Goitre
Goitre (occasionally)	Slow-relaxing reflexes
Umbilical hernia	Constipation
Delayed development	Short stature
	Delayed puberty
	Obesity
	Deterioration in school work
	Learning difficulties

JUVENILE HYPOTHYROIDISM

Autoimmune thyroiditis

This is the most common cause. Other autoimmune disorders, eg diabetes mellitus, may develop, particularly in children with Down or Turner syndrome. The clinical features are listed in Figure 22.6. Treatment is with thyroxine. It is more common in females. A goitre is often present but may also be physiological in pubertal girls. There is growth failure accompanied by delayed bone age. A slipped upper femoral epiphysis may be associated with secondary epiphyseal dysgenesis.

TSH deficiency

This is secondary to a pituitary or hypothalamic disorder, which is often accompanied by deficiencies of other pituitary hormones. However, this is the rarest of the pituitary hormone deficiencies.

Hyperthyroidism

Neonatal hyperthyroidism may occur in infants of mothers with Graves disease from the transplacental transfer of thyroid-stimulating immunoglobulins (TSI). Treatment is required, but the condition resolves spontaneously with the decline in transferred immunoglobulin.

JUVENILE HYPERTHYROIDISM

This usually results from Graves disease. It is most often seen in teenage girls. The clinical features are similar to those in adults (Figs 22.7 and 22.8). The levels of thyroxine and/or tri-iodothyronine are elevated and antithyroid antibodies are usually present. TSH levels are low.

The first line of treatment is medical, with drugs such as carbimazole or propylthiouracil which interfere with thyroid hormone synthesis. Initially, β-blockers can be added for symptomatic relief but should not be used on their own. Medical treatment is given for up to two years, which should control the thyrotoxicosis, but the eye signs may not resolve completely. When medical treatment is stopped, 40–75% relapse. A second course of drugs or surgery or radio-iodine is then given. Subtotal thyroidectomy will also usually result in permanent remission. Radio-iodine treatment is simple and is not considered to result in neoplasia or genetic damage. Follow-up is required as thyroxine replacement is often needed for subsequent hypothyroidism.

 An over-active thyroid can be easily missed; eye signs may be mild and thyrotoxicosis confused with nervousness.

Fig. 22.7 Clinical features of hyperthyroidism	
Systemic	**Eye signs** (not always present)
Anxiety, restlessness	Exophthalmos
Increased appetite	Ophthalmoplegia
Sweating	Lid retraction
Diarrhoea	Lid lag
Weight loss	
Rapid growth in height	
Advanced bone maturity	
Tremor	
Tachycardia	
Warm vasodilated peripheries	
Goitre (bruit)	
Learning difficulties/behaviour problems	

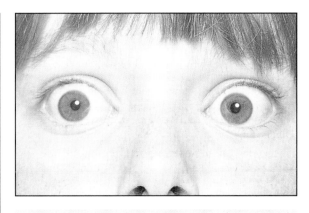

Fig. 22.8 Exophthalmos in hyperthyroidism.

Parathyroid disorders

Hypoparathyroidism is rare in childhood. It presents with hypocalcaemia, as parathormone (PTH) plays a key role in the mobilisation of calcium osteoclasts and the excretion of phosphate in the urine. In addition to a low serum calcium, there is a raised serum phosphorus and a normal alkaline phosphatase. The parathormone level is very low.

Hypoparathyroidism

In infants, this is usually due to a congenital deficiency (DiGeorge syndrome), associated with thymus aplasia, defective immunity, cardiac defects and facial abnormalities. There is often a deletion in chromosome 22q11. In older children, hypoparathyroidism is usually an autoimmune disorder and may be associated with chronic mucocutaneous candidiasis.

Pseudohypoparathyroidism

There is end organ resistance to the action of parathormone; serum calcium and phosphorus levels are abnormal but the parathormone levels are normal or high. The diagnosis may be confirmed by a poor urinary cyclic AMP response to a parathormone infusion. Other abnormalities are short stature, obesity, subcutaneous nodules, short fourth metacarpals (Fig. 22.9) and mild learning difficulties. There may be tooth enamel hypoplasia and calcification of the basal ganglia. There is often a positive family history.

Pseudopseudohypoparathyroidism

This term is used to describe a group of X-linked disorders with the physical characteristics of pseudohypoparathyroidism but the calcium, phosphorus and PTH are all normal.

Treatment

Treatment of acute symptomatic hypocalcaemia is with an intravenous infusion of calcium gluconate. The 10% solution of calcium gluconate must be diluted as extravasation of the infusion will result in severe skin damage. Chronic hypocalcaemia is treated with oral calcium and high doses of vitamin D analogues, adjusting the dose to maintain the plasma calcium concentration within the low normal range. Hypercalcaemia is to be avoided as it may cause nephrocalcinosis from hypercalcuria.

Adrenal cortical insufficiency

Primary adrenal cortical insufficiency (Addison disease) is rare in children. It may result from:
- an autoimmune process, sometimes in association with other autoimmune endocrine disorders, e.g. diabetes mellitus, hypothyroidism, hypoparathyroidism
- haemorrhage/infarction – neonatal, meningococcal septicaemia (usually fatal)
- adrenoleucodystrophy, a neurodegenerative disorder
- tuberculosis, now rare.

Adrenal insufficiency may also be secondary to hypopituitarism from hypothalamic-pituitary disease or from hypothalamic-pituitary-adrenal suppression from long-term corticosteroid therapy. An important cause of chronic

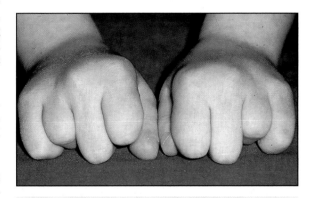

Fig. 22.9 Short fourth metacarpals in pseudo-hypoparathyroidism.

adrenal insufficiency is congenital adrenal hyperplasia (see Chapter 9).

Presentation
Infants present acutely (Fig. 22.10) with a salt-losing crisis and/or hypoglycaemia. Dehydration may follow a gastroenteritis-like illness, from which the child recovers until the next episode. In older children, presentation is usually with chronic ill health and pigmentation (Fig. 22.11).

Diagnosis
This is made by finding hyponatraemia and hyperkalaemia, often with a metabolic acidosis and hypoglycaemia. The plasma cortisol is low or normal and the plasma ACTH concentration high. With an ACTH (short synacthen) test, plasma cortisol concentrations remain low. A normal response excludes adrenal cortical insufficiency.

Management
An adrenal crisis requires urgent treatment with intravenous saline, glucose and hydrocortisone. Long-term treatment is with glucocorticoid and mineralocorticoid replacement. The dose of glucocorticoid needs to be increased three- to five-fold at times of illness or for an operation.

 A Medicalert bracelet is advisable for all children at risk of an adrenal crisis (congenital adrenal hyperplasia or Addison disease).

Fig. 22.10   Features of adrenal cortical insufficiency.

Acute	Chronic
Hyponatraemia	Vomiting
Hyperkalaemia	Lethargy
Hypercalcaemia	Brown pigmentation (gums, scars,
Hypoglycaemia	creases)
Dehydration	Growth failure
Hypotension	
Circulatory collapse	

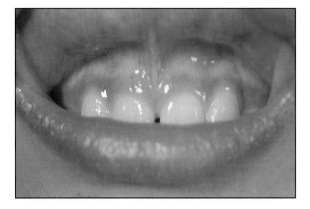

Fig. 22.11   Buccal pigmentation in adrenal cortical insufficiency (Addison disease) This 9-year-old male presented with salt craving and pigmentation. (Courtesy of Dr Steven Robinson.)

Cushing syndrome

Glucocorticoid excess in children is usually a side-effect of long-term glucocorticoid treatment for conditions such as nephrotic syndrome, asthma or bronchopulmonary dysplasia (Fig. 22.12). Corticosteroids are potent growth suppressors and prolonged use in high dosage will lead to reduced adult height. This unwanted side-effect is markedly reduced by taking corticosteroid medication in the morning on alternate days, though growth in puberty may still be affected. Rare causes of glucocorticoid excess are adrenocortical tumours, where there may also be accompanying masculinisation, and an ACTH-producing pituitary adenoma. Ectopic ACTH-producing tumours almost never occur in children.

The clinical features are shown in Fig. 22.13. A diagnosis of Cushing syndrome is often questioned in obese children. Most obese children are of above average height,

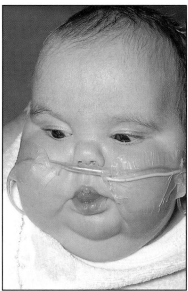

Fig. 22.12 Facial obesity from iatrogenic corticosteroid therapy for bronchopulmonary dysplasia in a preterm infant. Additional oxygen therapy is being given via nasal cannulae.

Fig. 22.13   Clinical features of Cushing syndrome

Short stature
Face and trunk obesity
Red cheeks
Hirsutism
Striae
Hypertension
Bruising
Carbohydrate intolerance
Muscle wasting
Osteoporosis
Psychological problems

in contrast to children with Cushing syndrome, who are short and have growth failure. The normal diurnal variation of cortisol (high in the morning, low at midnight) is lost in Cushing syndrome, the midnight concentration being high. In the dexamethasone suppression test there is failure to suppress plasma cortisol levels. Adrenal tumours are identified on CT or MR scan and a pituitary adenoma on an MR scan. Adrenal tumours are usually unilateral and are treated by adrenalectomy and radiotherapy if indicated. Pituitary adenomas are best treated by trans-sphenoidal resection but radiotherapy can be used in addition.

Inborn errors of metabolism

Many hundreds of enzyme defects have been identified, mostly with an autosomal recessive inheritance. Individually they are rare disorders and therefore often managed in specialist centres.

Presentation
An inborn error of metabolism may be suspected before birth from a positive family history or previous unexplained deaths in the family.

In the neonatal period, these disorders must be considered whenever infants become severely ill without an adequate explanation. Other modes of presentation are with:
- poor feeding, persistent or recurrent vomiting
- jaundice or hepatomegaly
- lethargy, convulsions or coma
- unusual smell of the body or urine.

There may be a severe metabolic acidosis, ketosis or raised plasma ammonia.

In older children, inborn errors of metabolism need to be considered as a cause of:
- unexplained learning difficulties, developmental delay or convulsions
- unusual odour of the body or urine
- intermittent unexplained vomiting, acidosis or coma
- jaundice or hepatomegaly.

Inborn errors should also be considered in children who develop coarse facies, dislocated ocular lens, abnormal hair, renal calculi and hypopigmentation.

DISORDERS OF AMINOACID METABOLISM

I. PHENYLKETONURIA
This occurs in 1 in 10 000–20 000 livebirths. It is either due to a deficiency of the enzyme phenylalanine hydroxylase or the synthesis or recycling of the biopterin cofactor for this enzyme. Untreated, it usually presents with infantile spasms or developmental delay at 6–12 months of age. There may be a musty odour due to the metabolite phenylacetic acid. Many affected children are fair-haired and blue-eyed and some develop eczema. Fortunately, most affected children are detected through the national biochemical screening programme. The raised plasma phenylalanine is detected at 5–7 days of age when milk feeding has been established. Many milder cases of hyperphenylalininaemia are also detected on screening.

Treatment is with restriction of dietary phenylalanine, while ensuring that there is sufficient for optimal physical and neurological growth. The blood plasma phenylalanine is monitored regularly. The recommendation is to continue some form of diet throughout life. This is particularly important during pregnancy, when high maternal phenylalanine levels may damage the fetus. The diet must be started before conception. Cofactor defects are treated with a diet low in phenylalanine and high in neurotransmitter precursors.

2. TYROSINAEMIA
Tyrosinaemia (type 1) is a rare, autosomal recessive deficiency of the enzyme fumarylacetoacetase. Accumulation of toxic metabolites may result in acute liver failure and renal tubular dysfunction in infancy and chronic liver disease in older children. There is a high incidence of hepatoma (probably 100%). The diagnosis is made by detecting elevated tyrosine in plasma and urine and confirming the enzyme deficiency.

Management consists of dietary restriction of tyrosine, which controls the metabolic features but not the progression to liver disease. Supplementation of the diet with calcium, phosphorous and vitamin D is required to prevent rickets. Definitive treatment is liver transplantation. Recently, therapy has been introduced with NTBC (2-[2-nitro-4-trifluoro-methybenzoyl] -3, 3-cyclohexanedione), which inhibits the tyrosine degradation pathway, preventing the build up of harmful metabolites. If started shortly after birth, NTBC appears to prevent the development of progressive liver disease and probably hepatoma.

3. HOMOCYSTINURIA
This is due to cystathionine synthetase deficiency. Presentation is with failure to thrive and developmental delay and subluxation of the ocular lens (ectopia lentis). There is progressive learning difficulty, psychiatric disorders and convulsions. Skeletal manifestations resemble Marfan syndrome. The complexion is usually fair with brittle hair. Thromboembolic episodes may occur at any age. Almost half respond to large doses of the coenzyme pyridoxine. Non-responders are treated with a low methionine diet supplemented with cysteine.

4. ALBINISM
This is due to a defect in biosynthesis and distribution of melanin. The albinism may be oculocutaneous, ocular or partial, depending on the distribution of depigmentation in the skin and eye (Fig. 22.14). The lack of pigment in the iris, retina, eyelids and eyebrows results in failure to develop a fixation reflex. There is pendular nystagmus and photophobia, which causes constant frowning. No treatment is available, but correction of refractive errors and tinted lenses may be helpful. In a few children, the fitting of tinted contact lenses from early infancy allows the development of

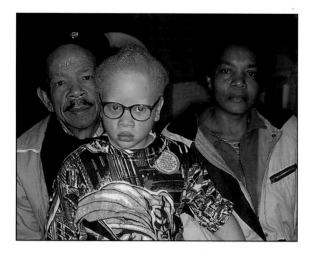

Fig. 22.14 A child with oculocutaneous albinism with her parents.

The management of the other organic acidaemias centres on the restriction of dietary protein. During acute decompensation, catabolism is limited by a high-carbohydrate, low-protein intake. Acidosis is corrected and hyperammonaemia treated by peritoneal dialysis or haemoperfusion. The outcome is often poor with significant developmental delay. Some disorders respond to large doses of vitamin co-factors e.g. vitamin B_{12}.

UREA CYCLE DEFECTS

Enzyme defects have been identified for all stages of the urea cycle. They tend to cause neonatal encephalopathy from high blood ammonia, but the onset may be delayed, when presentation is with coma associated with infection. Ornithine transcarbamylase deficiency is an X-linked disorder, but disorders of the other stages of the urea cycle are autosomal recessive.

DISORDERS OF CARBOHYDRATE METABOLISM

I. GALACTOSAEMIA

This rare, recessively inherited disorder results from deficiency of the enzyme galactose-1-phosphate uridyl transferase, which is essential for galactose metabolism. The inability to mobilise glucose from galactose may result in hypoglycaemia. When lactose-containing milk feeds such as breast or infant formula are introduced, affected infants feed poorly, vomit and develop jaundice and hepatomegaly and hepatic failure (see Chapter 17). Chronic liver disease, cataracts and developmental delay are inevitable if the condition is untreated. Management is with a lactose and galactose free diet. Even if treated early, severe learning difficulties are common.

2. GLYCOGEN STORAGE DISORDERS

These mostly recessively inherited disorders have specific enzyme defects which prevent mobilisation of glucose from glycogen. There is abnormal storage of glycogen. There are nine main enzyme defects (Figs 22.15 and 22.16). The disorder may predominantly affect muscle (e.g. types II, V) leading to skeletal muscle weakness.

normal fixation. The disorder is an important cause of severe visual impairment. The pale skin is prone to sunburn and skin cancer. In sunlight, a hat should be worn and high factor barrier cream applied to the skin.

THE ORGANIC ACIDAEMIAS

These are disorders of the catabolic pathways of several essential amino acids (the branched chain amino acids leucine, isoleucine and valine and odd chain aminoacids e.g. threonine) to cause maple syrup urine disease, methylmalonic acidaemia and propionic acidaemia, among others.

Maple syrup urine disease most often presents in the neonatal period with a severe metabolic acidosis, hypoglycaemia and seizures. There is increased excretion of the branched chain amino acids: leucine, isoleucine and valine. The urine has a characteristic maple syrup smell. If identified within 24 hours, outcome with dietary manipulation may be good but delay in diagnosis leads to learning difficulties and neurological dysfunction. There remains a high risk of early death during acute illnesses.

Fig. 22.15 Some of the glycogen storage disorders					
Type	**Enzyme defect**	**Onset**	**Liver**	**Muscle**	**Comments**
Type I (von Gierke)	Glucose-6-phosphatase	Infant	+++	-	See Fig. 22.16. Enlarged liver and kidneys. Growth failure. Hypoglycaemia. Prognosis good
Type II (Pompe)	Lysosomal α-glucosidase	Infant	++	+++	Hypotonia and cardiomegaly at several months. Death from heart failure
Type III (Cori)	Amylo-1,6-glucosidase	Infant	++	+	Milder features of Type I, but muscles may be affected. Good prognosis
Type V (McArdle)	Phosphorylase	Child	-	++	Temporary weakness and cramps in muscles after exercise. Myoglobinuria in later life

In type II (Pompe disease) there is generalised intra-lysosomal storage of glycogen. The heart is severely affected leading to death from cardiomyopathy. In other types (e.g. I, III) the liver is the main organ of storage and hepatomegaly and hypoglycaemia are prominent. Long-term complications of type I include hyperlipidaemia, hyperuricaemia, the development of hepatic adenomas and cardiovascular disease.

Management is to maintain blood glucose by frequent feeds or by carbohydrate infusion via a nasogastric tube in infancy. In older children glucose levels can be maintained using slow-release oligosaccharides (corn starch). In Type III disorder, a high-protein diet is required to prevent growth retardation and myopathy.

Hyperlipidaemia

Hyperlipidaemia is one of the main risk factors for coronary heart disease. Identification and treatment of hyperlipidaemia in childhood may delay the onset of cardiovascular disease in later life. Children should be screened for hyperlipidaemia if they are at increased risk – if a parent or grandparent has a history of coronary heart disease, peripheral vascular or cerebrovascular disease or sudden death before 55 years of age, or has a high serum cholesterol (>6.5 mmol/l). At present, screening of all children is not thought justifiable in view of the many uncertainties about selecting who should be treated,

what treatment should be given and its effect on outcome. If the serum cholesterol is high (>5.3 mmol/l) on random testing, fasting serum cholesterol, triglyceride and LHDL cholesterol are measured. Secondary causes of hypercholesterolaemia should be considered, such as obesity, hypothyroidism, diabetes mellitus, nephrotic syndrome and obstructive jaundice.

Familial hypercholesterolaemia (FH)
This autosomal dominant disorder of lipoprotein metabolism is due to a defect in the low-density lipoprotein (LDL) receptor. About 1 in 500 of the population are heterozygous and are affected. The serum LDL cholesterol concentration is markedly raised (>3.3 mmol/l). The condition is associated with premature coronary heart disease, which occurs in half by 50 years of age in males and by 60 years in females. Skin and tendon xanthomata (Fig. 22.16) may be present, but are uncommon in childhood. Homozygous disease is very rare and much more severe, causing xanthomata in childhood and clinical cardiovascular disease in the second decade.

Familial combined hypercholesterolaemia (FCH)
This autosomal dominant disorder may not cause raised lipid levels during childhood but is associated with an increased risk of premature coronary heart disease in adult life. Management involves attention to accompanying risk factors, such as obesity, hypertension, diabetes mellitus and smoking. Dietary management is by reducing the proportion of fat. Drug therapy may be considered for older

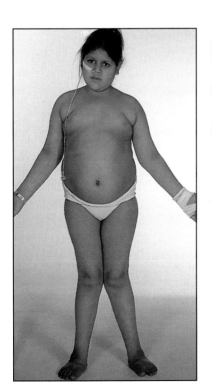

Fig. 22.16 Type I glycogen storage disease in a 12-year-old girl. There is:
• truncal obesity with a distended abdomen from an enlarged liver
• short stature and hypotrophic muscles
• 'doll' facies
• nasogastric feeding to maintain blood glucose levels overnight.

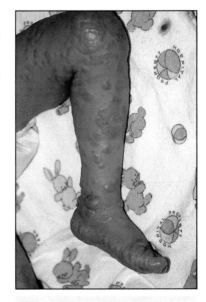

Fig. 22.17 Severe skin xanthomata. In this child it was secondary to liver failure and resolved within weeks of liver transplantation.

children (>10 years) if their serum LDL cholesterol concentration remains high. Drugs which sequester bile acid, e.g. cholestyramine or colestipol, are usually used. Results of treatment of children with simvastatin, an inhibitor of HMG CoA reductase, the rate-limiting enzyme in cholesterol synthesis, are awaited.

FURTHER READING

Brook CGD. *A Guide to the Practice of Paediatric Endocrinology.* Cambridge University Press, Cambridge, 1993. A short textbook.
Fernandes J, Sandubray JM, van den Berghe G (eds). *Inborn Metabolic Diseases.* Springer-Verlag, Berlin, 1995. Textbook.

CHAPTER 23

Bones and Joints

• Variations of normal posture • Disorders of the hip, knee and feet • Disorders of the back, spine and neck • The painful limb • Arthritis • Genetic skeletal dysplasias

Variations of normal posture

These are common and are noticed by parents or on routine developmental surveillance. Most resolve without any treatment but any that are severe, persistent, painful or asymmetrical should be referred for a specialist opinion.

BOW LEGS (GENU VARUM)
This is due to bowing of the tibiae causing the knees to be wide apart while standing with the feet together (Fig. 23.1). It is common in toddlers and children up to three years of age and seldom needs treatment. Severe bow legs may be caused by rickets which can be demonstrated on an X-ray of the metaphyses. Marked bow legs may also occur in Blount disease (infantile tibia vara), an uncommon condition seen predominantly in Afro-Caribbean children, where there is beaking of the proximal medial tibial epiphysis on X-ray, for which orthoses (splints and special footwear) and surgical correction may be required.

KNOCK-KNEES (GENU VALGUM)
In this condition, the feet are wide apart when standing with the knees held together (Fig. 23.2). It is seen in many children between two and seven years of age and usually resolves.

FLAT FEET (PES PLANUS)
Toddlers learning to walk usually have flat feet due to flatness of the medial longitudinal arch and the presence of a fat pad which subsequently disappears (Fig. 23. 3). Most people develop a medial longitudinal arch, but some do not and this is rarely troublesome. An arch can usually be demonstrated on standing on tiptoe. Marked flat feet can be the presentation of a collagen disorder such as Ehlers-Danlos syndrome. Some children with flat feet develop a prominence of the navicular bone on the medial aspect of the foot which resolves, but modification of the child's shoes or an arch support may be required. This will provide symptomatic relief but does not influence outcome. Surgery for flat feet is only indicated in symptomatic adolescents.

INTOEING
There are three main causes (Fig. 23.4):
*   *metatarsus varus* (Fig. 23.5a) – an adduction deformity of a highly mobile forefoot
*   *medial tibial torsion* (Fig. 23.5b) – at the lower leg, when the tibia is laterally rotated less than normal in relation to the femur
*   *persistent anteversion of the femoral neck* (23.5c) – at the hip, when the femoral neck is twisted forward more than normal.

OUT-TOEING
This is uncommon but may occur in infants between six and 12 months of age. When bilateral it is from lateral rotation of the hips and resolves spontaneously.

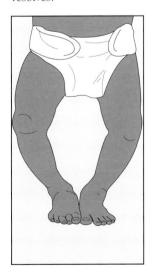

Fig. 23. 1 Bow legs.

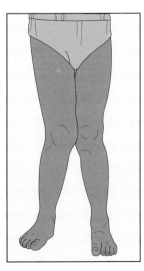

Fig. 23. 2 Knock-knees.

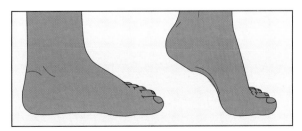

Fig. 23. 3 Pes planus showing the flat feet of toddlers. The medial longitudinal arch appears on standing on tiptoe

Fig. 23.4 Clinical features of intoeing in children

Metatarsus varus
- Occurs in infants
- Passively correctable
- Heel is held in the normal position
- No treatment required unless it persists beyond five years of age and is symptomatic

Medial tibial torsion
- Occurs in toddlers
- May be associated with bowing of the tibiae
- Self-corrects within about five years

Persistent anteversion of the femoral neck
- Presents in childhood
- Usually self-corrects by eight years of age
- May be associated with hypermobility of the joints
- Children sit between their feet with the hips fully internally rotated ('W' sitting)
- Most do not require treatment, but femoral osteotomy may be required if the anteversion persists

TOE WALKING

This is common in 1–3-year-old children. It may become persistent, usually from habit, but may be from mild cerebral palsy or else tight heel cords, when there is no neurological deficit but the feet cannot be dorsiflexed beyond a neutral position. In older boys, Duchenne muscular dystrophy should be excluded.

Disorders of the hip, knee and feet

LIMP

Congenital dislocation of the hip may be detected on routine examination of the newborn infant. Beyond infancy, hip disorders usually present with a limp, which may be painful or painless (Fig. 23.6).

 A limp in a child requires prompt evaluation.

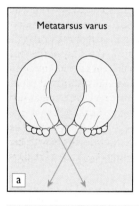
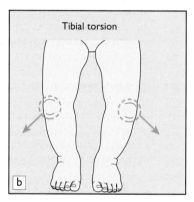
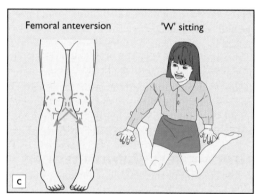

Fig. 23.5 Intoeing (a) at the feet, (b) lower leg, (c) hip, with 'W' sitting.

Fig. 23.6 Causes of limp

Age	Painful limp	Painless limp
1–3 years	Septic arthritis/osteomyelitis Transient synovitis Trauma – accidental/non-accidental	Congenital dislocation of the hip Neuromuscular e.g. cerebral palsy Unequal leg length JCA
3–10 years	Transient synovitis Septic arthritis/osteomyelitis Trauma JCA Perthes disease (acute) Malignant disease e.g. leukaemia	Perthes disease (chronic) Congenital dislocation of the hip Neuromuscular disorders e.g. Duchenne muscular dystrophy JCA
11–16 years	Slipped upper femoral epiphysis (acute) JCA Trauma Septic arthritis/osteomyelitis Bone tumours	Slipped upper femoral epiphysis (chronic) JCA Dysplastic hip

JCA = Juvenile Chronic Arthritis

CONGENITAL DISLOCATION OF THE HIP (CDH; *developmental dysplasia of the hip, DDH*)

This is a spectrum of disorders ranging from dysplasia to subluxation through to frank dislocation of the hip. Early detection is important as it usually responds to conservative treatment; late diagnosis is usually associated with hip dysplasia and more complex treatment often requiring surgery. Neonatal screening is performed as part of the routine examination of the newborn, checking if the hip can be dislocated posteriorly out of the acetabulum (Barlow manoeuvre) or can be relocated back into the acetabulum (Ortolani manoeuvre), as described on p. 81. These tests are repeated at routine surveillance at six weeks of age. Thereafter, presentation of the condition may be with detection of asymmetry of skin folds around the hip, limited abduction of the hip, shortening of the affected leg or a limp or waddling gait.

On neonatal screening an abnormality of the hip is detected in about 6 per 1000 live births. Most will resolve spontaneously; its true birth prevalence is about 1.5 per 1000 live births. Infants may be missed on neonatal screening, though, because of inexperience of the examiner, the abnormality may not yet be detectable clinically, for example, from a dysplastic hip where the acetabulum is shallow, or because it develops at a later age.

If congenital dislocation of the hip is suspected, a specialist orthopaedic opinion should be obtained. An ultrasound examination allows the hip to be assessed as normal or with increasing grades of dysplasia and subluxation to dislocation. This information helps in planning management and in avoiding unnecessary treatment. If the initial ultrasound is abnormal, the infant may be placed in a positioning device, which puts the hips in abduction (e.g. Craig splint), or in a restraining device (e.g. Pavlik harness (Fig. 23.7) or Von Rosen splint) for several months. Progress needs to be monitored by ultrasound or X-ray.

In most instances, a satisfactory response is obtained. If the hip has not stabilised or the condition is diagnosed late, the hip may be abducted using traction and a further period of splinting (in a plaster hip spica). If unsuccessful, MR or CT scans of the hip or an arthrogram may be performed to obtain more detailed information of the joint. Weight-bearing on a dislocated hip should be avoided as it causes damage to the femoral head and acetabulum. Open reduction and derotation femoral osteotomy is required if conservative measures fail.

TRANSIENT SYNOVITIS (TS, IRRITABLE HIP)

This is the most common cause of acute hip pain in children. It occurs in children of 2–12 years old. It often follows or is accompanied by a viral infection. Presentation is with sudden onset of pain in a hip or of a limp. There is no pain at rest, but there is decreased abduction and internal and external rotation. The pain may be referred to the knee. The child is afebrile or has a mild fever and does not appear ill.

This contrasts with septic arthritis, when the child has a high fever and looks unwell, there is pain at rest and minimal or no movement of the hip. In transient synovitis, the neutrophil count and acute phase reactants are normal or slightly raised, whereas they are markedly raised in septic arthritis. Blood cultures are negative, the X-ray of the joint is normal but there may be a small joint effusion on ultrasound. If there is any suspicion of septic arthritis, the joint is aspirated under ultrasound guidance. In a small proportion of children, the condition is found to be the presentation of Perthes disease or of slipped upper femoral epiphysis. Management of transient synovitis is with bed rest and skin traction. It usually responds within a few days.

PERTHES DISEASE

This is due to ischaemia of the femoral epiphysis, resulting in avascular necrosis, followed by revascularisation and reossification over 18–36 months. It mainly affects boys (male to female ratio of 5:1) of 5–10 years of age. Presentation is insidious with the onset of a limp or hip pain. The condition may initially be mistaken for transient synovitis. It is bilateral in 10–20 %. X-rays show increased density in the femoral head, which subsequently becomes fragmented and irregular (Fig. 23.8). Even if the initial X-ray is normal, a repeat may be

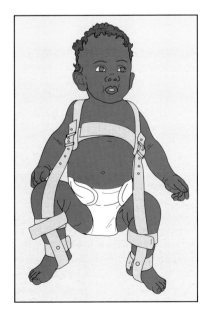

Fig. 23.7
Pavlik harness to keep the hip abducted in treating congenital dislocation of the hip.

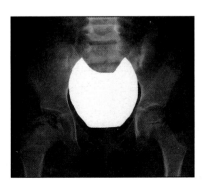

Fig. 23.8
Perthes disease, showing flattening with sclerosis and fragmentation of the right femoral capital epiphysis; the left hip is normal.

required if clinical symptoms persist. A bone scan and MR scan can be helpful in making the diagnosis.

In most children the prognosis is good, particularly in those below six years of age with less than half the epiphysis involved. When over half the epiphysis is affected and the child is older, deformity of the femoral head and metaphyseal damage is more likely, resulting in subsequent degenerative arthritis in adult life. If the condition is identified early and less than half the femoral head is affected, only bed rest and traction may be required. In more severe disease, the femoral head needs to be covered by the acetabulum to act as a mould for the reossifying epiphysis. This is done by maintaining the hip in abduction with plaster or calipers or by femoral or pelvic osteotomy.

SLIPPED UPPER FEMORAL EPIPHYSIS

There is displacement of the epiphysis of the femoral head postero-inferiorly. It is most common at 10–15 years of age, during the adolescent growth spurt, particularly in obese boys. Skeletal maturation may be delayed. Presentation is with a limp or hip pain, which may be referred to the knee. There is restricted abduction and internal rotation of the hip. The onset may be acute, following minor trauma. In 20 % it is bilateral. The diagnosis is confirmed on X-ray (Fig. 23.9), although a frog lateral view is sometimes required. Management is surgical, usually with pin fixation *in situ*. Severe slips may require subsequent, corrective realignment osteotomy once the epiphysis has fused or, rarely, open reduction of the hip, but this carries a risk of avascular necrosis.

THE PAINFUL KNEE

When assessing a painful knee, the hip must always be examined as hip pain is often referred to the knee.

Osgood-Schlatter disease

This is an overuse syndrome commonly occurring in physically active males around puberty, resulting in detachment of cartilage fragments from the tibial tuberosity (traction apophysitis). There is localised tenderness and swelling over the tibial tubercle. The disease is bilateral in 25–50 %. Most

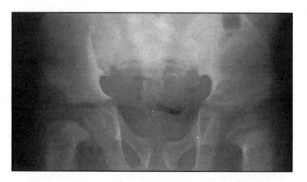

Fig. 23. 9 *Slipped upper femoral epiphysis of the right hip; the left hip is normal.*

resolve with reduced physical activity, trying to avoid over-restriction for a self-limiting disorder which remits when the tibial tubercle fuses to the diaphysis. A knee immobiliser splint may be helpful. In some patients the disorder fails to resolve over several months; a period of immobilisation or excision of the ossicle may then be required.

Chondromalacia patellae

In this condition there is softening of the articular cartilage of the patella. It most often affects adolescent females, causing pain when the patella is tightly apposed to the femoral condyles, as in standing up from sitting or on walking up stairs. Treatment is with rest and physiotherapy for quadriceps muscle strengthening.

Osteochondritis dissecans

Pain is caused by separation of bone and cartilage from the medial femoral condyle following avascular necrosis. Complete separation of articular fragments may result in loose body formation. Treatment is initially with rest and quadriceps exercises; sometimes arthroscopic surgery is required.

Subluxation and dislocation of the patella

Subluxation produces the feeling of instability or giving way of the knee. Treatment is with quadriceps exercises; surgery to realign the pull of the quadriceps on the patellar tendon is occasionally required. Dislocation of the patella laterally occurs suddenly. Reduction occurs spontaneously or on gentle extension of the knee. An X-ray is required to detect loose bodies from bone fracture. Immobilisation and sometimes surgery is required.

Injuries

Sporting injuries to the menisci and ligaments are common in adolescents. MR scans are helpful to determine the extent of damage. Management is usually conservative. In infants and young children, similar injuries are more likely to result in fractures as their ligaments are relatively stronger than their bones.

TALIPES EQUINOVARUS (CLUBFOOT)

Positional talipes from intrauterine compression is common. The foot is of normal size and the deformity is mild and can be corrected to a neutral position with passive manipulation. Often the baby's intrauterine posture can be recreated. If marked, parents can be shown passive exercises by the physiotherapist.

Talipes equinovarus is a complex abnormality (Figs 23.10 and 11). The entire foot is inverted and supinated and the forefoot is adducted. The heel is rotated inwards and in plantar flexion. The affected foot is shorter and the calf muscles thinner than normal. The position of the foot is fixed and cannot be corrected completely. It is often bilateral. The birth prevalence is 1.5 per 1000 live births, with a sex ratio of males to females of 2 to 1. It is of multifactorial inheritance, but may also be secondary to oligohydramnios during pregnancy, or a feature of a malformation syndrome or of a neuromuscular disorder such as spina bifida. It may be associated with congenital dislocation of the hip.

Treatment is started promptly, while the tissues are lax, with stretching and strapping or serial plaster casts. If this corrects the disorder, treatment can be discontinued or night splints used. If the condition is severe, corrective surgery is usually necessary. As the results of corrective surgery performed at a few weeks of age have been disappointing, surgery is increasingly delayed to 6–9 months of age. The condition needs to be differentiated from the rare *congenital vertical talus*, where the foot is stiff and rocker-bottom in shape. Many of these infants have other malformations. The diagnosis can be confirmed on X-ray. Surgery is usually required.

TALIPES CALCANEOVALGUS
The foot is dorsiflexed and everted (Fig. 23.12). It usually results from intrauterine moulding, and self-corrects. Passive foot exercises are sometimes advised. It is sometimes associated with dysplasia of the hip.

PES CAVUS
In pes cavus there is a high arched foot. When it presents in older children, it is often associated with neuromuscular disorders e.g. Friedreich ataxia and Type I hereditary motor

sensory neuropathy (peroneal muscular atrophy). Treatment is required if the foot becomes stiff or painful.

Disorders of the back, spine and neck

BACK PAIN
Back pain is uncommon in pre-adolescent children, becoming more common during adolescence. In contrast to adults, a cause can often be identified:
- **muscle spasm** or soft tissue pain from injury, often sport related
- **poor posture**, may accompany hypermobility of the joints
- **Scheuermann disease**, an osteochondritis of the thoracic vertebrae in adolescents resulting in a fixed kyphosis; diagnosed on X-ray
- **spondylolysis/spondylolisthesis** – stress fracture of the *pars interarticularis* of the vertebra, typically lower lumbar (spondylolysis); if the affected vertebral body moves anteriorly it produces a spondylolisthesis; diagnosis by X-ray
- **vertebral osteomyelitis/discitis** – presents with reluctance to walk or bear weight, with tenderness over the affected site; diagnosed on bone and CT scans
- **tumours** – may be benign or malignant
- **spinal cord/root compression** e.g. from a tumour or prolapsed intervertebral disc
- **idiopathic pain syndrome** – diagnosed when no physical cause is found; may be exacerbated by psychological stress.

SCOLIOSIS
Scoliosis is a lateral curvature in the frontal plane of the spine. In structural scoliosis, there is rotation of the vertebral bodies which causes a prominence in the back from rib asymmetry. It results in cosmetic problems and sometimes cardiorespiratory failure.

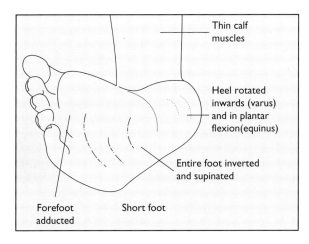

Thin calf muscles

Heel rotated inwards (varus) and in plantar flexion(equinus)

Entire foot inverted and supinated

Forefoot adducted

Short foot

Fig. 23.10 Abnormalities in talipes equinovarus.

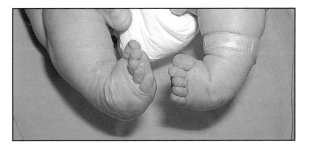

Fig. 23.11 Talipes equinovarus.

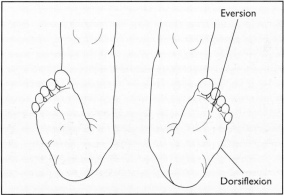

Eversion

Dorsiflexion

Fig. 23.12 Talipes calcaneovalgus.

Causes of scoliosis are:

- **idiopathic** – the most common, either early onset (less than five years old) or late onset
- **congenital** – from a congenital defect of the spine e.g. hemivertebrae, spina bifida, VATER association
- **secondary** – to other disorders, such as neuromuscular imbalance from cerebral palsy, muscular dystrophy, polio or disorders of bone such as neurofibromatosis or of connective tissues such as Marfan syndrome, or may be postural, such as secondary to leg length discrepancy.

Early onset idiopathic scoliosis usually resolves, but a few progress. Late onset idiopathic scoliosis is the most common type (85 %) and mainly affects girls of 10–14 years of age during their pubertal growth spurt.

The scoliosis can be identified on examing the child's back on forward bending (Fig. 23.13). This has been used as a screening test, but it identifies many minor degrees of curvature which resolve spontaneously and does not appear to reduce the need for surgery. For these reasons, routine screening is not currently recommended in the UK. If the scoliosis disappears on forward bending, it is postural and resolves, although leg lengths should be checked. The severity of the curvature of the spine can be determined by measuring the angle of curvature on an X-ray of the spine. Mild scoliosis usually resolves spontaneously. Treatment of severe scoliosis is with spinal braces, but their efficacy is questionable, and sometimes with specialist spinal surgery.

TORTICOLLIS

The most common cause of torticollis or wry neck in infants is a sternomastoid tumour (congenital muscular torticollis), which occurs in the first few weeks of life. It presents with a mobile non-tender nodule, which can be felt within the body of the sternocleidomastoid muscle. There may be restriction of head turning and tilting of the head. The condition usually resolves in 2–6 months. Passive stretching is performed, but its efficacy is unproven.

The painful limb

Episodes of generalised pain in the lower limbs, referred to as 'growing pains', or nocturnal idiopathic pain are common in pre-school children. The pain often wakes the child from sleep, and settles with massage or comforting. It occurs less often during the day, the child is otherwise healthy and there is no evidence of musculoskeletal disease. Children with hypermobility (thumbs and little fingers can be hyperextended onto the forearms, Fig. 23.14, elbows and knees can be hyperextended beyond 10°, hands can be placed flat on the floor with legs straight) often complain of generalised limb pain. In older children, limb pain may be related to psychological stress or result from over-protection of the limb following minor injury. The limb may be held in a splinted position, and in time localised tenderness, swelling and alteration in colour may develop (reflex sympathetic dystrophy) and eventually muscle atrophy (Sudeck atrophy) may occur.

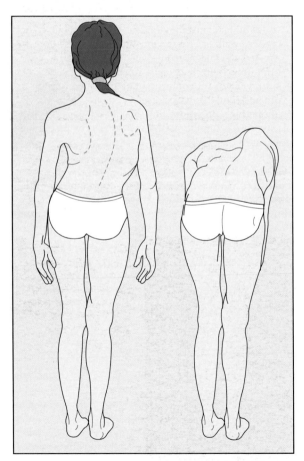

Fig. 23. 13 *Structural scoliosis with vertebral rotation shown by rib rotation on bending forward.*

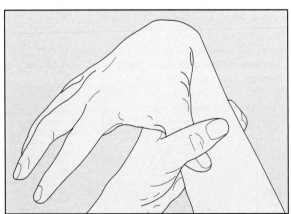

Fig. 23. 14 *Hypermobility syndrome, showing ability to hyperextend the thumb onto the forearm.*

Limb pain of acute onset has a number of causes. Trauma is the most common, usually accidental, often from sports injuries or falls, but occasionally non-accidental. Osteomyelitis and bone tumours are uncommon, but need urgent treatment.

OSTEOMYELITIS
In osteomyelitis, there is infection of the metaphysis of long bones. The most common sites are the distal femur and proximal tibia, but any bone may be affected (Fig 23.15). It is usually due to haematogenous spread of the pathogen, but may arise by direct spread from an infected wound. The skin is swollen directly over the affected site. Where the joint capsule is inserted distal to the epiphyseal plate, as in the hip, osteomyelitis may spread to cause septic arthritis. Most infections are caused by *Staphylococcus aureus*, but other pathogens include *Streptococci* and *H. influenzae*. In sickle cell anaemia, the risk is increased not only of staphylococcal but also of salmonella osteomyelitis. Chronic infection can cause a localised abscess in the bone (Brodie abscess) but is uncommon. Infection may be from tuberculosis, but this is rare in the UK.

Presentation
This is usually with a markedly painful immobile limb (pseudoparesis) in a child with an acute febrile illness. Directly over the infected site there is swelling and exquisite tenderness, and it may be erythematous and warm. Moving the limb causes severe pain. There may be a sterile effusion of an adjacent joint. Presentation may be more insidious in infants, in whom swelling or reduced limb movement is the initial sign. Beyond infancy, presentation may be with back pain in a vertebral infection or with a limp or groin pain in infection of the pelvis. Occasionally, multiple foci are affected (e.g. disseminated staphylococcal or *H. influenzae* infection).

Investigation
Blood cultures are usually positive, and the white blood count and acute phase reactants are raised. X-rays are initially normal, other than showing soft tissue swelling; it takes 7–10 days for subperiosteal new bone formation and localised bone rarefaction to become visible . The presence and site of infection can usually be identified on radionuclide bone scan (Fig. 23.16. Ultrasound may show periosteal elevation at presentation. The X-ray changes of chronic osteomyelitis are shown in figure 23.17.

Treatment
Prompt treatment with parenteral antibiotics is required for several weeks to prevent bone necrosis, chronic infection with a discharging sinus, limb deformity and amyloidosis.

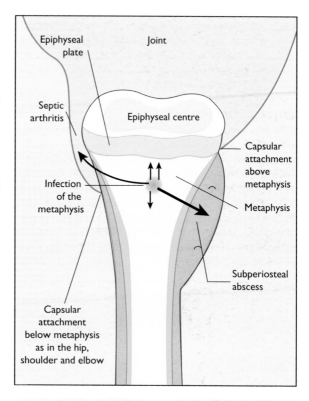

Fig. 23. 15 Possible spread of osteomyelitis. In children, the epiphyseal growth plate limits the spread of metaphyseal infection. In infants, before maturation of the growth plate, infection can spread directly to cause joint destruction and arrested growth.

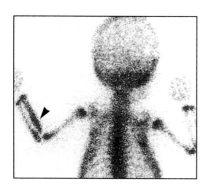

Fig. 23. 16 Bone scan of osteomyelitis with increased radionuclide uptake of the left radius. (Courtesy of Dr Carty.)

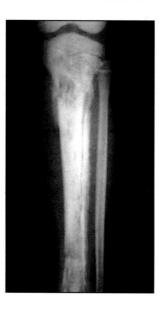

Fig. 23. 17 Chronic osteomyelitis, showing periosteal reaction along the lateral shaft of the tibia and multiple hypodense areas within the metaphyseal regions.

Antibiotics are given intravenously (e.g. flucloxacillin and sometimes fusidic acid; in young children a third-generation cephalosporin is added to cover *H. influenzae*) until there is clinical recovery and the acute phase reactants have returned to normal, followed by oral therapy for several weeks. Aspiration or surgical decompression of the subperiosteal space may be performed if the presentation is atypical or in immunocompromised children. Surgical drainage is performed if the condition does not respond rapidly to antibiotic therapy. The affected limb is initially rested in a splint and subsequently mobilised.

BONE TUMOURS

Malignant tumours, osteogenic sarcoma and Ewing tumour, are rare and present with pain or swelling or occasionally with a pathological fracture (*see* Chapter 18). Osteoid osteoma is a benign tumour affecting adolescents, especially boys, usually involving the femur or tibia. The pain, which is more severe at night, improves with salicylate therapy. There may be some localised tenderness. The X-ray is diagnostic, with a sharply demarcated radiolucent nidus of osteoid tissue surrounded by sclerotic bone, but if the X-ray is normal, a CT or MR scan may be required. Treatment is by surgical removal.

Arthritis

Presentation may be acute, with the sudden onset of joint pain, or chronic, with the insidious onset of early morning stiffness of the joints, 'gelling' after inactivity, or the development of a limp or slowness on walking. Initially, there may be only minimal evidence of joint swelling; but subsequently there may be swelling of the joint due to fluid within it (an effusion or pus or blood), inflammation and, in chronic arthritis, there may be proliferation (thickening) of the synovium and swelling of the periarticular soft tissues. Long term, there may be bone expansion from overgrowth, which in the knee may cause leg lengthening and in the wrist advancement of bone age.

In a monoarthritis of acute onset, septic arthritis or osteomyelitis must be diagnosed and treated urgently. Other conditions which need to be considered, using the hip as an example, are listed as causes of a painful limp in Figure 23.6 . The causes of a polyarthritis are listed in Figure 23.18.

SEPTIC ARTHRITIS

This is a serious infection of the joint space as it can lead to bone destruction. It is most common in children less than two years old. It usually results from haematogenous spread, but may also occur following a puncture wound or infected skin lesions e.g. chicken pox. In young children, it may result from spread from adjacent osteomyelitis into joints where the capsule inserts below the epiphyseal growth plate.

Beyond the neonatal period, the most common organism is *Staphylococcus aureus*, and usually affects a single joint. *H. influenzae* was an important cause in young children prior to Hib immunisation, and often affected multiple sites.

Presentation

This is usually with an erythematous, warm, acutely tender joint, with a reduced range of movement, in an acutely unwell, febrile child. Infants often hold the limb still (pseudoparesis, pseudoparalysis) and cry if it is moved. A joint effusion may be visible in peripheral joints but is difficult to detect in deep joints such as the hip.

The diagnosis of septic arthritis of the hip can be particularly difficult in toddlers, as the joint is well covered by subcutaneous fat (Fig. 23.19). Initial presentation may be with a limp or pain referred to the knee. In osteomyelitis, there may be a sympathetic joint effusion but the tenderness is over the bone.

Investigation

There is an increased white cell count and acute phase reactants. Ultrasound of deep joints, such as the hip, is helpful to identify an effusion. X-rays are used to exclude trauma and other bony lesions but are initially normal, other than showing widening of the joint space and soft tissue swelling. A bone scan may be helpful. Aspiration of the joint space may reveal organisms and a positive culture in some but not all instances. A prolonged course of antibiotics, initially intravenously (e.g. flucloxacillin, which

Fig. 23.18 Causes of polyarthritis	
Infection	Bacterial — septicaemia/septic arthritis, TB
	Viral — rubella, mumps, adenovirus, Coxsackie B, herpes, hepatitis, parvovirus
	Other — Mycoplasma, Lyme disease, rickettsia
	Reactive — gastrointestinal infection, streptococcal infection
	Rheumatic fever
Inflammatory bowel disease	Crohn disease, ulcerative colitis
Vasculitis	Henoch-Schönlein purpura, Kawasaki disease
Haematological disorders	Haemophilia, sickle cell disease
Malignant disorders	Leukaemia, neuroblastoma
Connective tissue disorders	Juvenile chronic arthritis (JCA), juvenile ankylosing spondylitis, systemic lupus eryhthematosis (SLE), dermatomyositis, mixed connective tissue disease
Other	Cystic fibrosis

in young children is combined with a third-generation cephalosporin to cover *H. influenzae*) should be given. Washing out of the joint or surgical drainage may be required if resolution does not occur rapidly or if it is a deep-seated joint such as the hip. The joint is initially immobilised in a functional position, but subsequently mobilised to prevent permanent deformity.

 Early treatment of septic arthritis is essential to prevent destruction of the articular cartilage and bone.

JUVENILE CHRONIC ARTHRITIS

Juvenile chronic arthritis (JCA) is a group of conditions in which there is chronic arthritis lasting, by definition, more than three months (six weeks in the US), presenting before 16 years of age. JCA is classified according to its presentation as systemic, polyarticular (more than four joints) and pauci/oligoarticular (up to and including four joints). Further classification according to the presence of antinuclear antibodies (ANA), HLA-B27 and rheumatoid factor and clinical examination has been proposed (Fig. 23.20). Infection and other causes of arthritis must be excluded.

Systemic (Still disease)

This usually affects young children. Clinical features are:
- acute illness, marked malaise
- high, spiking fever
- anorexia, weight loss
- salmon-pink rash at the height of the fever
- aches and pains in the joints and muscles (arthralgia/myalgia), but there is often no arthritis at presentation
- lymphadenopathy, hepatosplenomegaly and occasionally pericarditis
- anaemia, raised neutrophil and platelet count and markedly raised acute phase reactants.

Some children recover without developing chronic arthritis, others progress to a polyarthritis.

Polyarticular

This occurs at all ages, and in girls more than in boys. Any joint may be affected, but most often there is symmetrical involvement of the wrists and hands (Fig. 23.21), knees and ankles. The cervical spine, temporomandibular joint and jaw may also be affected.

A few children, usually females in the second decade, can be classified as having juvenile rheumatoid arthritis (JRA). They have a symmetrical polyarthritis and remain rheumatoid factor positive (seropositive polyarticular) and have a pattern of disease similar to adult rheumatoid arthritis. They may have or develop subcutaneous rheumatoid nodules, and over half develop chronic arthritis. Care needs to be taken on using the term 'rheumatoid arthritis' in children as it conjures a picture of a chronic crippling disease, whereas many children with juvenile chronic arthritis recover completely. In addition, rheumatoid factor may be transiently positive during acute illness in children. The term should be reserved

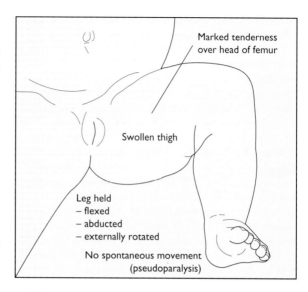

Fig. 23.19 *Septic arthritis of the hip in infants, showing the characteristic posture to reduce intracapsular pressure. Any leg movement is painful and is resisted.*

Fig. 23.20 *Revised classification of juvenile chronic arthritis (JCA)*
(proposed by the International League of Associations for Rheumatism, ILAR, 1994).

Systemic (9 %)
Polyarticular (> 4 joints) seronegative (16 %)
Polyarticular seropositive (3 %)
Pauciarticular or oligoarticular (≤4 joints) (49 %)
Enthesitis associated arthritis (usually B27-associated) (7 %)
Extended pauciarticular arthritis (8 %)
Juvenile psoriatic arthritis (7 %)
Unclassified (1%)

Percentages quoted are for the UK (ARC/British Paediatric Rheumatology Group)

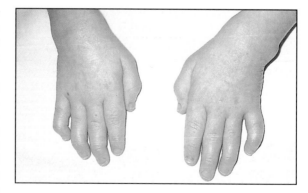

Fig. 23.21 *Polyarticular juvenile chronic arthritis, showing swelling of the wrists, metacarpal and interphalangeal joints and early swan-neck deformities of the the fingers.*

for those children with polyarticular disease who remain rheumatoid factor positive.

Pauciarticular

This usually occurs in young children, affecting the knees, less often the ankles and wrists. There is an increased risk of developing eye disease, a chronic anterior uveitis, especially in females who are antinuclear antibody (ANA) positive.

Enthesitis associated arthritis (juvenile spondyloarthropathy, B27-associated arthritis)

This predominantly affects older boys who present with a large joint arthritis, usually of the lower limbs and/or a swollen digit (sausage finger) and may have the HLA-B27 tissue type and a positive family history. In addition, there may be inflammation of the insertion of tendons into bone e.g. Achilles tendon, and of the plantar fascia (enthesitis). Subsequently there may be sacroiliac and spinal involvement. Acute symptomatic iritis may occur in these children and requires ophthalmological referral, but other complications are rare.

Juvenile psoriatic arthritis

Often involves the interphalangeal joints, and may present with a sausage-shaped swelling of a digit. It may occur before the onset of skin lesions or nail pitting.

Complications

Flexion contractures of the joints

Occur from holding the joint in the most comfortable position, which minimises intra-articular pressure (Fig. 23.22). Chronic disease can lead to joint destruction and the need for joint replacement in a few children.

Growth failure

May be generalised from anorexia and chronic disease, combined with the effects of steroid therapy.

Chronic anterior uveitis

Is asymptomatic but can lead to severe visual impairment. Regular ophthalmologic screening is indicated, especially in children with pauciarticular disease.

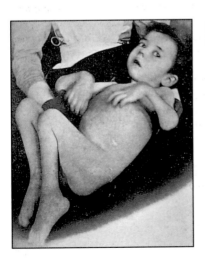

Fig. 23.22 Severe untreated polyarticular or systemic juvenile chronic arthritis, from Still's original description in 1897, showing severe misery, fused neck, flexion deformities and wasting of the muscles and subcutaneous tissue.

Amyloidosis

Is a rare but serious complication causing proteinuria and subsequent renal failure.

Management

A multi-disciplinary team approach is required for optimal treatment and to provide the child and family with information and psychosocial support. Successful management requires considerable compliance and motivation.

Physiotherapy is essential in order to encourage mobility and maintain a full range of joint movement and muscle strength. Daily exercise is usually required. Hydrotherapy is a helpful adjunct. Resting splints are used to prevent flexion contractures, and working splints for the wrists to maintain posture while writing.

Pain control and suppression of inflammation are provided by non-steroidal anti-inflammatory drugs (NSAIDs), such as naproxen or ibuprofen. Intra-articular corticosteroid therapy can be helpful in both pauciarticular and polyarticular disease. Multiple injections may be required.

Slow-acting anti-rheumatic drugs are used for persistent active polyarthritis not controlled by NSAIDs. Methotrexate is the drug of most benefit, but its short- and long-term side-effects need to be monitored. The place of therapy with gold, penicillamine, hydroxychloroquine and other agents is unproven. Systemic corticosteroids may be required for severe uveitis, pericarditis or severe systemic disease or immobility. They may also be needed to control polyarticular disease, using an alternate day regimen in the lowest dose that is efficacious. High-dose parenteral corticosteroids may be needed for an acute exacerbation of joint disease.

Genetic skeletal dysplasias

There are several hundred bone dysplasias, which are generalised developmental disorders of bone. They usually result in reduced growth and abnormality of bone shape rather than impaired strength, other than in osteogenesis imperfecta. The bones of the limbs and spine are often affected, resulting in short stature. Intelligence is usually normal. Improved knowledge of the molecular basis of collagen and its disorders is allowing better understanding and delineation of some of these disorders.

Achondroplasia

Inheritance is autosomal dominant, but about 50 % are new mutations. Clinical features are short stature from marked shortening of the limbs, a large head, frontal bossing and depression of the nasal bridge. The hands are short and broad. A marked lumbar lordosis develops. Hydrocephalus sometimes occurs.

Thanatophoric dysplasia

This results in stillbirth. The infants have a large head, extremely short limbs and a small chest. The appeearence

Case history

SYSTEMIC-ONSET JUVENILE CHRONIC ARTHRITIS

A two-year-old boy presented with a high fever (Fig. 23.23a) and malaise. A salmon-coloured rash was present at times of fever (Fig. 23.23b). Acute investigation showed markedly raised acute phase reactants. A diagnosis of systemic onset juvenile chronic arthritis was made on the basis of the clinical presentation and exclusion of other disorders (Fig. 23.23c).

Shortly afterwards, he developed polyarthritic joint disease. He required high-dose alternate-day corticos-teroid therapy as well as other disease-modifying drugs. He developed marked short stature. In his teens he required bilateral hip replacements. He is now at university, drives his own car and is fiercely independent.

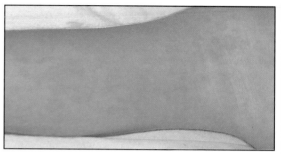

Fig. 23. 23b Salmon-pink rash.

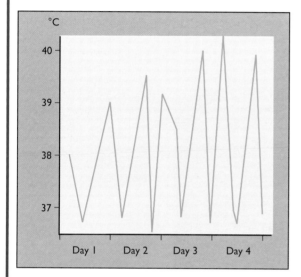

Fig. 23. 23a Temperature chart.

Fig. 23.23c Differential diagnosis of systemic onset of juvenile chronic arthritis.
Infection – bacterial/viral/protozoal (e.g. malaria), Mycoplasma and other (e.g. Lyme disease)
Kawasaki disease
Rheumatic fever
Reactive arthritis – post-streptococcal, post-enteric, post-viral
Malignancy – leukaemia/neuroblastoma
Connective tissue disorders – systemic lupus erythromatosis (SLE), polyarteritis nodosa (PAN)

of the bones on X-ray are characteristic. The importance of the correct diagnosis of this disorder is that, in contrast to achondroplasia, its inheritance is sporadic. It may be identified on antenatal ultrasound.

Cleidocranial dysostosis

In this autosomal dominant disorder there is absence of part or all of the clavicles and delay in closure of the anterior fontanelle and of ossification of the skull. The child is often able to bring the shoulders together in front of the chest to touch each other as a trick manoeuvre. Short stature is usually present.

Arthrogryposis

This is a heterogeneous group of congenital disorders in which there is stiffness and contracture of joints. Its cause is usually unknown, but it may be associated with oligohydramnios or with widespread congenital anomalies or chromosomal disorders. It is usually sporadic. Marked flexion contractures of the knees, elbows and wrists, dislocation of the hips and other joints, talipes equinovarus and scoliosis are common, but the disorder may be localised to the upper or lower limbs. The skin is thin, subcutaneous tissue is reduced and there is marked muscle atrophy proximal and distal to the affected joints. Intelligence is usually unaffected. Management is with physiotherapy and correction of deformities where possible by splints, plaster casts or surgery. Walking ability is related to the severity of the disorder.

Osteogenesis imperfecta (brittle bone disease)

This is a group of disorders of collagen metabolism causing bone fragility, with bowing and frequent fractures.

In the most common form (Type I), which is autosomal dominant, fractures occur during childhood. Affected children also have blue sclerae and may develop hearing loss. The prognosis is variable. It is autosomal dominant. Fractures require splinting to minimise joint deformity. There is a severe, lethal form (Type II) with multiple fractures already present before birth (Fig. 23.24). Many affected infants are stillborn. Inheritance may be autosomal dominant with new mutations or autosomal recessive. In other types, scleral discolouration may be minimal. The condition is often considered in the evaluation of unexplained fractures in suspected child abuse.

Osteopetrosis (marble bone disease)

In this rare disorder the bones are dense but brittle. The severe autosomal recessive disorder presents with failure to thrive, hypocalcaemia, anaemia and thrombocytopenia and infection. Prognosis is poor, but bone marrow transplantation can be curative. A less severe autosomal dominant form may present during childhood with fractures.

Marfan sydrome

This is an autosomal dominant disorder associated with tall stature, long thin digits (arachnodactyly), hyperextensible joints, a high arched palate and dislocation of the lenses of the eyes and severe myopia. The body proportions are altered, the long, thin limbs resulting in a greater distance between the pubis and soles (lower segment) than from the crown to the pubis (upper segment). The arm span, measured from the extended fingers, is greater than the height. There may be chest deformity and scoliosis. The major problems are cardiovascular, from degeneration of the media of vessel walls resulting in a dilated, incompetent aortic valve and mitral valve prolapse and regurgitation. Aneurysms of the aorta may dissect or rupture. Monitoring by echocardiography is required.

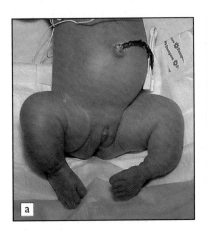
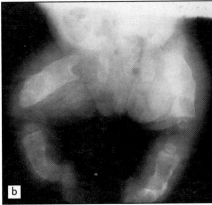

Fig. 23.24 Osteogenesis imperfecta (Type II).
a) Shortened deformed lower limbs.
b) X-ray showing gross deformity of the bones of the lower limbs with multiple healing fractures.

FURTHER READING

Ansell BM, Rudge S, Schaller JG. Color Atlas of Paediatric Rheumatology. London, Wolfe Medical Publications, 1991.

Muller M (ed) Pediatric clinics of North America. Ped Rheum. 1995;**42**:3.

Southwood TR, Malleson PN. Arthritis in children and adolescents. In: Clinical Paediatrics 1(3). Baillière Tindall, London, 1993. A short multi-author book.

CHAPTER 24

Neurological Disorders

• *Meningitis* • *Encephalitis* • *Headache* • *Seizures* • *Cerebral palsy* • *Ataxia* • *Cerebral haemorrhage* • *Neural tube defects and hydrocephalus* • *Neuromuscular disorders* • *Neurocutaneous syndromes* • *Neurodegenerative disorders*

Key facts about neurological disorders in children are:
- bacterial meningitis predominantly affects children
- headaches are common in older children and adolescents
- febrile convulsions occur in 3% of children
- cerebral palsy usually requires multidisciplinary and multi-agency care
- the birth prevalence of neural tube defects has markedly declined
- neuromuscular and neurodegenerative disorders are more accurately diagnosed with modern technology such as DNA analysis, MR spectroscopy and advanced biochemical techniques and enzyme assays.

Meningitis

BACTERIAL MENINGITIS

Over 80% of all patients with bacterial meningitis in the UK are younger than 16 years old. Bacterial meningitis remains a serious infection in children, with a 5–10% mortality. Over 10% of survivors are left with long-term neurological impairment.

Pathophysiology
Bacterial infection of the meninges usually follows bacteraemia. It is now thought that much of the damage caused by meningeal infection results from the host response to infection and not from the organism itself. The release of inflammatory mediators and activated leucokines together with endothelial damage leads to cerebral oedema, raised intracranial pressure and decreased cerebral blood flow.

Organisms
The organisms which commonly cause bacterial meningitis vary according to the child's age (Fig. 24.1).

Presentation
The early signs and symptoms of meningitis are non-specific, which makes early diagnosis problematic. Infants and young children may present with any combination of fever, poor feeding, vomiting, irritability, lethargy, drowsiness, seizures, reduced consciousness or coma. A bulging fontanelle, neck stiffness (Fig. 24.2) and the child lying with an arched back are late signs. Once children can talk, they are likely to describe the classical features of headache, neck stiffness and photophobia. Neck stiffness may also be seen in some children with tonsillitis and cervical lymphadenopathy. Meningococcal infection should be seriously considered in any febrile child with purpura, even if the child does not appear unduly ill at the time. As children with meningitis may also be septicaemic, signs of shock, including tachycardia, poor capillary refill, oliguria and hypotension, may be present.

Investigations
The essential investigations are listed in Chapter 4. The non-specific early clinical features of meningitis in infants and young children necessitates a low threshold for doing a diagnostic lumbar puncture (Fig. 24.3)to obtain cerebrospinal fluid (CSF) to confirm the diagnosis and identify the organism responsible and its antibiotic sensitivity. However, if there is raised intracranial pressure, a lumbar puncture carries a risk of coning of the cerebellum through the foramen magnum and should not be performed (Fig. 24.4). Instead, a blood culture, which will frequently reveal the causative organism, a rapid antigen screen and a throat swab should be taken and antibiotics and supportive therapy given immediately.

It is imperative that there is no delay in the administration of antibiotics. If necessary, a lumbar puncture can be performed once the child's condition has stabilized.

Fig. 24.1 Organisms which commonly cause bacterial meningitis according to age

Neonatal–3 months	Group B streptococcus
	E. coli and other Gram-negative organisms
	Listeria monocytogenes
1 month–6 years	Neisseria meningitidis (meningococcus)
	Streptococcus pneumoniae (pneumococcus)
	Haemophilus influenzae
> 6 years	Streptococcus pneumoniae
	Neisseria meningitidis

Fig. 24.2 Signs associated with neck stiffness

Brudzinski sign	Flexion of the neck with the child supine causes flexion of the knees and hips.
Kernig sign	With the child lying supine and with the hips and knees flexed, there is pain on extension of the knee.

Fig. 24.3 *Typical changes in the cerebrospinal fluid (CSF) in meningitis beyond the neonatal period*

Aetiology	Appearance	White blood cells	Protein	Glucose
Normal	Clear	0–5/mm³	0.15–0.4 g/l	>50% blood glucose
Bacterial	Turbid	↑↑Polymorphs	↑↑	↓
Viral	Clear	↑Lymphocytes, initially may be more polymorphs	↓	Normal
TB	Clear/viscous	Lymphocytes	↑↑↑	↓↓

Fig. 24.4 *Contraindications to lumbar puncture*

Cardiorespiratory instability
Focal neurological signs
Clinical signs of raised intracranial pressure (including coma or papilloedema)
Coagulopathy
Local infection at site of needle insertion
If it causes undue delay in the administration of antibiotics

Although the organism will rarely be grown following antibiotic therapy, biochemical and cytological abnormalities will still indicate bacterial meningitis for up to 48 hours after starting treatment.

Management
This is described in Chapter 4. The choice of antibiotics will depend on the likely pathogen. A third-generation cephalosporin, e.g. cefotaxime or ceftriaxone, has become the preferred antibiotic. Ampicillin with chloramphenicol is an acceptable alternative, but resistance to these drugs means that they cannot be relied upon when used as single agents, and the side-effects of chloramphenicol makes it undesirable as first-line treatment. Below three months of age, ampicillin should be included to cover *Listeria monocytogenes* infection. Dexamethasone is given when antibiotics are started as it may reduce the risk of vasculitis.

Cerebral complications
Local vasculitis. This may lead to cranial nerve pareses (usually VIth or VIIIth nerve). All children who have had meningitis should have an audiological assessment at follow-up.

Local cerebral infarction. Results in focal or multifocal seizures, which may result in subsequent epilepsy.

Subdural effusion. Particularly associated with *Haemophilus influenzae* meningitis. This is confirmed by CT scan. Most resolve spontaneously.

Hydrocephalus. May result from impaired resorption of CSF. A ventricular shunt may be required.

Cerebral abscess. The child's clinical condition deteriorates, with the emergence of signs of a space-occupying lesion. The temperature will continue to fluctuate. It is confirmed on CT scan. Aspiration of the abscess is required.

Prophylaxis
Prophylactic treatment with rifampicin is given to all household contacts for meningococcal meningitis and for young children in the household for *Haemophilus influenzae* infection. It is also given to the patient for 48 hours before discharge to eradicate nasopharyngeal carriage.

SPECIFIC CAUSES

Meningococcal infection
In the UK, *Neisseria meningitidis* (meningococcus) is the most common cause of meningitis and its incidence has increased over the last five years. There have been winter peaks and small outbreaks. In countries where it remains endemic, larger outbreaks occur. Meningococcal infection is a disease that strikes fear into both parents and doctors as it can kill perfectly healthy children within hours. While meningitis is the main clinical form of infection with this organism, septicaemia alone carries a worse prognosis. Characteristically, the infection is accompanied by a purpuric rash which may start anywhere on the body and then spreads. Characteristic lesions are irregular in size and outline and have a necrotic centre (Fig. 24.5). Any febrile child who develops a purpuric rash should be treated immediately with systemic antibiotics such as penicillin when seen at home or in the general practitioner's surgery before urgent transfer to hospital. Although there is a vaccine against Groups A and C meningococcus, there is no effective vaccine for Group B meningococcus, which accounts for more than 60% of isolates in the UK.

 Meningococcal septicaemia and meningitis can kill children in hours.

Haemophilus meningitis
Before the introduction of Hib vaccine, *H. influenzae* type b was the second most common cause of meningitis in the UK and the most common in the US. Immunisation has been remarkably effective and should almost eradicate this organism as a cause of meningitis.

Pneumococcal meningitis
While this organism was responsible for only 10% of meningitis before Hib vaccine was introduced, its prominence will increase as *H. influenzae* meningitis declines. It is associated with a high mortality (10%) and morbidity, with more than 30% of survivors having neurological sequellae.

Tuberculous meningitis
Tuberculous meningitis, although uncommon, is still seen

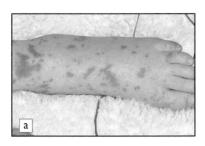
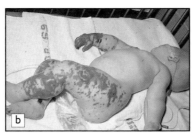

Fig. 24.5 (a) Characteristic lesions in meningococcal infection are irregular in size and outline and have a necrotic centre. (b) The lesions may be very extensive, when it is called 'purpura fulminans'.

in the UK. The onset of the illness is often insidious, over 2–3 weeks. Meningism may be minimal. There may be a history of TB contact. Most, but not all, affected children have a positive Mantoux test and abnormal chest X-ray. The acid-fast bacilli may be identified on Ziehl–Nielsen staining of the CSF or in early morning urine samples or gastric aspirates. As there are few organisms, they are easily missed. Rapid diagnostic tests, e.g. based on polymerase chain reaction (PCR), are under development but not widely available. As the cultures may take 2–3 months, treatment will need to be started empirically. This condition is associated with a high mortality and morbidity.

Partially treated bacterial meningitis

Children are frequently given oral antibiotics for a non-specific febrile illness. If they have early bacterial meningitis this partial treatment with antibiotics may cause diagnostic problems. CSF examination usually shows a raised number of white cells, but cultures are usually negative. Latex agglutination is sometimes helpful in these circumstances. Where the diagnosis is suspected clinically, a full course of antibiotics should be given.

Viral meningitis

Overall, two-thirds of CNS infections are viral. Causes include enteroviruses, Epstein–Barr virus, adenoviruses

and mumps. Mumps was the most commonly identified viral cause of meningitis, but should become less common with the wide uptake of MMR vaccine. The illness is usually much less severe than bacterial meningitis and a full recovery can be anticipated. Poliomyelitis has fortunately become rare in the UK, but is still a problem in many developing countries.

Uncommon pathogens

Where the clinical course is atypical or there is failure to respond to antibiotic and supportive therapy, unusual organisms, e.g. Mycoplasma or *Borrelia burgdorferi* (Lyme disease), or fungal infection need to be considered. Uncommon pathogens are particularly likely in children who are immunocompromised. Fistulae from a congenital midline sinus may cause recurrent bacterial meningitis.

Encephalitis

Whereas in meningitis there is inflammation of the meninges, in encephalitis there is inflammation of the brain substance.

Case history

MENINGOCOCCAL SEPTICAEMIA AND MENINGITIS

This 7-month-old boy presented with a 12-hour history of a purpuric rash, which was spreading, and lethargy. On admission to hospital he required immediate resuscitation and transfer to a paediatric intensive care unit for multi-organ failure (Fig. 24.6a). The gross oedema is from capillary leak. He required colloid and inotropic support and peritoneal dialysis for renal failure. He made a full recovery (Fig. 24.6b).

 A febrile child with a purpuric rash should be given systemic antibiotics immediately and transferred urgently to hospital.

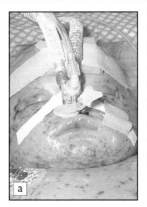
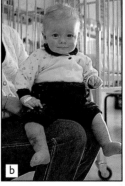

Fig. 24.6 (a) A boy with meningococcal septicaemia receiving intensive care.
(b) After full recovery

There may be:
- direct invasion of the cerebrum by a neurotoxic virus (encephalitis)
- delayed brain swelling following a disordered neuro-immunological response to an antigen, usually a virus (post-infectious encephalopathy), such as following measles
- slow virus infection such as HIV infection or subacute sclerosing panencephalitis (SSPE) following measles.

In an encephalopathy (e.g. Reye syndrome, inborn errors of metabolism) there are neurological features suggestive of encephalitis, but brain inflammation is absent.

The major causes of viral encephalitis in the UK are herpes simplex virus 1 and 2, enteroviruses, varicella and mumps. The clinical features, investigations and treatment are described in Chapter 4. Of particular importance is the early recognition and treatment of herpes simplex encephalitis, in which the characteristic feature is the development of focal seizures and neurological signs. The EEG and CT or MR brain scan may show temporal lobe abnormalities (Fig. 24.7). Untreated, the mortality rate is about 70% and those who survive often have permanent neurological damage.

Treatment with acyclovir improves the prognosis and should be given promptly whenever the diagnosis is suspected. Confirmation of the diagnosis is made retrospectively from CSF viral culture, detection of viral DNA in the CSF by polymerase chain reaction (PCR), or elevated antibody titres to the organism. Most affected children do not have outward signs of herpes infection such as herpetic gingivostomatitis or skin lesions.

Neonatal meningitis. See Chapter 8.
Septicaemia. See Chapter 4.
Bacterial meningitis. See Chapter 4.
Viral encephalitis. See Chapter 4.

Headache

Headaches are common in children. At least 95% of school children will experience one or more headaches each year, 10% have recurrent tension headaches and 6% migraine. Headaches occur infrequently in young children but become more common with age. They affect females slightly more often than males. The causes of acute headache are listed in Figure 24.8. The causes of recurrent headache are considered below.

TENSION HEADACHE

This is a symmetrical headache of gradual onset, often described as a tightness, band or pressure. There are usually no other symptoms, but it may be accompanied by abdominal pain and behaviour problems. It may occur every day.

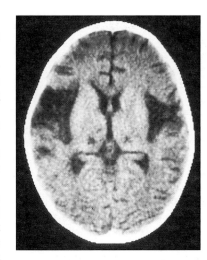

Fig. 24.7 Herpes simplex encephalitis. The CT scan shows gross atrophy from loss of neural tissue in the temporo-parietal regions.

MIGRAINE

This periodic disorder is characterised by paroxysmal headache, often unilateral, accompanied by visual or gastro-intestinal disturbance and, rarely, unilateral sensory or motor symptoms. The visual disturbances (aura) include:
- hemianopia (loss of half the visual field)
- scotoma (small areas of visual loss)
- fortification spectra (seeing zigzag lines).

The gastrointestinal features may be:
- nausea
- vomiting
- abdominal pain.

The attacks usually last for a few hours, during which time the child prefers to lie down in a quiet, dark place and are relieved by sleep.

Migraine is classified as:
- common – without aura
- classical – with an aura (visual, sensory or motor) which precedes the migraine; this type is present in about 10% of sufferers
- complicated – associated with neurological phenomena such as ophthalmoplegia, hemiparesis, parasthesiae or hemidysaesthesia (altered sensation down one side of the body).

At times, aura may not be accompanied by a headache. Complicated migraine occurs in only 1–2% of cases and, rarely, recurrent bouts may lead to permanent neurological deficit.

Fig. 24.8 Causes of acute headache
Febrile illness
Meningitis/encephalitis
Acute sinusitis
Subarachnoid or intracerebral haemorrhage
Head injury
Benign intracranial hypertension
Drugs including alcohol
Migraine
Stress

Rarely, vertebro-basilar migraine may give rise to cerebellar signs, including nystagmus and vomiting with retching.

Tension-like headache and migraine may be part of the same pathophysiological spectrum, as symptoms often overlap, making it difficult to separate the diagnoses. Half the children with recurrent headaches have an affected first- or second-degree relative. In young children, episodes of nausea, vomiting and recurrent abdominal pain may precede the development of recurrent headaches (abdominal migraine). Stressful situations at home or school may trigger headaches or make them more difficult to cope with. In some people, migraine occurs at times of relaxation, e.g. weekends. Certain foods may trigger headaches – cow's milk, cheese, chocolate, eggs, coffee and the colouring tartrazine. In some girls, headaches are related to menstruation.

RAISED INTRACRANIAL PRESSURE

It is the fear of a brain tumour that leads many parents to take their child with headaches to see a doctor. The cardinal feature of an intracranial space-occupying lesion is that the headache is worse when lying down (in contrast to migraine and other headaches when lying down helps) and morning vomiting is characteristic. Changes in personality and school performance may be present. Headache from raised intracranial pressure is often accompanied by abnormal localising neurological signs and particular attention should be given to looking for these during the physical examination. Growth and visual fields may be affected in craniopharyngioma. Cerebellar signs are present in posterior fossa tumours, and cranial nerve abnormalities in brainstem tumours. Cranial bruits may be heard in arteriovenous–venous malformations, but these lesions are rare. Papilloedema is a late and serious sign, but can also represent benign intracranial hypertension, a syndrome of raised intracranial pressure without any space-occupying lesion or obstruction to the CSF pathways.

OTHER CAUSES

Acute sinusitis may cause facial pain. Percussion over the affected sinus causes discomfort. Chronic sinusitis may cause 'fuzzy headedness' in the presence of chronic rhinorrhoea.
Temporomandibular pain is a muscle contraction headache. Discomfort is worse on chewing. It is due to dental malocclusion or dislocation of the joint.
Ocular headaches are associated with refractive errors.
Head trauma, even if relatively minor, may be followed by recurrent headaches, particularly in those who are prone to headaches.
Solvent or drug abuse in adolescents, or environmental poisoning such as from lead intoxication (very uncommon in the UK) can sometimes cause headaches.
Subclinical seizures may cause headaches.
Hypertension in children does not cause headaches unless severe enough to cause encephalopathy.

Management of headaches

The mainstay of management is a thorough history and examination and detailed explanation and advice. Investigations are rarely indicated. EEGs are not usually diagnostic and generally do not help with patient management. If there are symptoms or signs of raised intracranial pressure or growth failure, a CT or MR scan is the essential investigation.

Children and parents should be informed that recurrent headaches are common. There are likely to be good and bad patches, over months or years, but they cause no long-term harm. Written information for the child and parents to take home is helpful. Children should be advised on how to live with and control the headaches rather than the headaches controlling them. Steps should be taken to reduce stress due to factors such as bullying, anxiety over exams or illness in friends or family. It is usually impossible or difficult to identify specific food triggers, so exclusion diets are rarely helpful and usually unpopular with the child.

Minor analgesics should be taken as early in the headache as possible. When nausea is troublesome, older children may take anti-emetics such as metoclopramide or prochlorperazine. The latter may be used rectally. Prophylactic therapy should only be used if the above measures are unsuccessful and headaches have become troublesome and intrusive for the young person. Pizotifen – a serotonin (5-HT) antagonist, is useful but may cause sleepiness. An alternative is to use β-blockers, such as propranolol, but the dose needs to be higher than for cardiac use and may result in feelings of lightheadedness or nightmares. It is contraindicated in children with asthma. For the acute disabling bout of migraine, sumatriptan, a serotonin (5-HT$_1$) agonist, curtails the period of vasodilatation and associated symptoms, but is not licensed for use in young children.

Seizures

A seizure or fit is a clinical event in which there is a sudden disturbance of neurological function, usually in association with an abnormal or excessive neuronal discharge.

A febrile convulsion is a seizure associated with fever in the absence of another cause and not due to intracranial infection from meningitis or encephalitis.

Epilepsy is recurrent seizures other than febrile convulsions in the absence of an acute cerebral insult.

The causes of seizures are listed in Figure 24.9.

FEBRILE CONVULSIONS

These occur in about 3% of children, usually between six months and three years, but up to six years of age. There is a genetic predisposition, with 10–20% of relatives having a seizure disorder, including febrile convulsions. The seizure usually occurs early in a viral infection, when the temperature is rising rapidly. The seizures are usually brief, lasting 1–2 minutes, and are generalised tonic or tonic–clonic. They need to be differentiated from rigors, triggered by a fever, and from reflex anoxic seizures. In about 15% of cases, seizures recur in the same illness. The overall risk of a further febrile convulsion is 1 in 3, and of these a further third will have three or more seizures. The recurrence risk is higher if the onset occurs before the age of one year and if there is a positive family history.

Febrile convulsions usually have a benign prognosis; only 2–4% of children with febrile convulsions develop epilepsy by seven years of age, and there is little evidence that this is caused by the febrile convulsion. The risk of later seizures is 7% up to 25 years of age. Risk factors for the subsequent development of partial epilepsy are a prolonged seizure (longer than 30 minutes), if the seizure is focal or if seizures recur in the same illness. The risk of partial epilepsy if there is one of these risk factors is about 3%, but with two or more it is about 10%. The risk factors for the subsequent development of generalised epilepsy are a first-degree relative with epilepsy or five or more febrile convulsions.

Management

The immediate management of seizures is described on p. 35. In caring for a child with a febrile convulsion it is essential to be certain that the child does not have meningitis or another serious bacterial infection requiring treatment. Where this cannot be decided with certainty on clinical examination the child will need an infection screen, including lumbar puncture for CSF examination and a urine sample to identify a urinary tract infection. An EEG is not indicated if the history and clinical findings are typical, as it is not a useful guide for treatment or predictor for recurring seizures or for the subsequent development of epilepsy.

The aim is to prevent febrile convulsions, especially if pro-longed, as occurs in 6% of all febrile convulsions. However, 80% of prolonged convulsions occur during the first convulsion.

During febrile illnesses, parents should be advised to try to keep the child's temperature low by removing warm clothing, by tepid sponging and giving an antipyretic, e.g. paracetamol. Parents of children with an increased risk of seizure recurrence should be supplied with rectal diazepam to give for any seizure lasting longer than five minutes. Prophylactic anticonvulsant therapy has been used but there is no good evidence that it lowers the risk of recurrence or the subsequent development of epilepsy. Parents should receive written as well as verbal advice on the first aid management of a further convulsion.

 Febrile convulsions occur between six months and six years of age.

EPILEPSY

The diagnosis of epilepsy is based on a detailed history, preferably from both an eye witness of the seizures and the child's own account, as well as clinical examination and EEG findings. A home video of a seizure or suspected seizure is very helpful, if available. Epilepsy needs to be distinguished from other seizure disorders (Fig. 24.9). The seizure type needs to be classified as to whether it is generalised or partial, and any particular epilepsy syndrome identified (Fig. 24.10).

Epilepsy affects 5 per 1000 school-age children, in 10% of whom the disorder is severe. Most epilepsy is idiopathic.

Epilepsy

Fig. 24.9 Causes of seizures.

Epilepsy	Idiopathic (70–80%)
	Secondary
	Cerebral dysgenesis/malformation,
	e.g. porencephalic cyst, hydrocephalus
	Cerebral damage, e.g. congenital infection,
	hypoxic-ischaemic encephalopathy,
	intraventricular haemorrhage/ischaemia
	Cerebral tumour
	Neurodegenerative disorders
	Neurocutaneous syndromes
Non epileptic	Febrile convulsions
	Metabolic
	Hypoglycaemia
	Hypocalcaemia/hypomagnesaemia
	Hypo/hypernatraemia
	Head trauma
	Meningitis/encephalitis
	Poisons/toxins

Fig. 24.10 Classification of epilepsy.

Generalised seizures	Absence
	Myoclonic seizures
	Tonic
	Tonic–clonic
	Atonic
Partial seizures	Simple partial
	(consciousness not impaired)
	Complex partial
	(consciousness impaired)
	Partial seizures becoming
	secondarily generalised
	Unclassified
Epilepsy syndromes	Generalised epilepsies:
	Infantile spasms
	Lennox-Gastaut syndrome
	Typical (petit mal) absences
	Myoclonic epilepsy of
	adolescence (juvenile myoclonic
	epilepsy)
	Partial epilepsies:
	Benign rolandic epilepsy

Generalised seizures

Generalised seizure disorders always involve loss of consciousness, there is no warning and the seizure discharge is bilaterally synchronous on the EEG. The seizures are symmetrical and their onset is in central cerebral structures. Generalised seizures comprise:

- absence seizures – where there is a transient loss of consciousness, with an abrupt onset and termination, unaccompanied by motor phenomena except for some flickering of the eyelids and minor alteration in muscle tone
- myoclonic seizures – repeated, brief, usually isolated jerks of the limbs, neck or trunk
- tonic seizures involving a generalised increase in tone
- tonic–clonic seizures involving rhythmical contraction of muscle groups following the tonic phase
- atonic seizures, (which are often preceeded by a myoclonic jerk) in which a transient loss of muscle tone causes a sudden fall to the floor or drop of the head.

Absences may be typical (petit mal) or atypical (more prolonged than petit mal) and can often be precipitated by hyperventilation, which is a useful diagnostic test. Non-epileptic myoclonic movements are seen physiologically in hiccoughs (myoclonus of the diaphragm) or on passing through stage II sleep. The atonic and myoclonic seizures often accompany cerebral dysgenesis or a neuro-degenerative disorder and have a poor prognosis.

In the tonic phase of tonic–clonic seizures, children may fall to the ground, sometimes injuring themselves. They do not breathe and become cyanosed. This is followed by the clonic phase, with jerking of the limbs. There may be biting of the tongue and incontinence of urine. Breathing is irregular, cyanosis persists and saliva may accumulate in the mouth. The seizure usually lasts for a few seconds to minutes, and is followed by unconsciousness or deep sleep for up to several hours. Status epilepticus, multiple seizures without recovery of consciousness in between, may result in hypoxic brain damage and death. Its management is described in Chapter 4. The tonic or tonic–clonic seizure disorders may remit.

Partial seizures

Partial seizures begin locally, presumed to be reflecting focal structural dysfunction, though this may not be demonstrable on imaging. The seizures may be heralded by an aura. Symptoms reflect the seizure's site of origin. The seizures may or may not be associated with change in consciousness or more generalised motor jerking. Partial seizures comprise:

- simple partial seizures – when the child will retain awareness with consciousness unimpaired
- complex partial seizures – when there is an altered conscious state or confusion due to the abnormal electrical discharge spreading from the originating site to become generalised
- partial seizures with secondary generalisation – when there is a focal seizure manifest clinically or on an ictal EEG followed by a generalised tonic clonic seizure.

If seizure activity in simple partial seizures begins in the motor cortex, tonic-clonic movements may 'march' proximally up the arm, known as a Jacksonian seizure. A post-ictal (Todd) paresis may follow.

As partial seizures may arise from anywhere in the brain, there may be a wide range of symptoms. The most common symptoms in complex partial seizures are abnormal sensations of taste or smell, distortion of vision or sounds, or autonomic symptoms and signs. There may be psychomotor phenomena with lip smacking, repetitive stereotyped movements such as pulling at clothes, walking in a non-purposeful manner (automatisms), '*déjà vu*' or '*jamais vu*' phenomena (intense feelings of having or never having been in the same situation before) or fright. Consciousness may be impaired. The episodes usually last a few minutes. The child may not recall the seizure.

The diagnosis is suspected from the characteristic history. The EEG can be helpful in looking for abnormal electrical discharges arising particularly from the temporal lobes, though these cannot always be demonstrated. About a third of affected children will enter adult life free of attacks and off medication, a third will be prone to seizures but will be controlled on medication, while the remainder will continue to have seizures in spite of medication.

Some common epilepsy syndromes

Generalised epilepsies

1. Infantile spasms (West syndrome)

Onset is usually between four and six months of age with violent flexor spasms of the head, trunk and limbs followed by extension of the arms (so called 'salaam spasms'). The flexor spasms last 1–2 seconds and are often multiple, occurring in bursts of 20–30, frequently on waking. The spasms may occur many times a day. The diagnosis may be delayed by misinterpreting these episodes as colic. Two-thirds of the children are neurologically abnormal before the onset of the seizures, some with tuberous sclerosis. Developmental progress is often arrested by the seizure disorder and social interaction impaired, which may cause parents to suspect that their baby cannot hear.

The EEG shows hypsarrhythmia, a chaotic pattern of high voltage dysrhythmic slow wave activity with sharp components (Fig. 24.11). Until recently, treatment with high-dose ACTH or prednisolone for 4–6 weeks was the treatment of choice. This results in a good response in 30–40% of cases, but is associated with a high risk of side-effects. First-line treatment is now the anticonvulsant vigabatrin, which has a lower risk of side-effects and high clinical efficacy. Many infants will subsequently show loss of skills and developmental delay, and later develop learning disability or epilepsy.

2. Lennox Gastaut syndrome

This affects children of 1–3 years of age who have myoclonic episodes with single jerks, atonic drop attacks

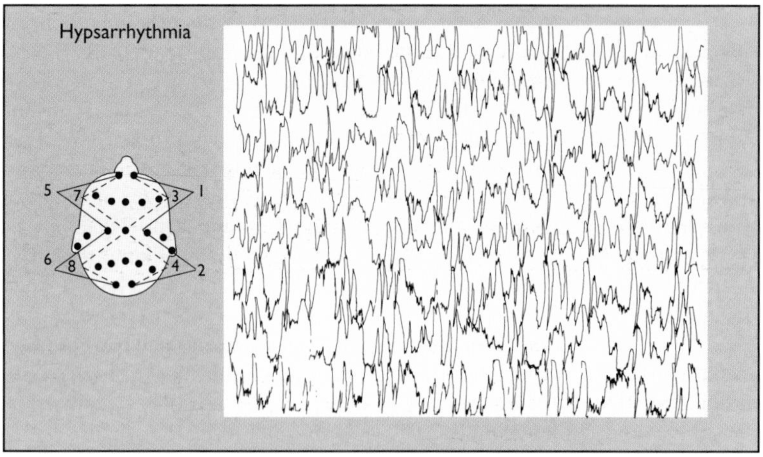

Hypsarrhythmia

Fig. 24.11 EEG of hypsarrhythmia in infantile spasms. There is a chaotic background of slow wave activity with sharp components.

or atypical absences. The latter have a less abrupt onset and termination. There is neurodevelopmental arrest or regression followed by learning and behaviour difficulties. The seizures subsequently tend to be replaced by generalised tonic–clonic seizures confined to sleep or the first few hours after waking and carry a poor prognosis.

3. Typical (petit mal) absence seizures

This accounts for 1–2% of childhood epilepsy. Onset is between four and 12 years of age. It is rarely associated with developmental problems. Affected children momentarily stare, become pale and stop moving, although they may twitch their eyelids or a hand minimally. The episodes last only a few seconds and certainly not longer than 30 seconds. Afterwards the child is able to continue immediately the conversation or action which was interrupted by the seizure. Affected children have no recall of the seizure except that they may realise that they have missed something during the absence and so many say 'pardon' on regaining consciousness, or look puzzled.

The episodes may be induced by hyperventilation, which is a useful test in the outpatient clinic. The EEG shows three per second spike and wave discharge which

is bilaterally synchronous during and sometimes between attacks (Fig. 24.12). The prognosis is good, with seizures stopping in adolescence in 95%.

4. Myoclonic epilepsy of adolescence (juvenile myoclonic epilepsy)

This usually presentsbetween the ages of 10 and 20 years, with females affected twice as often as males. There may be a family history. Myoclonic seizures predominate but absences and tonic–clonic seizures also occur. They are most evident shortly after waking. Learning is unimpaired. The response to treatment is usually good.

Partial epilepsies

1. Benign rolandic epilepsy of childhood

This is the most common benign epilepsy in childhood. It is important to recognise as the seizures usually stop by the mid-teens and may not require treatment. Seizures often occur during sleep when they are generalised tonic–clonic; they may start with distortion of the face and arm on one side associated with an abnormal feeling on the tongue. Rolandic spike wave activity is seen in the centrotemporal area on the EEG.

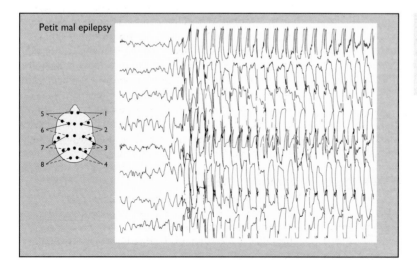

Petit mal epilepsy

Fig. 24.12 EEG in a typical absence (petit mal) seizure. There is 3/sec spike and wave discharge which is bilaterally synchronous during and sometimes between attacks.

Fig. 24.13 Choice of anticonvulsants		
Seizure type	**1st choice**	**2nd choice**
Generalised epilepsies:		
Tonic–clonic	Valproate, carbamazepine	Lamotrigine
Absence	Valproate	Lamotrigine, ethosuximide
Myoclonic	Valproate	Clobazam, clonazepam
Partial epilepsies	Carbamazepine, valproate	Vigabatrin, gabapentin

Investigation

An EEG is indicated whenever epilepsy is suspected. If the standard EEG is normal, an abnormality may be revealed from a sleep-deprivation recording, an EEG within an hour of a clinical seizure or a 24-hour ambulatory recording.

CT or MR brain scans may be indicated in young children (less than five years old) or where seizures are drug resistant, when a demonstrable localised brain abnormality is more likely. If there are interictal neurological signs, especially if these are focal, a brain scan should be carried out to exclude a tumour or vascular lesion which could be treatable.

Metabolic and neuroimmunological investigation may complement the brain scan to help identify the aetiology.

Management

A diagnosis of epilepsy does not automatically mean that the child requires anticonvulsant therapy. This should be based on the frequency and nature of the seizures and the social or educational consequences of having further seizures. If there is no demonstrable cause for the first seizure, it is usual to wait before starting anticonvulsant therapy. There are differences of opinion about the choice of anticonvulsant therapy; a scheme for particular seizure types is shown in Figure 24.13. All anticonvulsant drugs have side-effects (Fig. 24.14), but these can be kept to a minimum through knowledge of how to introduce, use and modify dosages. Single drug therapy, using the minimum dose, is used where possible.

Fig. 24.14 Some side-effects of anticonvulsants	
Drug	**Side-effects**
Valproate	Increased appetite and weight
	Transient hair loss
	Idiosyncratic liver failure
Carbamazepine	Lupus erythematosis syndrome
	Dizziness, visual disturbance
Vigabatrin	Behaviour disturbance
	Confusion, sleepiness, weight gain
Lamotrigine	Rash, behaviour disturbance, irritability
Ethosuximide	Blood dyscrasia

All the above may cause drowsiness and occasional skin rashes. Liver enzyme induction, which can interfere with other medication, may occur with carbamazepine.

Sometimes two or more anticonvulsants are required. Sugar-free preparations are used. Serum anticonvulsant levels can be measured for some drugs and are useful:
- if toxicity is suspected
- to check compliance
- when high drug doses are used
- with multiple drug therapy
- in children who are severely disabled, when toxicity is difficult to recognise.

However, serum levels do not necessarily reflect those in the brain. In general, anticonvulsant therapy is withdrawn slowly after two years free of seizures.

Seizures may be provoked by sleep, alcohol, drugs, excitement, anxiety, menstruation or too rapid withdrawal of anticonvulsant drugs. Children with photosensitive epilepsy should watch TV from a distance, in a well-lit room and with one eye covered when approaching the set. In children with intractable seizures, cure or considerable improvement can occasionally be achieved by a ketogenic diet or, if the seizures are partial in type, by surgical removal of the epileptic focus.

The aim should be to help children with epilepsy live as normal a life as possible. Young children should only swim under adult supervision, and teenagers ideally with the knowledge of a life-guard and friend. They should avoid cycling along busy roads, climbing and other situations where a seizure could cause serious injury. Some children with epilepsy and their families need psychological help to adjust to the disability. The school needs to be aware of the child's problem and teachers advised on the management of seizures. Unrecognised absences may interfere with learning, which is an indication for being vigilant about 'odd episodes' which may represent seizures, in order to achieve better seizure control. Some children require educational help for associated learning difficulties. Two-thirds of children with epilepsy go to a mainstream school; one-third attend a special school, but they often have multiple disabilities. A few children require residential schooling where there are facilities and expertise in monitoring and treating intractable seizures.

FUNNY TURNS

There are a number of benign paroxysmal disorders which may mimic epilepsy. A detailed history, preferably from a person who has witnessed the event in question, is crucial in distinguishing epilepsy from other disorders. The causes are listed in Figure 24.15.

Fig. 24.15 Causes of funny turns

Breath-holding attacks

These occur in some toddlers when they are upset. The child cries, holds his breath and goes blue. Sometimes children will briefly lose consciousness but rapidly recover fully. Drug therapy is unhelpful. Attacks resolve spontaneously but behaviour modification therapy with avoidance of confrontation may help.

Reflex anoxic seizures

These occur in infants or toddlers. Many have a first-degree relative with a history of faints. The most common triggers are pain or discomfort, particularly from minor head trauma, cold food (such as ice cream or cold drinks) or fright. Fever is another common trigger. Some children with febrile convulsions may have experienced this phenomenon. After the triggering event, the child becomes very pale and falls to the floor. The hypoxia may induce a generalised tonic–clonic seizure. The episodes are due to cardiac asystole from vagal inhibition. The seizure is brief and the child rapidly recovers. Ocular compression under controlled conditions often leads to asystole and paroxysmal slow wave discharge on the EEG.

Syncope

Children may faint if in a hot and stuffy environment, on standing for long periods or from fear.

Migraine

May sometimes lead to paroxysmal headache involving unsteadiness or lightheadedness as well as the more common visual or gastro-intestinal disturbance. In some young people these episodes occur without headache.

Benign paroxysmal vertigo

This is characterised by recurrent attacks of vertigo, lasting from one to several minutes, associated with nystagmus, unsteadiness or even falling. The cause is often not identified, but a viral labyrinthitis should be excluded.

Other causes

Cardiac arrhythmias	Prolonged Q–T interval may rarely cause syncopal attacks which may be related to exercise
Tics, daydreaming, night terrors	
Masturbation	Young children may stimulate their genitalia in order to achieve a feeling of comfort
Pseudoseizures	When children feign seizures
Munchausen by proxy	Seizures are fabricated or induced e.g. from hypoglycaemia from injecting insulin

---

Cerebral palsy

Cerebral palsy is defined as a disorder of movement and posture due to a non-progressive lesion of the motor pathways in the developing brain. Although the lesion is non-progressive, the clinical manifestations evolve with cerebral maturation. It is the most common cause of motor impairment in children, affecting about 2 per 1000 live births. In addition to disorders of movement and posture, children with cerebral palsy often have other problems, reflecting more widespread damage to the brain. These include:

- learning impairment in about 60%, although some children, especially those with dyskinetic cerebral palsy, may have normal intelligence
- visual impairment in 20% from errors of refraction and cortical damage
- squints in 30%
- hearing loss in 20%
- speech and language disorders due to a combination of hearing loss, muscle incoordination and learning impairment
- behaviour disorders
- epilepsy in 40%.

Causes

The main causes of cerebral palsy are shown in Figure 24.16. Most are antenatal in origin from cerebral dysgenesis or cerebral malformations.

Only about 10% are thought to be due to birth asphyxia and this proportion has remained relatively constant over the last decade. The rise in the number of preterm infants of early gestation surviving has been associated with a substantial increase in the number of these children with cerebral palsy.

Clinical presentation

Many children who develop cerebral palsy are identified as being at risk in the neonatal period because of dysmorphic features, neonatal encephalopathy, seizures, abnormal neurological signs, symptomatic hypoglycaemia or a gross abnormality on cranial ultrasound.

Cerebral palsy usually presents with:

- abnormal tone and posturing in early infancy
- delayed motor milestones
- abnormal gait once walking is achieved
- feeding difficulties with oromotor incoordination, slow feeding, gagging and vomiting
- developmental delay particularly in language and social skills.

Hand preference in those less than 12 months old often signifies the emergence of a hemiparesis.

In cerebral palsy primitive reflexes, which facilitate the emergence of normal patterns of movements, may persist and become obligatory rather than facultative (Fig. 24.17).

The diagnosis is made by clinical examination with particular attention to assessment of the pattern of tone, posturing and observation of gait. There are three main clinical types of cerebral palsy, each reflecting damage to a specific motor pathway, as well as a mixed pattern.

Spastic (70%)

In this type, there is damage to the upper motor neurone (pyramidal) pathway. Limb tone is abnormally increased (spasticity), with associated brisk deep tendon reflexes and extensor plantar responses. The increased limb tone may suddenly yield under pressure in a 'clasp knife' fashion. Before spasticity appears there may be hypotonia of the trunk and limbs which gradually changes to include increased tone. The distribution of signs may be in the form of:

- hemiparesis – unilateral involvement of the arm and leg (Fig. 24.18)
- diplegia – all four limbs are affected but the legs to a much greater degree than the arms, so that hand function may appear to be relatively normal (but is still compromised)
- quadriparesis – all four limbs are affected to a fairly similar degree, often severely, though the arms may be affected more than the legs with poor axial tone.

In **hemiparesis**, the arm may be affected more than the leg or vice versa, usually sparing the face. Affected children often present at 4–12 months of age with fisting of the affected hand, a pronated flexed forearm, or tiptoe walk on the affected side. The limb may initially be flaccid and hypotonic, but increased tone soon emerges as the predominant sign. The past medical history, including the birth history, has usually been normal.

In **diplegia**, it is with functional use of the hands that motor difficulties in the arms are most apparent.

In **quadriparesis**, the trunk is often involved, with extensor posturing and poor head control (Fig. 24.19). Despite limb spasticity there may be hypotonia of the trunk and limbs which predisposes to the development of scoliosis. This form of cerebral palsy is often associated with seizures and moderate or severe intellectual impairment. There may have been a history of severe birth asphyxia.

Ataxic hypotonic (10%)

Signs are usually symmetrical. There is early hypotonia, poor balance and delayed motor development. Later, incoordinate movements and intention tremor may be evident, reflecting damage to the cerebellum or its pathways.

Dyskinetic (10%)

There is dyskinesia (fluctuating muscle tone) leading to involuntary movements (athetosis and dystonia) and poor postural control. Intellect may be relatively unimpaired.

Fig. 24.16 Causes of cerebral palsy	
Antenatal (80%)	Cerebral dysgenesis
	Cerebral malformation
	Congenital infection – rubella, toxoplasmosis, cytomegalovirus
Intrapartum (10%)	Birth asphyxia/trauma
Postnatal (10%)	Intraventricular haemorrhage/ischaemia
	Meningitis/encephalitis/encephalopathy
	Head trauma/non-accidental injury
	Symptomatic hypoglycaemia
	Hydrocephalus
	Hyperbilirubinaemia

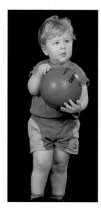

Fig. 24.18
A child with a right spastic hemiplegia. His right arm is hyper-pronated.

Fig. 24.17 Some primitive reflexes present at birth–6 months of age	
Reflex	**Description**
Moro	Sudden head extension causes symmetrical extension followed by flexion of all limbs
Grasp	Flexion of the fingers of the hand when an object is placed in the palm at the base of the fingers
Rooting	Turning of the head towards a stimulus near the mouth
Placing	With the infant held vertically and the dorsum of the feet brought into contact with a surface, the infant lifts first one foot, placing it on the surface, followed by the other
Atonic neck reflex	On lying supine, when the head is turned to one side, the infant adopts a 'fencing' posture, with the arm outstretched on the side to which the head is turned

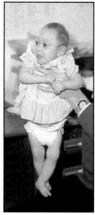

Fig. 24.19
A child with spastic quadriplegia showing scissoring of the legs from excessive adduction of the hips, pronated forearms and 'fisted' hands. (Courtesy of Dr Diane Smyth.)

Affected children often present with floppiness and delayed motor development in infancy, with abnormal movements sometimes not appearing before one year of age. The signs are due to damage to the basal ganglia or their associated pathways (extrapyramidal).

Mixed pattern of the above types (10%)
There are features of several clinical types.

Management
Parents should be given early and accurate details of the diagnosis and prognosis. However, during infancy it can be very difficult to predict severity until the pattern of evolving signs and the child's developmental progress have been observed over several months, or even the first few years of life. Children with cerebral palsy are likely to have a wide range of medical, psychological and social problems, making it essential to adopt a multidisciplinary approach to assessment and management. This is described in Chapter 25.

Ataxia

The commonest cause of ataxia in children results from damage to the cerebellum or its connections. In cerebellar ataxia, there is an unsteady gait, difficulty in performing repetitive and alternating movements, overshooting of target directed movement and an intention tremor which becomes more pronounced when the child puts more effort into trying to hold a posture. The gait has a wide base to provide stability and to compensate for the truncal ataxia. There may be associated wobble of the head, nystagmus and a scanning dysarthria. Cerebellar ataxia may be:

- acute, from drugs including alcohol and solvent abuse
- a manifestation of viral encephalitis following varicella or other viral infections
- from a cerebellar tumour.

Ataxia may also be part of a chronic neurological condition such as ataxic cerebral palsy, ataxia telangiectasia and Friedreich ataxia.

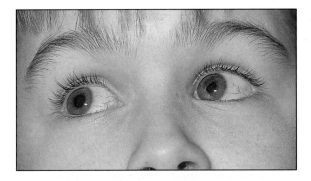

Fig. 24.20 Telangiectasia of the conjunctivae are present from about four years of age in ataxia telangiectasia.

ATAXIA TELANGIECTASIA
This disorder of DNA repair is an autosomal recessive condition. There may be mild delay in motor development in infancy, but difficulty with balance and coordination and oculomotor problems (oculomotor dyspraxia) become evident at school age. There is subsequent deterioration, with many children wheelchair-bound in early adolescence. Telangiectasia develop in the conjunctivae (Fig. 24.20), neck and shoulders from about four years of age. The children:

- have an increased susceptibility to infection, principally from an IgA surface antibody defect
- may develop malignant disorders, principally acute lymphoblastic leukaemia (about 10%)
- have a raised serum alphafetoprotein
- have an increased white cell sensitivity to irradiation which can be used diagnostically and to identify heterozygotes.

FRIEDREICH ATAXIA
This is the most common of the spinocerebellar degenerations. It is an autosomal recessive condition which presents with progressive clumsiness. Ataxia of the limbs and trunk, distal wasting in the legs, diminished reflexes, pes cavus and dysarthria may develop. This is similar to the hereditary motor sensory neuropathies, but in Friedreich ataxia there is impairment of joint position and vibration sense and there is often optic atrophy. The cerebellar component becomes more apparent with age, as also the onset of scoliosis and cardiomyopathy. The latter often causes death at 40–50 years of age.

Cerebral haemorrhage

EXTRADURAL HAEMORRHAGE
This usually results from arterial or venous bleeding into the extradural space following direct head trauma. It usually accompanies a skull fracture. In young children there is often a lucid interval until the conscious level deteriorates and seizures occur, secondary to the space-occupying lesion formed by the enlarging haematoma. There may be focal neurological signs with dilatation of the ipsilateral pupil, paresis of the contralateral limbs and a false localising uni- or bilateral VIth nerve paresis. In young children initial presentation may be with anaemia and shock. The diagnosis is confirmed on a CT scan. Immediate management is to correct hypovolaemia. Surgical evacuation of the haematoma with arrest of the bleeding may be required.

SUBDURAL HAEMATOMA
This results from tearing of the veins as they cross the subdural space. In children it is seen almost exclusively in infants or toddlers due to non-accidental injury caused by shaking (see Chapter 5). Retinal haemorrhages are usually

present. Subdural haematomas are occasionally seen following a fall from a considerable height.

SUBARACHNOID HAEMORRHAGE
Presentation is usually with acute onset of head pain, neck stiffness and occasionally fever. Retinal haemorrhage is usually present. Seizures and coma may develop. A CT scan of the head usually identifies hyperdense blood in the CSF. A lumbar puncture is best avoided as haemorrhage may extend following the release of intracranial pressure. Angiography is performed to identify the aetiology, which is often an aneurysm or arteriovenous malformation. Treatment may be by interventional radiography or surgery.

Neural tube defects and hydrocephalus

NEURAL TUBE DEFECTS
Neural tube defects result from failure of normal fusion of the neural plate to form the neural tube during the first 28 days following conception. They used to be one of the most common serious malformations detected at birth. In the 1970s its birth prevalence in the UK was 4–8 per 1000 live births. This was the highest prevalence in the world, with a peak level in Ireland, declining towards the south-east of England. Since then the birth prevalence in the UK has fallen dramatically (Fig. 24.21). This is mainly because of a natural decline, as well as antenatal screening.

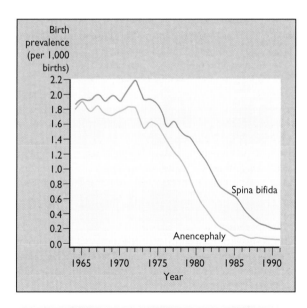

Fig. 24.21 The decline in the number of infants born with neural tube defects. This has resulted from a natural decrease together with antenatal diagnosis and termination of pregnancy.

The reason for the natural decline is uncertain, but may be associated with improved maternal nutrition. It is well recognised that mothers of a fetus with a neural tube defect have a tenfold increased risk of having a second affected fetus. It has been shown that supplementing these mothers' diet with high doses of folic acid markedly reduces this risk. It is now recommended that women planning a pregnancy should have a high-dose folic acid intake periconceptually if they have had a previously affected infant; low-dose folic acid supplementation is recommended to be taken for all pregnancies.

Anencephaly
This is failure of development of most of the cranium and brain. Affected infants are stillborn or die shortly after birth. It is detected on antenatal ultrasound screening and termination of pregnancy is usually performed.

Encephalocele
There is extrusion of brain and meninges through a midline skull defect, which can be corrected surgically. However, there are often underlying associated cerebral malformations.

Spina bifida occulta
This failure of fusion of the vertebral arch (Fig. 24.22) is often an incidental finding on X-ray, but there may be an associated overlying skin lesion such as a tuft of hair, lipoma, birth mark or small dermal sinus, usually in the lumbar region. There may be an associated underlying tethering of the cord (diastomyelia) which, with growth, may cause neurological deficits of bladder function and lower limbs. The extent of the underlying lesion can be delineated using ultrasound and/or MR scans. Neurosurgical release of tethering is usually indicated.

Meningocele and myelomeningocele
Meningoceles (Fig. 24.22) usually have a good prognosis following surgical repair. The main problems associated with myelomeningoceles (Figs 24.22 and 24.23) include:
- variable paralysis of the legs
- muscle imbalance which may cause dislocation of the hip and talipes
- sensory loss
- bladder denervation (neuropathic bladder)
- bowel denervation (neuropathic bowel)
- scoliosis
- hydrocephalus from the Arnold-Chiari malformation (herniation of the cerebellar tonsils through the foramen magnum), leading to disruption of CSF flow.
Physiotherapy is required to prevent joint contractures and strengthen paralysed muscles. Walking aids may be required to permit mobility but some children are wheelchair bound. With sensory loss, skin care is required to avoid the development of skin damage and ulcers.

An indwelling catheter may be required for bladder denervation, or intermittent urinary catheterisation may be performed by parents or by older children themselves. Urine

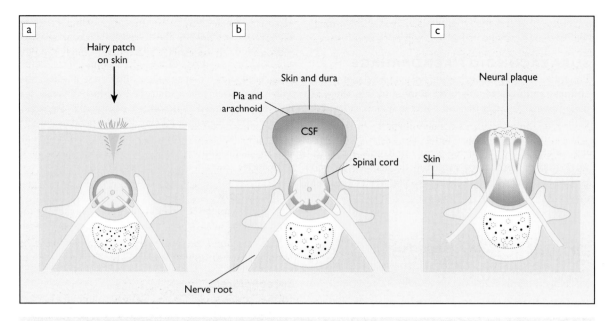

Fig. 24.22 Neural tube defects: (a) spina bifida occulta; (b) meningocele; (c) myelomeningocele.

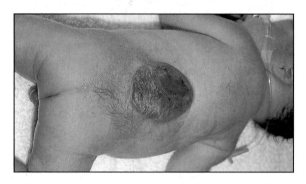

Fig. 24.23 Myelomeningocele showing the exposed neural tissue and the patulous anus from neuropathic bowel.

samples should be checked regularly for infection. Continuous prophylactic antibiotics may be necessary. The child should be monitored for early evidence of hypertension and renal failure. Medication (such as ephedrine or oxybutinin) may improve bladder function and improve urinary dribbling. Bowel denervation requires regular toiletting, and laxatives and suppositories are likely to be necessary.

Scoliosis is monitored and may require surgical treatment. Ventricular dilatation from the Arnold-Chiari malformation is often present at birth and 80% of affected infants require a shunt for progressive hydrocephalus during the first few weeks of life.

Those children destined to be the most severely disabled have at birth a spinal lesion above L3. This is likely to result in inability to walk, scoliosis, neuropathic bladder, hydronephrosis and often an associated hydrocephalus.

In the 1970s, follow-up studies of severely affected children showed that many had severe physical and intellectual impairment. Many had to undergo multiple operations. In adolescence and adulthood, they and their families faced many problems – psychological, sexual, finding employment and being cared for. As a consequence, many advocated a non-interventionist conservative approach, in which surgery was not performed to repair the meningeal lesion and overlying skin and supportive care only was provided. Most died from meningitis and ventriculitis, progressive hydrocephalus or renal failure. Subsequent studies have shown that with modern medical care, the quality of life for severely affected children is much better than in the past. Most affected infants are now treated with closure of the lesion of the back soon after birth. Their care is managed by a specialist multidisciplinary team.

HYDROCEPHALUS

Hydrocephalus is due to excess CSF causing accelerated head enlargement. It is usually secondary to obstruction of CSF flow in the ventricular system (non-communicating) or failure of CSF re-absorption (communicating). The main causes are shown in Figure 24.24.

Clinical features

In infants with hydrocephalus, the head circumference is disproportionately large or its rate of growth is excessive, the sutures become separated and the scalp veins congested. The anterior fontanelle pressure, with the infant relaxed, will feel increased on palpation, and will subsequently bulge. If left untreated, the eyes deviate downwards (setting-sun sign) (Fig. 24.25). The infant subsequently develops symptoms and signs of raised intracranial pressure. Using ultrasound ante- or postnatally, ventricular dilatation is increasingly recognised before the infant becomes symptomatic. In older children, clinical features are from raised intracranial pressure.

Management

Assessment of ventricular dilatation is with cranial ultrasound (*see* Chapter 8) and/or CT or MR scan. Treatment is required for symptomatic relief of raised intracranial pressure to minimise the risk of neurological damage. The mainstay is the insertion of a ventricular shunt (Fig. 24.26). Shunt revision is only required if there is symptomatic malfunction from obstruction, infection (usually with coagulase-negative *Staphylococcus*) if it is unresponsive to antibiotics or overdrainage of fluid.

Neuromuscular disorders

Any part of the lower motor pathway can be affected so that anterior horn cell disorders, peripheral neuropathies, disorders of neuromuscular transmission and primary muscle diseases can all occur. The causes of neuromuscular disorders are shown in Figure 24.27.

The key clinical feature of a neuromuscular disorder is weakness, which may be progressive or static. Affected children may present with:
- floppiness
- delayed motor milestones
- muscle weakness
- unsteady/abnormal gait
- fatiguability.

Older children often show the waddling gait of proximal muscle weakness, muscle wasting, generalised hyptonia and absent or reduced deep tendon reflexes. Gower sign is the need to rise from supine by turning prone and then climbing 'up the legs with the hands' to gain the standing position (Fig. 24.28). A pattern of distal wasting and

weakness, particularly in the presence of pes cavus, is usually due to one of the hereditary motor sensory neuropathies. Increasing fatiguability through the day, often with ptosis, suggests myasthenia gravis.

Investigations

These include:
- serum creatine phosphokinase – markedly elevated in Duchenne and Becker dystrophies
- electromyography and nerve conduction studies
- muscle and nerve biopsies – needle muscle biopsy is usually sufficient, and modern histochemical techniques often enable a definitive diagnosis to be made
- recombinant DNA studies
- ultrasound, CT and MR imaging of muscles – allow accurate documentation of specific muscle disorders.

Muscle fatiguability on repetitive nerve stimulation can be demonstrated in myasthaenia gravis. The tests help in

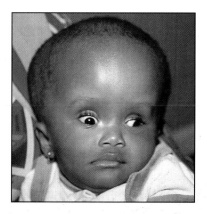

Fig. 24.25 Grossly enlarged head and downward deviation of the eyes ('setting sun' sign) from untreated hydrocephalus.

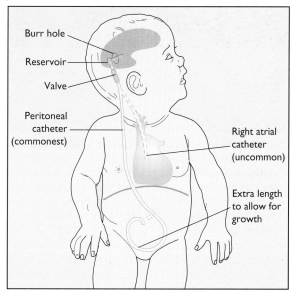

Fig. 24.26 Ventriculo-peritoneal shunt for drainage of symptomatic hydrocephalus. A sufficient length of shunt tubing is left in the peritoneal cavity to allow for the child's growth. Right atrial catheters require revision with growth.

Fig. 24.24 Causes of hydrocephalus
Non-communicating (obstruction in the ventricular system)
Congenital malformation
Aqueduct stenosis
Atresia of the outflow foramina of the fourth ventricle
(Dandy–Walker malformation)
Post-haemorrhagic in preterm infant
Post-intracranial infection
Neoplasm or vascular malformation
Communicating (failure to reabsorb cerebrospinal fluid)
Subarachnoid haemorrhage
Tuberculous meningitis
Arnold–Chiari malformation

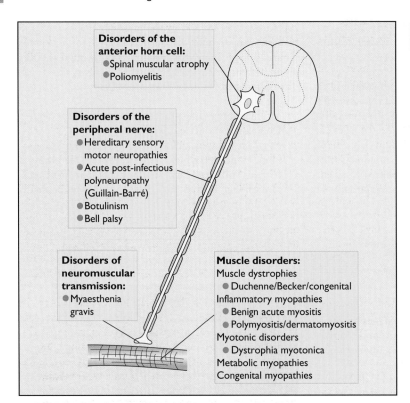

Fig. 24.27 Neuromuscular disorders.

Disorders of the anterior horn cell:
- Spinal muscular atrophy
- Poliomyelitis

Disorders of the peripheral nerve:
- Hereditary sensory motor neuropathies
- Acute post-infectious polyneuropathy (Guillain-Barré)
- Botulinism
- Bell palsy

Disorders of neuromuscular transmission:
- Myaesthenia gravis

Muscle disorders:
Muscle dystrophies
- Duchenne/Becker/congenital
Inflammatory myopathies
- Benign acute myositis
- Polymyositis/dermatomyositis
Myotonic disorders
- Dystrophia myotonica
Metabolic myopathies
Congenital myopathies

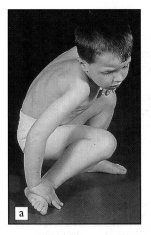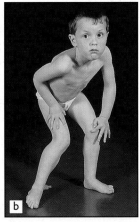

Fig. 24.28 (a, b) Gower sign. The child needs to turn prone to rise, then uses his hands to climb up on his knees before standing, because of poor hip girdle fixation and/or proximal muscle weakness. Any child continuing to do this after three years of age is likely to have a neuromuscular condition.

differentiating myopathic from neuropathic disorders but should be used selectively in children as the nerve conduction studies cause a tingling sensation and electromyography requires insertion of fine needle electrodes.

Identification of the specific gene defect for a number of neuromuscular disorders allows accurate antenatal diagnosis. Genetic counselling and advice can then be offered.

DISORDERS OF THE ANTERIOR HORN CELL

Presentation is with weakness, wasting and absent reflexes. The features of poliomyelitis are described in Chapter 12.

Spinal muscular atrophy

This disorder is usually autosomal recessive and due to degeneration of the anterior horn cells. It leads to progressive weakness and wasting of skeletal muscles. This is the second most common cause of neuromuscular disease in the UK after Duchenne muscular dystrophy.
Spinal muscular atrophy Type I (Werdnig-Hoffmann disease)
A very severe progressive disorder presenting in early infancy (Fig. 24.29). Diminished fetal movements are often noticed during pregnancy and there may be arthrogryposis (positional deformities of the limbs) at birth. Typical signs include:
- fasciculation of the tongue
- intercostal recession
- lack of antigravity power in hip flexors
- absent deep tendon reflexes.

Death is from respiratory failure by about 12 months of age. There are milder forms of the disorder with a later onset and clinical course lasting a few or many years, but still leading to early death.

It is now thought that the spinal muscular atrophies and muscular dystrophies account for most of the scapuloperoneal, facio-scapulo-humeral or predominantly distal patterns of wasting and weakness. These were formerly thought to be separate conditions.

DISORDERS OF PERIPHERAL NERVE

The hereditary motor sensory neuropathies (HMSN)

This group of disorders typically leads to symmetrical, slowly progressive muscular wasting which is distal rather than proximal. Type I, formerly known as peroneal muscular atrophy (Charcot-Marie-Tooth disease), is usually dominantly inherited. Affected nerves may be hypertrophic due to demyelination followed by attempts at remyelination. Nerve biopsy typically shows 'onion bulb formation' due to these two processes. Onset is in the first decade with distal atrophy and pes cavus, the legs being affected more than the arms. Rarely, there may be distal sensory loss and the reflexes are diminished. The disease is chronic. None of those affected lose the ability to walk. The presentation of Friedreich ataxia can be similar.

Acute post-infectious polyneuropathy (Guillain–Barré)

This disorder is probably due to the formation of antibody attaching itself to protein components in myelin. Presentation is typically 2–3 weeks after an upper respiratory tract infection. There may be fleeting abnormal sensory symptoms in the legs but the prominent feature is an ascending symmetrical weakness with autonomic involvement. Sensory symptoms are less striking than the paresis. Involvement of bulbar muscles leads to difficulty with chewing and swallowing and the risk of aspiration. Respiratory depression may require artificial ventilation. The maximum muscle weakness may occur only 2–4 weeks after the onset of illness. Although full recovery may be expected in 95% of cases, this may take up to two years.

The CSF protein is characteristically markedly raised, but this may not be seen if the lumbar puncture is done at the beginning of the illness. The CSF white cell count is not raised. Nerve conduction velocities are reduced.

Management of post-infectious polyneuropathy is supportive, particularly of respiration. Steroids have been shown to have no beneficial effect or may even delay recovery. Controlled trials have shown that the ventilator-dependent period can be significantly reduced by the use of immunoglobulin infusion, which is preferable to plasma exchange.

Bell palsy

This is an isolated lower motor neurone paresis of the VIIth cranial nerve leading to facial weakness (Fig. 24.30). If symptoms of an VIIIth nerve paresis are also present, then the most likely diagnosis is a compressive lesion in the cerebello-pontine angle. Although the aetiology is unclear in Bell palsy, it is probably post-infectious. The herpes virus may invade the geniculate ganglion and give painful vesicles on the tonsillar fauces and external ear, along with a facial nerve paresis. Hypertension should be excluded as there is an association between Bell palsy and coarctation of the aorta. Sarcoidosis should be suspected if facial weakness is bilateral.

Corticosteroids may be of value in reducing oedema in the facial canal during the first week. Recovery is complete in the majority of cases, but may take some months. The main complication is conjunctival infection due to incomplete eye closure on blinking. This may require the eye to be protected with a patch or even tarsorrhaphy.

DISORDERS OF NEUROMUSCULAR TRANSMISSION

Myasthenia gravis

This presents as abnormal muscle fatiguability which improves with rest or anticholinesterase drugs.

Transient neonatal myasthenia is described in Chapter 7, 'Perinatal Medicine'.

Juvenile myasthenia is similar to adult autoimmune myasthenia and is due to binding of antibody to acetylcholine receptors on the post-junctional synaptic membrane. This gives a reduction in the number of functional receptors. Presentation is usually after 10 years of age.

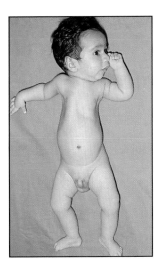

Fig. 24.29 Spinal muscular atrophy (Werdnig–Hoffmann disease) showing proximal muscle wasting, chest deformity from weakness of the intercostal muscles and thighs held abducted because of hypotonia.

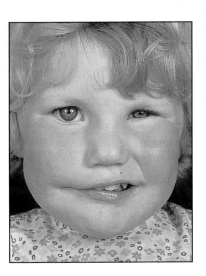

Fig. 24.30 Bell palsy. There is right facial weakness of both the upper and lower face.

The initial symptoms are often bulbar, but in approximately half they are ocular. Presentation is usually with ptosis, loss of facial expression and difficulty chewing (Fig. 24.31). General, especially proximal, weakness may be seen.

Diagnosis is made by observing improvement following the administration of edrophonium. Treatment is with the use of anticholinesterases such as neostigmine or pyridostigmine. In the longer term, immunosuppressive therapy with prednisolone or azathioprine has been shown to be of value. Plasma exchange is used for crises. Thymectomy is performed if a thymoma is present or if the response to medical therapy is unsatisfactory.

MUSCLE DISORDERS
The muscular dystrophies
This is a group of inherited disorders with muscle degeneration, often progressive.

1. Duchenne muscular dystrophy
This is the most common muscular dystrophy, affecting 1 in 4000 male infants. It is inherited as an X-linked recessive disorder, though about a third are new mutations. It results from a deletion of chromosome material on the short arm of the X chromosome (at the Xp21 site). This site is now known to code for a protein called dystrophin which maintains the integrity of the muscle cell wall. Where it is deficient, there is an influx of calcium ions, a breakdown of the calcium calmodulin complex and an excess of free radicals. These lead eventually to irreversible destruction of the muscle cells. The serum creatine phosphokinase is markedly elevated.

Children present with a waddling gait. They lack a spring to their step and have to mount stairs one by one. The average age of diagnosis remains 5.5 years, although the children are often first referred for a medical opinion when much younger, highlighting the importance of interpreting Gower sign correctly. There may be selective atrophy of muscle, in particular of the sternal head of the pectoralis major and brachioradialis. There is pseudohypertrophy of the calves because of replacement of muscle fibres by fat and fibrous tissue.

In the early school years affected boys just tend to be slower and more clumsy than their peers, but the progressive atrophy and weakness leads them to become non-ambulant and in need of a wheelchair by the age of about 10–14 years. Death ensues in the late teens or early 20s from respiratory failure or the associated cardiomyopathy. About a third of affected children have learning difficulties. Scoliosis is a common complication.

Management
Contractures, particularly at the ankles, should be prevented by passive stretching and the provision of night splints. Appropriate exercise helps maintain muscle power and mobility and delays the onset of scoliosis. Walking can be prolonged with the provision of orthoses, in particular those which allow ambulation by the child leaning from side to side. Lengthening of the Achilles tendon may be

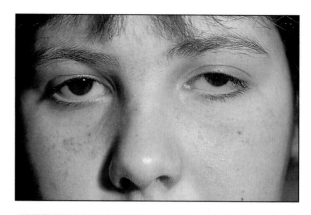

Fig. 24.31 Myasthenia gravis showing ptosis from ocular muscle fatigue which improved with edrophonium.

required to facilitate ambulation. Attention towards maintaining a good sitting posture helps minimise the risk of scoliosis. The emergence of scoliosis is managed with a truncal brace, a moulded seat and occasionally surgical insertion of a metal rod into the spine. Later in the illness, episodes of nocturnal hypoxia secondary to weakness of the intercostal muscles may present with lassitude or irritability. Respiratory aids may be provided to improve the quality of life. As with all chronic disabling conditions, parent self-help groups are a useful continuing source of information and support for families. Affected children should be reviewed periodically at a specialist regional centre.

It may be possible to identify female carriers if they have a mildly raised creatine phosphokinase or if the gene deletion can be detected on DNA analysis. Antenatal diagnosis is then possible.

2. Becker muscular dystrophy
The clinical features of this muscular dystrophy are similar to those of Duchenne muscular dystrophy but the disease progresses more slowly. The average age of onset is 11 years, there is inability to walk in the late 20s, with death in the early 40s, though this varies widely from 20–50 years of age.

3. Congenital muscular dystrophies
This is a heterogeneous group of disorders which present with muscle weakness at birth or early infancy. Unlike Becker and Duchenne dystrophies they have an autosomal recessive inheritance. These disorders are often nonprogressive. The muscle biopsy shows histological changes similar to those seen in muscular dystrophy.

The inflammatory myopathies
1. Benign acute myositis
This is assumed to be a post-viral phenomenon as it often follows an upper respiratory tract infection. Pain and weakness occur in affected muscles.

2. Dermatomyositis

This tends to be more benign than the adult illness. It is probably due to a vasculitis. There is ascending symmetrical muscle weakness with an insidious onset over some weeks. The anterior neck flexors and trunk muscles are typically involved as may be the bulbar muscles affecting chewing and swallowing. Post-exercise pain and aching are seen in the majority of cases and there may be tenderness of the muscles. Classically there is a violaceous hue to the eyelids with periorbital oedema (Fig. 24.32). Extensor surfaces of joints may also be affected by the rash. More rarely subcutaneous calcification may occur, leading to palpable induration. Although the ESR and creatine phosphokinase are often raised, they may be normal. Muscle biopsy reveals an inflammatory cell infiltrate. The mainstay of management is corticosteroid therapy, which usually needs to be continued for at least six months. If the response to therapy is poor, immunoglobulin, azathioprine or cyclosporin may be tried. Over half the children recover fully.

Myotonic disorders

Myotonia is delayed relaxation after sustained muscle contraction. It can be identified clinically and on electromyography.

1. Dystrophia myotonica

This is a dominantly inherited disorder. When presentation occurs in the newborn period, there is profound hypotonia, feeding difficulty and intermittent respiratory difficulty. These infants have an affected mother.

More typically, it presents with learning difficulties associated with a somewhat expressionless face (Fig. 24.33), distal wasting and myotonia. The latter usually first appears in late adolescence or the early 20s. Cataracts and, in males, baldness and testicular atrophy are common later associations. Death is usually due to an associated cardiomyopathy.

Metabolic myopathies

These present with floppiness in infancy or, in older children, with muscle weakness or cramps on exercise. The main causes are:

- glycogen storage disorders (see Chapter 22)

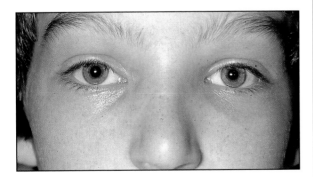

Fig. 24.32 Heliotrope rash in dermatomyositis.

- muscle lipid disorders, affecting oxidation of fatty acids, a major source of energy for skeletal muscle, particularly during prolonged low intensity exercise or fasting
- mitochondrial cytopathies, rare disorders which are coded as maternally inherited mitochondrial DNA.

Myopathy may be the major manifestation of a mitochondrial cytopathy, or the disorder maybe multisystem with lactic acidosis and encephalopathy.

Congenital myopathies

These present at birth or in infancy with generalised hypotonia and muscle weakness. They are categorised according to the appearance of the muscle biopsy on electron microscopy. They do not show the morphological changes of muscular dystrophy. Disease types are:

- central core disease
- multicore disease
- nemaline myopathy
- congenital fibre-type disproportion.

Creatine phosphokinase levels are normal or only mildly elevated.

THE 'FLOPPY INFANT'

Persisting hypotonia in infants may be central or peripheral in origin (Fig. 24.34). The hypotonia can be readily felt on

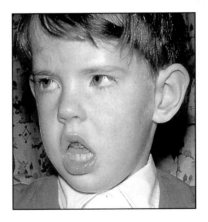

Fig. 24.33 Dystrophia myotonica in an eight-year-old boy who has marked facial weakness and moderately severe learning difficulties.

Fig. 24.34 Causes of the floppy infant
Central
Cerebral
– causes of developmental delay e.g. Down syndrome, Prader–Willi syndrome
– evolving cerebral palsy
Hypothyroidism
Hypocalcaemia
Drug therapy
Peripheral
Spinal muscular atrophy
Myopathy
Myasthenia gravis

picking up the infant: there is marked head lag when traction is applied to the arms and the infant feels as if he is slipping through the examiner's hands when held vertically. If there is associated peripheral (lower motor neurone) weakness, affected infants have poor antigravity movements of the arms and legs which causes them to adopt a froglike posture when lying supine (Fig. 24.29); when suspended prone they slump over the examiner's hand, with their arms and legs extended under the pull of gravity. With central (brain) hypotonia, the muscles are not weak and antigravity movements of the arms and legs are normal.

Neurocutaneous syndromes

NEUROFIBROMATOSIS (VON RECKLINGHAUSEN DISEASE)

This is dominantly inherited, but up to 50% are new mutations. It affects about 1 in 4000 live births. The cutaneous features consist of six or more café-au-lait patches (Fig. 24.35), axillary freckling and firm nodular neurofibromata which may be palpable on peripheral nerves. The cutaneous features tend to become more evident after puberty.

In neurofibromatosis Type I (NF-I, peripheral), which is coded for on chromosome 17, neurofibromata appear in the course of any peripheral nerve, including cranial nerves. They may look unsightly or cause neurological signs if they occur at a site where a peripheral nerve

passes through a bony foramen. Visual or auditory impairment may result if there is compression of the II or VIII cranial nerve. Megalencephaly with learning difficulties and epilepsy are seen in a few cases.

Neurofibromatosis Type II (NF-II, bilateral acoustic or central) is coded for on chromosome 22. Bilateral acoustic neuromata are the predominant feature and present with deafness and sometimes a cerebello-pontine angle syndrome with a facial (VII) nerve paresis and cerebellar ataxia.

There may be an overlap between the features of NF-I and NF-II. Other associations are phaeochromocytoma, pulmonary hypertension, retinal artery stenosis with hypertension, and gliomatous change particularly in central nervous system lesions. Rarely, the benign tumours undergo sarcomatous change. However, most people with the disorder carry no features other than the cutaneous stigmata.

TUBEROUS SCLEROSIS

This disorder is dominantly inherited but 80% are new mutations. The cutaneous features consist of:

* depigmented 'ash leaf'-shaped patches which fluoresce under ultraviolet light (Woods light)
* roughened patches of skin (Shagreen patches) usually over the lumbar spine
* adenoma sebaceum (angiofibromata) in a butterfly distribution over the bridge of the nose and cheeks, which are unusual before the age of three (Fig. 24.36).

Neurological features are:

* developmental delay with infantile spasms

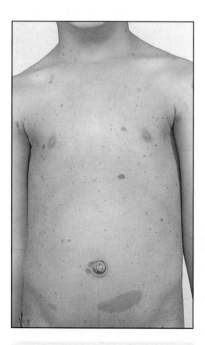

Fig. 24.35 Café-au-lait patches in neurofibromatosis.

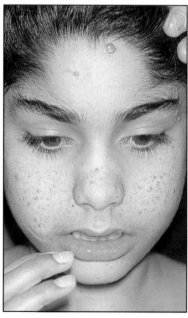

Fig. 24.36 Adenoma sebaceum in tuberous sclerosis.

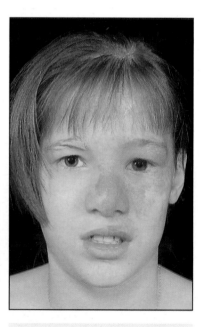

Fig. 24.37 Sturge–Weber syndrome. There is a port wine stain in the distribution of the trigeminal nerve.

- epilepsy – often partial
- intellectual impairment.

These children invariably have severe learning difficulties and often have autistic features to their behaviour when older.

Other features are:

- fibromata beneath the nails (subungual fibromata)
- dense white areas on the retina (phakomata) from local degeneration
- rhabdomyomata of the heart which are identifiable in the early weeks on echocardiography but often resolve
- polycystic kidneys.

As with neurofibromatosis, gliomatous change can occur in the brain lesions. Many people who carry the gene have no stigmata other than the cutaneous features.

A characteristic feature on the skull X-ray is 'railroad track calcification', usually after the first year of life. These calcified subependymal nodules can be identified earlier on CT or MR brain scans.

STURGE–WEBER SYNDROME

This is a sporadic disorder with a haemangiomatous facial lesion (a port-wine stain) in the distribution of the trigeminal nerve associated with a haemangiomatous lesion of the brain. The ophthalmic division of the trigeminal nerve is always involved (Fig. 24.37). In the most severe form, it may present with epilepsy, learning difficulties and hemiplegia. Children presenting with intractable epilepsy in

early infancy may benefit from hemispherectomy. For children who are less severely affected, deterioration is unusual after the age of five years though there may still be seizures and learning difficulties.

Neurodegenerative disorders

The cardinal feature of these disorders is developmental regression with the evolution of abnormal neurological signs. For some, the specific enzyme defect responsible has been identified. A wide variety of these inherited disorders has been described, such as the lysosomal enzyme storage disorders, which include the mucopolysaccharidoses and lipid storage disorders (Fig. 24.38). Developmental regression occurs in subacute sclerosing panencephalitis (SSPE) following measles and in Wilson disease.

MUCOPOLYSACCHARIDOSES

These are progressive multisystem disorders which may affect the neurological, ocular, cardiac and skeletal systems (Fig. 24.39). Hepatosplenomegaly is usually present. Most children present with developmental delay following a period of essentially normal growth and development up to 6–12 months of age. Developmental attainment then slows and children may show some loss of skills. It is only

Disorder	Enzyme defect	Clinical features
Tay–Sachs disease	Hexosaminidase A	Autosomal recessive disorder
		Most common among Ashkenazi Jews
		Developmental regression in late infancy, exaggerated startle response to noise, visual inattention and social unresponsiveness
		Severe hypotonia, enlarging head
		Cherry red spot at the macula
		Death by 2–5 years
		Diagnosis – measurement of the specific enzyme activity
		Carrier detection in high-risk couples is practised
		Antenatal detection is possible
Gaucher disease	Betaglucosidase	Occurs in 1 in 500 Ashkenazi Jews
		Chronic childhood form – splenomegaly, bone marrow suppression, bone involvement, normal IQ
		Splenectomy may alleviate hypersplenism. Enzyme replacement therapy has recently become available, but is extremely expensive
		Acute infantile form – splenomegaly, neurological degeneration with seizures
		Carrier detection and antenatal diagnosis are possible
Niemann–Pick disease	Sphingomyelinase	At 3–4 months, feeding difficulties and failure to thrive, hepatosplenomegaly, developmental delay, hypotonia and deterioration of hearing and vision
		Cherry-red spot at macula affects 50%
		Death by 4 years

Fig. 24.38 Lipid storage disorders

in the second six months of life that the characteristic facies begins to emerge, with coarsening of the facial features and prominent forehead due to frontal bossing (Fig. 24.40).

The characteristics of five of the varieties are shown in Figure 24.41. The diagnosis is made by identifying the enzyme defect and the excretion in the urine of the major storage substances, the glycosaminoglycans (GAGs). Treatment is supportive according to the child's needs. Enzyme replacement by bone marrow transplantation has been performed for the most severe variety, Hurler syndrome.

Mucopolysaccharidoses

Fig. 24.39 Clinical features of mucopolysaccharidoses

Eyes	Corneal clouding
	Retinal degeneration
	Glaucoma
Skin	Thickened skin
	Coarse facies
Heart	Valvular lesions
	Cardiac failure
Neurology	Developmental regression
Skeletal	Thickened skull
	Broad ribs
	Claw hand
	Thoracic kyphosis
	Lumbar lordosis
Other	Hepatosplenomegaly
	Carpal tunnel syndrome
	Conductive deafness
	Umbilical and inguinal hernias

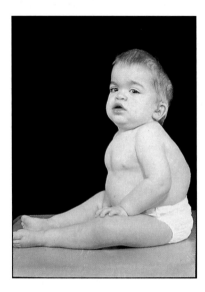

Fig. 24.40 Hurler syndrome showing the characteristic facies and skeletal dysplasia.

Fig. 24.41 Types of mucopolysaccharidoses

Type	Inheritance	Cornea	Heart	Brain	Skeletal
MPS I (Hurler)	AR	+++	++	+++	++
MPS II (Hunter)	X-linked	–	+	++	+
MPS III (Sanfilippo)	AR	+/–	–	+	+
MPS IV (Morquio)	AR	+	+	–	+
MPS VI (Morateaux-Lamy)	AR	+++	++	–	++

AR = autosomal recessive

FURTHER READING

Brett EM. *Paediatric Neurology.* Churchill Livingstone, Edinburgh, 1991. A comprehensive textbook.
Newton RW. *Colour Atlas of Paediatric Neurology.* Mosby-Wolfe, London, 1995. A well-illustrated book.

The Child with Special Needs

While many children with a chronic illness or medical condition will have additional health, social and educational requirements, the concept of special needs is used for children with neurodevelopmental disabilities which are long lasting and complex. These children may have:

- an impairment – any loss or abnormality of physiological function or anatomical structure
- a disability – any restriction or lack of ability due to the impairment
- a handicap – a disadvantage from a disability which limits or prevents the fulfilment of a normal role. However, the term handicap gives the impression of a dependent person, often the object of pity and charity, and its use has fallen out of favour. The term 'impairment' or 'disability' is used instead.

The current approach in assessing a child with special needs is to identify what the child can do and what the difficulties are. Functional skills can be categorised according to:

- hand function, mobility
- vision, hearing
- language and communication,
- behaviour and emotion
- physical health
- social
- self-care including continence
- learning.

Once the child's abilities and difficulties are identified, it is possible to formulate a plan to help the child's full potential to be achieved. Multidisciplinary clinical teams have been established to fulfil this role, for example a child development team, school health team, learning disability team and sometimes a young adult disability team. However, needs cannot always be met by health-based services. They frequently require the integrated support of health and social services, local education authorities and voluntary agencies (Fig. 25.1). In England and Wales, social services departments are required (by the 1989 Children Act) to maintain a register of children with disabilities and special needs to facilitate the provision of care.

Presentation

Children with special needs may present at any time in childhood or adolescence, but particular times and modes of presentation are listed below.

Antenatal period:
- identified from biochemical screening tests e.g. Tay–Sachs disease, or family history
- chromosomal abnormalities or structural anomalies of the central nervous system, such as spina bifida and hydrocephalus, identified on antenatal screening.

Newborn infants:
- chromosomal abnormality or syndrome identified at birth
- abnormal neurological behaviour – poor feeding, abnormal axial and/or limb tone and movement, including a floppy infant, visual inattention, seizures. There may be a history of birth asphyxia or neonatal encephalopathy.
- preterm infant with a large intraventricular haemorrhage, periventricular leucomalacia or hydrocephalus on cranial ultrasound.

Infancy:
- motor delay such as with sitting and walking, persistent fisting, poor motor function or hand preference before 1 year of age. Spastic quadriplegia is usually evident in early infancy, but hemiplegic cerebral palsy often presents in late infancy.

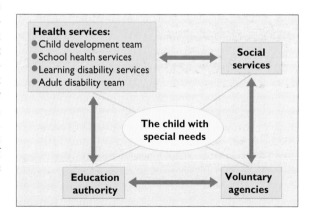

Fig. 25.1 Children with special needs often require care from multidisciplinary clinical teams integrated with social services, local education authorities and voluntary agencies.

- severe visual or auditory impairment noted by parents or by screening.

Pre-school:
- speech and language delay – as specific deficit or part of global developmental delay
- odd gait from mild cerebral palsy, neuromuscular conditions or skeletal dysplasias
- general developmental delay. This may require investigation (Fig. 25.2) but often no cause is identified. Specific clinical features may become apparent in late infancy or even later e.g. the facial features in mucopolysaccharidoses or cutaneous stigmata in neurocutaneous disorders
- loss of skills from a neurodegenerative disorder.

School age:
- poor dexterity, balance or coordination – may only become evident when the child is compared with peers
- general learning difficulties
- clumsiness – these children often retain a degree of hypotonia, with poor fixation of proximal girdle musculature, which causes difficulty in performing fine movements
- specific learning difficulties e.g. dyslexia. Children with specific learning difficulties require neuropsychological assessment. The child can be assisted by using appropriate reading material and the advice of a remedial therapist.

Any age:
- following a serious illness e.g. meningitis, or a head injury, the child may be left with permanent disability.

The multidisciplinary team

The multidisciplinary child development team can be organised in a number of different ways. It may be based in the community or hospital, but preferably should work flexibly in both. The professionals constituting the child development team may differ, but those usually included are listed in Figure 25.3. The paediatrician provides

---

Fig 25.2 Investigation of undiagnosed delayed development

Basic screening investigations
Plasma urea and electrolytes, calcium, liver function tests
Urine amino and organic acids
Muco- and oligopolysaccharide screen
Thyroid function tests
Chromosomes and DNA analysis for fragile X

Further investigations if indicated
CT/MR brain scan
EEG
Blood gases
Creatine phosphokinase
Plasma lactate, capillary pH
Serology/urine for congenital infection
Blood lead, copper
White blood cell enzymes
Nerve conduction and electromyography
Nerve and muscle biopsy
Maternal aminoacids for raised phenylalanine

Fig 25.3 Child development team members

Paediatricians
Have special medical expertise in neurodevelopmental problems and management of complex handicap.

Physiotherapists
Assess patterns of movement. Offer advice to children and parents on play and activities that promote the development of good patterns of movement and balance, thereby limiting skeletal deformity. Help with the provision of mobility aids.

Occupational therapists
Work in conjunction with the physiotherapists. Assess fine motor skills and functional tasks involving hand use, such as dressing, toiletting and feeding. Provide aids to improve hand and manipulation skills and advise on appropriate seating and mobility aids including wheelchairs. They also advise on how to adapt houses to make them more suitable for a disabled person.

Speech and language therapists
Assess speech, language and other communication disorders. Advise parents how to encourage the child's language development. This may include using an alternative means of communication such as the Makaton sign language and Bliss symbols board, which are suitable for children with severe learning difficulties (Fig. 25.4). In conjunction with occupational therapists, speech and language therapists may help children with feeding difficulties.

Psychologists
Perform detailed developmental assessments using standardised tests. They also help combat disordered behaviour by advising on structured behaviour modification programmes. Educational psychologists assess learning ability and advise on suitable educational resources to meet the child's special needs. The developmental assessments help in advising parents about their child's progress and future skills.

Social workers
Act as advocates for individual families and children and advise on resources available e.g. allowances, day nursery placements, housing. Social workers can also help parents formulate questions they may have about their child's disorder and, as with other team members, offer psychological support. Social services departments have statutory duties e.g. maintaining a register of children with special needs.

Community nurses/specialist health visitors
Help coordinate care between professionals in the community and hospital, enabling as much care as possible to be carried out in the community. Provide detailed information and advice and psychological support for the family. May advise parents on play which can be incorporated into the child's everyday activities to attain further developmental progress. This can be done in a structured way e.g. the Portage scheme.

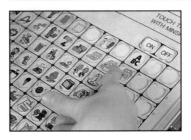

Fig. 25.4
A touch pad communication system using symbols. This child with dystonic posturing can still press the desired key.

medical assessment and investigation of the child and usu-ally coordinates the input of different therapists or other health professionals, who may be consulted as appropriate. Many teams now also nominate a family advocate, usually a team member, to help families resolve their anxieties and gain access to the resources they need.

The services required will vary according to the child's age. Pre-school children with special needs are predomi-nantly supported by the health-led multidisciplinary child development team, with educational professionals playing a role in assessment and provision of support. Families should be provided at an early stage with information on available financial benefits, voluntary support agencies and respite care.

For school age children, the key input is likely to be from the education authority and therapists working in the schools and with the doctors in the community health service.

For school leavers and young adults, social services bev-comes the key agency. Young adults with learning or physical disabilities are provided for by community disability teams.

However, there is a need for all three statutory services – health, education and social services to be available to a greater or lesser extent at all stages of the child's life, and for the accent to be on coordinated care. Ideally a proliferation of professionals and overlap of activity should be avoided while still meeting the child's needs.

Parental reaction to disability

The diagnosis of a disability may be the culmination of months of parental concern about their child's develop-ment or it may be sudden, as with the diagnosis of a chro-mosomal abnormality in the immediate postnatal period. Either way, the parents are likely to be left feeling shocked, with their expectations of having a normal child shattered. The initial interview, when the diagnosis is discussed, is extremely important and has to be handled very sensitively in order that the relationship between the parents, doctors and other professionals can remain constructive. This requires honesty and trust on all sides. The importance of seeing both parents together and the need to present the facts simply, honestly and as early as possible have been described in Chapter 3.

Some of the greatest resentment arises if doctors are subsequently seen to have been withholding information on the grounds that the family were not 'ready to receive it'.

Because of anxiety, parents are often not able to assim-ilate information given at the initial meeting and further meetings are required. It is often helpful to have an advo-cate for the parents present, such as their social worker or health visitor, who will help them in subsequent more private discussions and in formulating questions they may later wish to ask.

Some disabilities, e.g. cerebral palsy, may become appar-ent only gradually over the first months of life. Consider-able experience and fine clinical judgement are needed in the early recognition of disabilities and determining their likely prognosis.

Parents' initial reaction to the news that their child may have a disabling condition is usually grief accompanied by anger, guilt, despair or denial. Realisation and acceptance often follow, with psychological adaptation to the new circum-stances when parents start to plan and organise for the future. The father, mother and other family members may all react differently to the news about the disability. Par-ents may find counselling and support helpful during this period.

The grief parents feel is centred on losing the image of the child they dreamt of and its replacement by imagery based on previous experience and the common view of a particular handicap.

Doctors, too, may harbour their own prejudice or nat-ural revulsion of disabilities. They can learn how to deal with these emotions by listening to families with children with disabilities and from the literature on the subject. Often, no curative treatment is available, but health pro-fessionals have much to offer children and families, allow-ing a realistic but positive approach, even when the disability is severe.

Continuing medical care

Many children with special needs have active medical prob-lems which require regular assessment (Figs 25.5).

Special problems of consent

Rarely, parents of children with a severe disability will not consent to life-saving operative procedures. For example, they may decline the repair of duodenal atresia in Down syn-drome. In an emergency, doctors are legally entitled to inter-vene in the best interests of the child without the consent of parents, but, where there is more time, legal advice should be obtained about seeking judgement in court. The ques-tion may arise about whether it is lawful for doctors to with-hold life-saving treatment from a child with severe disabilities. In the UK, it has been found to be 'not unlaw-ful' to allow a child to die where severe disabilities exist and where suffering would be avoided. Individual judgement in court is required.

In the UK, children may give consent to a medical pro-cedure if their understanding of the situation appears ade-quate. Where a person is incapable of understanding the issues involved but is over 16 years old, and when the treat-ment is controversial, e.g. sterilisation, leave of the court should be sought.

If the treatment is not controversial, doctors can proceed with the agreement (but not the consent) of the parents or the person's usual caretakers, provided this can be defend-ed as being in the child's best interests.

Fig 25.5 Medical problems commonly encountered by children with special needs

Vision and hearing
These need to be regularly reviewed. Their assessment in children with disabilities can be difficult.

Epilepsy
Adjustment of anticonvulsant therapy may be required.

Skeletal deformity
Central nervous system and neuromuscular disorders can lead to skeletal deformity. Regular physiotherapy, adequate seating and the provision of appropriate aids is required (Fig. 25.6). Mobility should be maintained for as long as possible. Postural deformity can be minimised by physiotherapy, footwear, callipers, orthoses and serial bracing if required. Permanent skeletal deformity may be ameliorated with surgery.

Behaviour
Many children with central nervous system abnormalities have behaviour disorders. They may be a part of the disorder or environmentally determined. The clinical psychology or child psychiatry service can help parents by analysing the situation and advising on appropriate behaviour modification programmes.

Feeding problems
These are often associated with cerebral palsy, particularly spastic quadriplegia, and may be secondary to pseudobulbar involvement. Calorie intake may be increased with advice from the dietician, speech and language therapist and occupational therapist. Positioning of the head and trunk during feeding is important in infants, as is diet and food texture. If the child's food intake is inadequate because of impaired oromotor function, or if oral feeding is complicated by significant risk of inhalation, insertion of a gastrostomy tube needs early consideration.

Chest infections
These are common in the non-ambulant child, particularly those with feeding difficulties. Aspiration pneumonia and wheezing may be due to immobility or secondary to gastro-oesophageal reflux.

Renal function and urinary incontinence
In children with a neurogenic bladder, the anatomy and physiology of the renal tract will need to be determined radiologically and by pressure monitoring, and renal function monitored. Urinary catheterisation or bypass surgery may be required.

Constipation and faecal incontinence
This is a problem for many children with cerebral palsy, particularly if they are immobile. Attention needs to be paid to diet, while laxatives and intermittent enemas may be required..

Education

In England and Wales the 1981 and 1993 Education Acts were devised to provide adequate rights and safeguards for children with disabilities and learning difficulties, and to ensure their right to integration into mainstream school whenever possible. Education authorities have a duty to identify children whose special educational needs will require additional resources. Parents can request such an assessment and doctors who identify such children have a statutory responsibility to inform the education authority. Notification generates a more detailed assessment of the child's educational needs which may result in a 'statement' of special educational needs. Although children are integrated into mainstream education where practicable, special schools are usually more suitable for children with severe learning difficulties and sometimes for those with severe physical, communication and behaviour problems. Many special educational placements will have a need for therapy input (physiotherapy, occupational and speech/language therapy).

Young adults

Young adults with physical and mental disability have their own special needs for medical support, therapy, assistance with social problems (housing, employment, mobility, finance, leisure, etc.) and sexual and genetic counselling. Unfortunately this service is still poorly developed compared to the multidisciplinary services available for young children with complex disabilities

FURTHER READING

Hall D, Hill P, Elliman D. *The Child Surveillance Handbook.* Radcliffe Medical Press, Oxford, 1994. A practical handbook.

Harvey D, Miles M, Smyth D. *Community Child Health and Paediatrics.* Butterworth–Heinemann, Oxford, 1995. A comprehensive textbook.

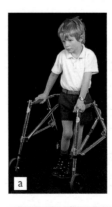
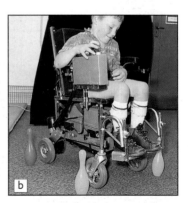

Fig. 25.6 (a) A boy with athetoid cerebral palsy is able to walk with the help of a frame. **(b)** A six-year-old boy with four-limb spasticity is able to steer this electric wheelchair.

Appendix

- *Growth charts* • *Blood pressure chart* • *Peak flow chart* • *Gestational age assessment of newborn infants*
  • *Normal ranges: Clinical chemistry and Haematology*

Growth charts

These are examples of growth charts used in the UK (Figs 1a, b and c).

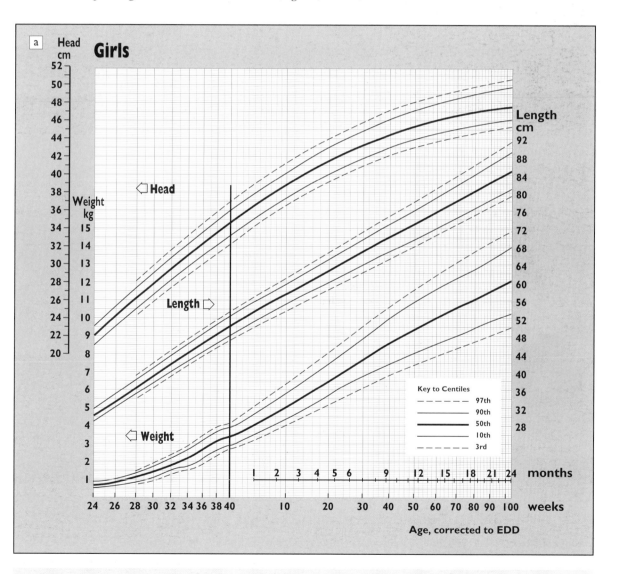

Fig. 1(a) Growth chart for female infants from 24 weeks gestation to 2 years of age. It includes measurements of weight, length and head circumference. (Courtesy of Castlemead Publications.)

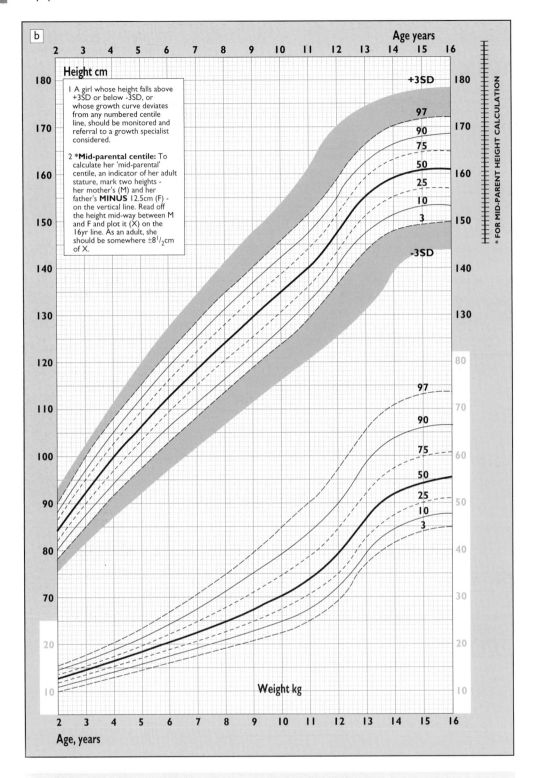

Fig. 1(b) Growth chart for females from 2 to 16 years for weight and length. The lowest centile lines are the 3rd, the highest the 97th. For height, the range for ±3 SD (Standard Deviation) is shown. The mid-parental height centile can also be determined. (Courtesy of Castlemead Publications.)

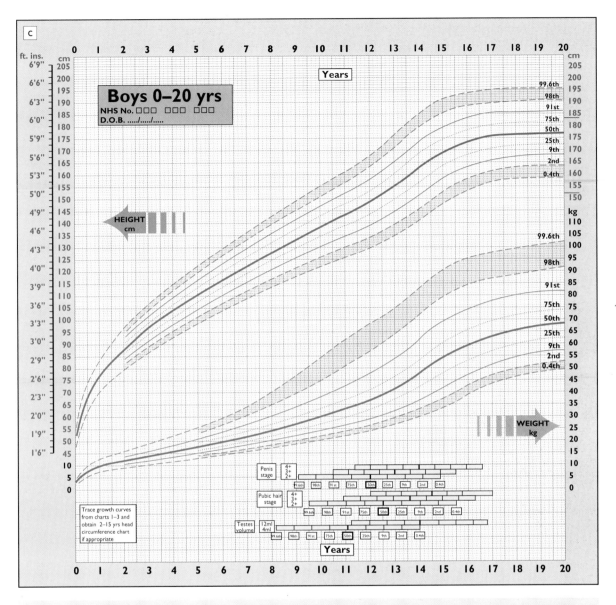

Fig. 1(c) Growth chart for males from birth to 20 years using the 1990 nine centile UK chart. This shows the 0.4 and 99.6 centile lines. The interval between each pair of centiles lines is the same − $^2/_3$ SD (Standard Deviation).
(Courtesy of Child Growth Foundation.)

Blood pressure chart

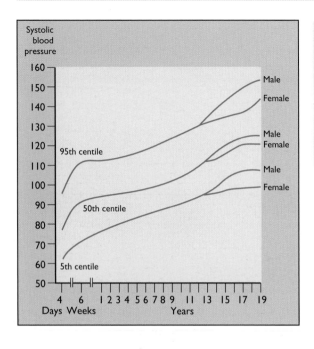

Fig. 2 Systolic blood pressure according to age. Blood pressure charts are also available according to height. (Data from de Swiet M, Fayers P, Shinebourne EA. Systolic Blood Pressure in a Population of Infants in the First Year of Life: The Brompton Study. Pediatrics *1980; 65:1028–1035 and de Man SA, Andre J, Bachmann H, Grobbe DE, Ibsen KK, Laaser U, Lippert P, Hofman A. Blood pressure in childhood: pooled findings of six European studies.* Journal of Hypertension *1991;9:109–114).*

Peak flow chart

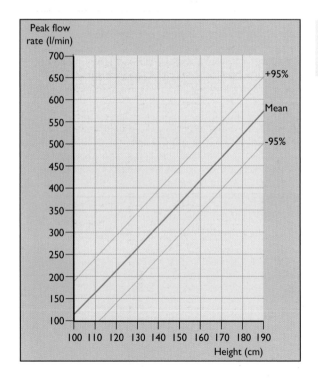

Fig. 3 The normal range of peak flow measurements according to height. (Reproduced with permission from Godfrey S. Br J Dis Chest *1970;64:15.)*

Gestational age assessment of newborn infants

(a) External appearance.

External sign	0	1	2	3	4
Oedema	Obvious oedema of hands and feet; pitting over tibia	No obvious oedema of hands and feet; pitting over tibia	No oedema		
Skin texture	Very thin gelatinous	Thin and smooth	Smooth; medium thickness. Rash or superficial peeling	Slight thickening. Superficial cracking and peeling especially of hands and feet	Thick and parchment-like; superficial or deep cracking
Skin colour	Dark red	Uniformly pink	Pale pink; variable over body	Pale; only pink over ears, lips, palms, or soles	
Skin opacity (trunk)	Numerous veins and venules clearly seen, especially over abdomen	Veins and tributaries seen	A few large vessels clearly seen over abdomen	A few large vessels seen indistinctly over abdomen	No blood vessels seen
Lanugo (over back)	No lanugo	Abundant; long and thick over whole back	Hair thinning especially over lower back	Small amount of lanugo and bald area	At least half of back devoid of lanugo
Plantar creases	No skin creases	Faint red marks over anterior half of sole	Definite red marks over > anterior 1/2; indentations over < anterior 1/3	Indentations over >anterior 1/3	Definite deep indentations over >anterior 1/3
Nipple formation	Nipple barely visible; no areola	Nipple well defined; areola smooth and flat, diameter <0.75cm	Areola stippled, edge not raised, diameter <0.75cm	Areola stippled, edge raised, diameter >0.75cm	
Breast size	No breast tissue palpable	Breast tissue on one or both sides, <0.5cm diameter	Breast tissue both sides; one or both 0.5-1.0cm	Breast tissue both sides; one or both >1cm	

(b) Neurological examination.

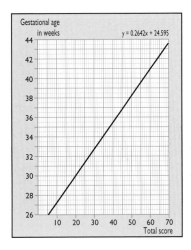

Neurological sign	Score					
	0	1	2	3	4	5
Posture						
Square window	90°	60°	45°	30°	0°	
Ankle dorsiflexion	90°	75°	45°	20°	0°	
Arm recoil	180°	90-180°	<90°			
Leg recoil	180°	90-180°	<90°			
Popliteal angle	180°	160°	130°	110°	90°	<90°
Heel to ear						
Scarf sign						
Head lag						
Ventral suspension						

Fig. 4 (a) and (b) Scoring system for assessment of gestational age in newborn infants (Dubowitz examination). This is a method of assessing gestational age according to external appearance and neurological examination. The infant's gestational age (±2 weeks) is determined from the total score using a conversion graph.
Adapted from Dubowitz LMS, Dubowitz V & Goldberg C. Clinical assessment of gestational age in the newborn infant. Journal of Pediatrics 1970; 77:1–10.

(c) Graph for reading gestational age from total score.

Normal ranges: Clinical chemistry

As the normal range for tests varies between laboratories, this must be checked with the local laboratory. (Values adapted with permission from Addy, D P. *Investigations in Paediatrics.* WB Sanders, London, 1994 and other sources.)

Test		Normal range (plasma or serum)	
Alanine aminotransferase (ALT)		<40 U/l	
Albumin	Neonate*	25–35 g/l	
	Child	35–55 g/l	
Alkaline Phosphatase (ALP)	Neonate*	150–700 U/l	
	1m–1yr	250–1000 U/l	
	2–9 yr	250–850 U/l	
	Yr	Females	Males
	10–11	250–950 U/l	250–730 U/l
	14–15	170–460 U/l	170–970 U/l
	>18	60–250 U/l	50–200 U/l
Ammonia	Neonate	< 100 µmol/l	
	Infant/Child	< 40 µmol/l	
Amylase	Neonate	< 50 IU/l	
	1–3m	< 100 IU/l	
	>1yr	100–400 IU/l	
Aspartate amino transferase (AST)		< 50 U/l	
Blood gas (arterial, not preterm)	pH	7.35–7.45 (Hydrogen ion 35–44 nmol/l)	
	pO_2	11–14 kPa (82–105 mmHg)	
	pCO_2	4.5–6 kPa (32–45 mmHg)	
	Bicarbonate	18–25 mmol/l	
	Base excess	–3 to +3 mmol/l	
Calcium (total)	24–48h	1.8–3.0 mmol/l	
	>1 week	2.15–2.60 mmol/l	
Calcium (ionised)	24–48h	1.00–1.17 mmol/l	
	>1 week	1.18–1.32 mmol/l	
Chloride		96–110 mmol/l	
Creatinine kinase	Infant/child	60–300 U/l	
Creatinine	Infant*	20–65 µmol/l	
	1–10yr	20–80 µmol/l	
Creatinine clearance	1–3 months	27–69 ml/min/1.73m^2	
	3–6 months	61–84 ml/min/1.73m^2	
	6–12 months	77–126 ml/min/1.73m^2	
	>2 yrs	110–200 ml/min/1.73m^2	
C–reactive protein		< 10 mg/l	
Ferritin	Child	<150 µg/l	
Gammaglutaryl transferase (GGT)	1–12m	<80 U/l	
Glucose	1d*	2.2–3.3 mmol/l	
	>1d	2.6–5.5 mmol/l	
	Child	3.0–6.0 mmol/l	
Glycosylated haemoglobin (HbA_{1c})	5–16y	3–6%	
17–Hydroxyprogesterone (17–OHP)	>2d	0.7–12nmol/l	
	Child	0.4–4 nmol/l	

Cont'd.

Clinical chemistry (continued)

Test		Normal range (plasma or serum)
Iron	Infant	5– 25 μmol/l
	Child	10–30 μmol/l
Lactate (fasting)		0.5–2.0 mmol/l
Magnesium		0.6–1.0 mmol/l
Osmolality		275–295 mosm/kg
Phosphate	Neonate*	1.4–2.6 mmol/l
	Infant	1.3–2.1 mmol/l
	Child	1.0–1.8 mmol/l
Potassium	Infant	3.5– 6.0 mmol/l
	Child	3.3–5.0 mmol/l
Protein (total)	Neonate *	54–70 g/l
	Infant	59–70 g/l
	Child	60–80 g/l
Pyruvate		40–70 μmol/l
Sodium		133–145 mmol/l
Thyroid stimulating hormone (TSH)	>1week	0.3– 4.5 mU/l
Thyroxine (T4, total)	Child	85– 180 nmol/l
Urea	Neonate*	1.0–5.0 mmol/l
	Infant	2.5–8.0 mmol/l
	Child	2.5–6.5 mmol/l
Urate		120–350 μmol/l

*Depends on gestational age

Normal ranges: Haematology

Age	Hb (g/dl)	MCV (fl)	WBC ($\times 10^9$/l)	Platelets ($\times 10^9$/l)
Birth	14.5–21.5	100–135	10–26	150–450 at all ages
2 weeks	13.4–19.8	88–120	6–21	
2 months	9.4–13.0	84–105	6–18	
1 year	11.3–14.1	71–85	6–17.5	
2–6 years	11.5–13.5	75–87	5–17	
6–12 years	11.5–15.5	77–95	4.5–14.5	
12–18 years				
Male	13.0–16.0	78–95	4.5–13	
Female	12.0–16.0	78–95	4.5–13	

Index